Dietary Bioactives and Bone Health

Special Issue Editor
Taylor C. Wallace

MDPI • Basel • Beijing • Wuhan • Barcelona • Belgrade

MDPI

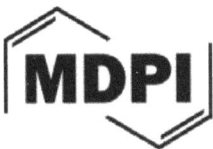

Special Issue Editor
Taylor C. Wallace
George Mason University
USA

Editorial Office
MDPI AG
St. Alban-Anlage 66
Basel, Switzerland

This edition is a reprint of the Special Issue published online in the open access journal *Nutrients* (ISSN 2072-6643) from 2016–2017 (available at: http://www.mdpi.com/journal/nutrients/special_issues/dietary_bioactives_bone_health).

For citation purposes, cite each article independently as indicated on the article page online and as indicated below:

Lastname, F.M.; Lastname, F.M. Article title. *Journal Name*. **Year**. Article number, page range.

First Edition 2018

ISBN 978-3-03842-845-9 (Pbk)
ISBN 978-3-03842-846-6 (PDF)

Table of Contents

About the Special Issue Editor

Taylor C. Wallace, PhD, CFS, FACN is Principal and CEO at the Think Healthy Group and a Professor in the Department of Nutrition and Food Studies at George Mason University. Prior to founding the Think Healthy Group, Dr. Wallace served as the Senior Director of Science Policy and Government Relations at the National Osteoporosis Foundation and previously in senior leadership roles at the Council for Responsible Nutrition and the North American Branch of the International Life Sciences Institute. He has extensive experience in developing and implementing comprehensive and evidence-based science, policy and legislative programs in the fields of nutrition and food science. His academic research interests are in nutritional interventions (micronutrient and dietary bioactive components) to promote health and prevent the onset of chronic disease. Dr. Wallace's background includes a PhD and an MS in Food Science and Nutrition from The Ohio State University and a BS in Food Science and Technology from the University of Kentucky. Dr. Wallace is a fellow of the American College of Nutrition (ACN), the 2015 recipient of the Charles A. Regus Award, given by the ACN for original research in the field of nutrition, and the Deputy Editor of the Journal of the American College of Nutrition. Dr. Wallace is an editor of five academic textbooks and has authored over 40 peer reviewed manuscripts and book chapters.

Preface to "Dietary Bioactives and Bone Health"

Osteoporosis, low bone mass and other age-related degenerative bone diseases are common debilitating conditions that effect millions of individuals worldwide. There are an estimated 2 million new osteoporotic-related fractures each year in the USA and 9 million globally, with an estimated economic impact burden of over $100 billion.

Dietary bioactives, have been previously defined by the U.S. National Institutes of Health as "compounds that are constituents in foods and dietary supplements, other than those needed to meet basic human nutritional needs, which are responsible for changes in health status." They have promise in protecting against bone loss, likely related to their anti-inflammatory properties. Dietary bioactives are generally thought to be safe in food at normal consumption levels. Their biological activities may be dependent of the presence of a single compound or class of compounds for which optimal effects may be achieved through consumption of mixtures where the exact identity and composition are often unknown. Classes of related compounds are commonly found in similar types of plants; however, their ratios and relative concentrations can vary significantly because of environmental factors such as cultivation, soil, altitude, and weather conditions. Food processing may also influence the types and amounts of dietary bioactives present.

Critical to the field of nutrition science will be the development of intake recommendations for dietary bioactives, likely to be based on chronic disease endpoints. Several limitations relating to absorption, distribution, metabolism and excretion of certain dietary bioactives still exist and must be better understood in the scientific literature for this to occur. The purpose of this book is to effectively and accurately communicate modern-day research to a large group of scientific audiences ranging from university classrooms to industry product developers and basic researchers in the fields of nutrition and food science. The search for an international assortment of expert scientists working in the field of bioactives and bone health who were qualified to contribute manuscripts to this book was indeed an exciting editorial challenge. The interdisciplinary range of content that is covered by the various manuscripts made this work particularly intellectually stimulating. I would like to personally thank each contributing author for their dedication to producing a high-quality manuscript for this book (a reproduction of a Special Edition of the journal Nutrients). The unique expertise of each distinguished scientist in their particular field makes this book both authoritative and cutting-edge.

It is my hope that this book will strengthen our understanding of how many dietary bioactive compounds may influence long-term maintenance of bone health.

Taylor C. Wallace
Special Issue Editor

![nutrients logo] *nutrients*

MDPI

Article

Germinated Pigmented Rice (*Oryza Sativa* L. cv. Superhongmi) Improves Glucose and Bone Metabolisms in Ovariectomized Rats

Soo Im Chung [1], Su Noh Ryu [2] and Mi Young Kang [1,*]

[1]   Department of Food Science and Nutrition, Brain Korea 21 Plus, Kyungpook National University, Daegu 41566, Korea; zizibe0312@nate.com
[2]   Department of Agricultural Science, Korea National Open University, Seoul 03087, Korea; ryusn@knou.ac.kr
*   Correspondence: mykang@knu.ac.kr; Tel.: +82-53-950-6235

Received: 21 September 2016; Accepted: 19 October 2016; Published: 21 October 2016

Abstract: The effect of germinated Superhongmi, a reddish brown pigmented rice cultivar, on the glucose profile and bone turnover in the postmenopausal-like model of ovariectomized rats was determined. The ovariectomized Sprague-Dawley rats were randomly divided into three dietary groups ($n = 10$): normal control diet (NC) and normal diet supplemented with non-germinated Superhongmi (SH) or germinated Superhongmi (GSH) rice powder. After eight weeks, the SH and GSH groups showed significantly lower body weight, glucose and insulin concentrations, levels of bone resorption markers and higher glycogen and 17-β-estradiol contents than the NC group. The glucose metabolism improved through modulation of adipokine production and glucose-regulating enzyme activities. The GSH rats exhibited a greater hypoglycemic effect and lower bone resorption than SH rats. These results demonstrate that germinated Superhongmi rice may potentially be useful in the prevention and management of postmenopausal hyperglycemia and bone turnover imbalance.

Keywords: pigmented rice; germination; Superhongmi; bone metabolism; glucose

1. Introduction

Germination is considered as a simple, effective, and inexpensive method of improving the nutritional quality of rice [1]. The soaking of rice grains in water for a few days induces slight germination which causes an increase in nutrient bioavailability and absorption [2]. During germination, biochemical changes occur including the release of free and bound materials and the activation of dormant enzymes which break down large molecular substances, resulting in the generation of bioactive compounds and an increase in nutrients [3]. Germinated rice has been found to have higher amounts of bioactive compounds such as γ-oryzanol, γ-aminobutyric acid (GABA), tocopherols, and tocotrienols than non-germinated rice [4,5]. Moreover, it has been shown to possess strong antidiabetic, antihyperlipidemic, and antioxidative properties [1,6].

Pigmented rice cultivars with black, purple, red, or brown pericarp are known for their higher nutritional value and greater antioxidant potential than non-pigmented cultivars [7,8]. They contain high amounts of anthocyanins, phenolic compounds and bioactive components [9,10] and their consumption has been associated with a reduced risk of diabetes and cardiovascular disease [11]. Investigations on various pigmented cultivars revealed that ingestion of pigmented rice could improve the lipid and glucose profiles in mice, delay the starch and sugar absorption in rats, and suppress postprandial blood sugar elevation in human subjects [12,13].

Menopause, the permanent cessation of menstruation, promotes metabolic syndromes and increases the risk of diabetes, dyslipidemia, and obesity in women [14]. An elevation in the concentrations of glucose, insulin, cholesterol, and triglyceride has been observed in postmenopausal women relative to premenopausal ones [14–16]. Menopause is also believed to be associated with the pathogenesis of osteoporosis, a metabolic bone disorder characterized by enhanced bone fragility and increased fracture risk, in elderly women [17]. The rapid decrease of the ovarian hormone estrogen after menopause is regarded as the primary cause of these metabolic dysfunctions [14]. The surgical removal of ovaries, known as ovariectomy, mimics the estrogen-deficient condition in postmenopausal women. Hence, ovariectomized animal models are widely used in investigating the pathophysiological changes associated with menopause and in developing therapeutic strategies against menopause-induced metabolic disorders [18].

Superhongmi is a new pigmented rice cultivar with a reddish brown pericarp developed in Korea. Recent studies have shown that germinated Superhongmi rice has a strong antioxidant capacity and could improve the lipid metabolism in ovariectomized rats [19,20]. To further explore the therapeutic potential of Superhongmi rice against metabolic dysfunctions, particularly those caused by menopause, the present study investigated the effect of germinated Superhongmi rice on the glucose metabolism and bone turnover in the postmenopausal-like model of ovariectomized rats.

2. Materials and Methods

2.1. Rice Samples and Chemicals

Whole grains of Superhongmi rice were obtained from the department of Agricultural Science, Korea National Open University. They were grown from May to October 2014 in Dangjin, Chungcheongnam-do, South Korea. All chemicals and standards used in this study were of analytical grade and purchased from Merck KGaA (Darnstadt, Germany) and Sigma-Aldrich, Inc. (Steinhein, Germany).

2.2. Rice Germination

Dehusked whole rice grains were germinated following the method of Wu et al. [21] with slight modifications. The grains (50 g) were washed twice with distilled water to remove any dirt and placed evenly in a tray overlaid with cotton pads and cheesecloth. Distilled water (100 mL) was added and the whole tray was covered with a clean transparent plastic wrap with holes to allow for ventilation and incubated at 30 °C in an oven. The grains were regularly checked every 12 h to ensure there was no foul odor and fungal growth. After 72 h, the germinated rice grains, including the emerged radicles, were dried at 50 °C for 2 h, ground and pulverized (200–300 μm) using a grinding machine (HMF-3250S, Hanil Electronics, Seoul, South Korea), packed in hermetically sealed Ziploc plastic bags, and stored at −20 °C until further analysis. For the non-germinated samples, 50 g rice grains were washed, dried, ground (200–300 μm), and stored using the same method described above for the germinated grains. Both the germinated and non-germinated rice samples were analyzed for their bioactive compounds γ-oryzanol, GABA, phytic acid, tocols (tocopherols and tocotrienols), and policosanol, based on previously described methods [22–26] and for their proximate compositions using the methods of AOAC [27]. The results are shown in Table 1.

2.3. Animals and Diet

Thirty female ovariectomized Sprague-Dawley rats (10-week-old), weighing approximately 229 g each, were purchased from Central Laboratory Animal Inc. (Seoul, Korea). The animals were individually housed in a hanging stainless steel cage in a room (25 ± 2 °C, 50% relative humidity) with 12/12 h light-dark cycle and fed initially with a pelletized chow diet and distilled water ad libitum for 1 week. They were then randomly divided into three dietary groups (*n* = 10): normal control diet (NC) and NC diet supplemented with either 20% (w/w) non-germinated Superhongmi (SH) or germinated Superhongmi (GSH) rice powder. They were fed for 8 weeks and allowed free access to distilled water. The composition of the experimental diet (Table 2) was based on the AIN-93M diet [28]. At the end of the experimental period, the rats were anaesthetized with carbon dioxide by inhalation following a 12-h fast. The blood samples were drawn from the inferior vena cava into a heparin-coated tube and centrifuged at $1000 \times g$ for 15 min at $4\,^\circ$C to obtain the plasma. The liver, heart, kidney, and white adipose tissues (perirenal and inguinal) were removed, rinsed with physiological saline, weighed, and stored at $-70\,^\circ$C until analysis. The current study protocol was approved by the Ethics Committee of Kyungpook National University for animal studies (approval No. 2015-0087).

Table 1. Bioactive components and proximate composition of Superhongmi rice powder.

Bioactive Compound	Non-Germinated	Germinated
γ-Oryzanol (mg/100 g rice)	33.21 ± 2.66	51.96 ± 1.99 [1],*
GABA (mg/100 g rice)	98.54 ± 3.96	1102.02 ± 11.63 *
Phytic acid (mg/100 g rice)	2.01 ± 0.09	4.02 ± 0.14 *
Tocols (µg/100 g rice)	133.69 ± 8.62	256.79 ± 6.98 *
Policosanol (mg/100 g rice)	21.69 ± 1.02	26.51 ± 1.24 *
Proximate composition (% dry basis)		
Carbohydrates	76.58 ± 0.91 *	53.92 ± 0.98
Crude protein	7.11 ± 0.12 *	5.71 ± 0.41
Crude fat	2.31 ± 0.19	3.58 ± 0.17 *
Crude ash	1.34 ± 0.04 *	1.11 ± 0.02
Moisture	12.66 ± 0.32	35.68 ± 0.61 *

[1] Values are means $\pm$ standard error ($n = 3$); * indicates significant difference ($p < 0.05$) between germinated and non-germinated samples.

Table 2. Composition of experimental diets (%).

	NC [1]	SH	GSH
Casein	14.0	12.4	12.2
Sucrose	10.0	10.0	10.0
Dextrose	15.5	15.5	15.5
Corn starch	46.6	28.7	29.1
Cellulose	5.00	5.00	5.00
Soybean oil	4.00	3.50	3.24
Mineral mix	3.50	3.50	3.50
Vitamin mix	1.00	1.00	1.00
L-Cystine	0.18	0.18	0.18
Choline bitartrate	0.25	0.25	0.25
Non-germinated rice	-	20.0	-
Germinated rice	-	-	20.0
Total	100	100	100
Kcal	380	380	380

[1] NC, normal control diet (AIN-93M); SH, normal diet + non-germinated Superhongmi rice powder; GSH, normal diet + germinated Superhongmi rice powder.

2.4. Determination of Glucose Profile and Plasma Adipokine Levels

The levels of blood glucose and plasma insulin were determined using Accu-Chek Active Blood Glucose Test Strips (Roche Diagnostics, Berlin, Germany) and enzyme-linked immunosorbent assay (ELISA) kits (TMB Mouse Insulin ELISA kit, Shibayagi Co., Gunma, Japan), respectively. The hepatic glycogen level was determined using the anthrone-H_2SO_4 method with glucose as standard [29]. The homeostasis model assessment of insulin resistance (HOMA-IR) index was calculated using the equation described by Vogeser et al. [30]. The following plasma adipokines were analyzed using commercial assay kits: adiponectin (Shibayagi Co., Gunma, Japan), leptin (Cayman Chemical, Ann Arbor, MI, USA), resistin (B-Bridge International Inc., Santa Clara, CA, USA), and tumor necrosis factor (TNF)-α (Abcam, Cambridge, MA, USA).

2.5. Determination of Hepatic Glucose-Regulating Enzymes Activities

The liver tissue was homogenized in a buffer solution containing triethanolamine, EDTA, and dithiothreitol and centrifuged at $1000\times g$ at 4 °C for 15 min [31]. The pellet was removed and the supernatant was centrifuged at $10,000\times g$ at 4 °C for 15 min. The resulting precipitate served as the mitochondrial fraction and the supernatant was further centrifuged at $105,000\times g$ at 4 °C for 1 h. The resulting precipitate and supernatant served as the microsome and cytosol fractions, respectively. The protein content was measured using the Bradford protein assay [32]. The phosphoenolpyruvate carboxykinase (PEPCK) activity was determined based on the method of Bentle and Lardy [33]. The absorbance of the assay mixture was measured at 340 nm. The glucokinase (GK) activity was measured following the method described by Davidson and Arion [34]. The reaction mixture was incubated at 37 °C for 10 min and the change in absorbance at 340 nm was recorded. The glucose-6-phosphatase (G6pase) activity was determined using the method of Alegre et al. [35]. The reaction mixture was incubated at 37 °C for 4 min and the change in absorbance at 340 nm was recorded. The enzyme activities were expressed as μmol/min/mg protein.

2.6. Measurement of Bone Metabolism Biochemical Markers

The levels of calcium and alkaline phosphatase (ALP) were measured using Ca and ALP assay kits (Cobas, Indianopolis, IN, USA), respectively. The levels of 17-β-estradiol, intact parathyroid hormone (PTH), osteocalcin, N-terminal telopeptide of type 1 collagen (NTx-1) and C-terminal telopeptide of type 1 collagen (CTx-1) were analyzed using commercial assay kits (MyBiosource Inc., San Diego, CA, USA).

2.7. Statistical Analysis

All data are presented as the mean $\pm$ standard error (SE). The data were evaluated by one-way ANOVA using a Statistical Package for Social Sciences software program version 19.0 (SPSS Inc., Chicago, IL, USA) and the differences between the means were assessed using Tukey's test. An independent t-test was used to assess the difference between the germinated and non-germinated rice samples. Statistical significance was considered at $p < 0.05$.

3. Results

3.1. Body and Organ Weights

The final body weight markedly decreased in both SH (389 g) and GSH (374 g) groups relative to that of the control group (403 g) (Table 3). The feed intake and feed efficiency ratio were lowest in the GSH group and highest in the NC group. The white adipose tissue weight was lowest in GSH rats (8.56 g), followed by the SH group (9.04 g), then the NC group (10.26 g). The weights of liver and heart were significantly lower in the SH and GSH groups compared to that of the NC group.

3.2. Glucose Profile

As shown in Table 4, the final blood glucose level was lowest in the GSH group (5.04 nmol/L), followed by the SH group (5.61 nmol/L), then the NC group (6.98 nmol/L). The plasma insulin level was also lowest in the GSH group (3.39 mU/L) and highest in the NC group (4.93 mU/L). Accordingly, the HOMA-IR index was highest in the NC group (1.49), followed by the SH group (0.97), then the GSH group (0.78). Both the SH and GSH groups showed significantly higher hepatic glycogen level (149–153 mg/g) than the NC group (94.7 mg/g).

Table 3. Body weight gain and weights of organs and adipose tissue in ovariectomized rats fed with germinated Superhongmi rice powder.

Parameter	NC	SH	GSH
Initial weight (g)	229.24 ± 1.25	228.32 ± 1.18	228.14 ± 0.79
Final weight (g)	402.65 ± 5.33 [c]	388.69 ± 4.92 [b]	374.25 ± 5.41 [a]
Weight gain (g)	174.68 ± 5.63 [c]	160.24 ± 4.72 [b]	148.32 ± 3.30 [a]
Feed intake (g/week)	181.58 ± 4.32 [c]	162.25 ± 3.20 [b]	149.44 ± 3.41 [a]
Feed efficiency ratio	0.16 ± 0.00 [c]	0.14 ± 0.00 [b]	0.12 ± 0.00 [a]
White adipose tissue weight (g)	10.26 ± 0.19 [c]	9.04 ± 0.19 [b]	8.56 ± 0.12 [a]
Organ weight (g)			
Liver	2.88 ± 0.01 [c]	2.57 ± 0.02 [b]	2.50 ± 0.01 [a]
Heart	0.26± 0.01 [b]	0.23 ± 0.01 [a]	0.22 ± 0.01 [a]
Kidney	0.40 ± 0.01	0.39 ± 0.02	0.39 ± 0.04

[a–c] Values are means ± SE (*n* = 10). Means in the same row not sharing a common superscript are significantly different at $p < 0.05$. NC, normal control diet (AIN-93M); SH, normal diet + non-germinated Superhongmi; GSH, normal diet + germinated Superhongmi rice.

Table 4. Glucose profile, adipokine level, and glucose-regulating enzyme activity in ovariectomized rats fed with germinated Superhongmi rice powder.

Parameter	NC	SH	GSH
Initial blood glucose (mmol/L)	4.98 ± 0.02	5.01 ± 0.02	5.08 ± 0.02
Final blood glucose (mmol/L)	6.98 ± 0.05 [c]	5.61 ± 0.03 [b]	5.04 ± 0.03 [a]
Plasma insulin (mU/L)	4.93 ± 0.03 [c]	3.91 ± 0.05 [b]	3.39 ± 0.01 [a]
Hepatic glycogen (mg/g liver)	94.68 ± 2.26 [a]	149.25 ± 2.78 [b]	152.88 ± 3.07 [b]
HOMA-IR index	1.49 ± 0.00 [c]	0.97 ± 0.02 [b]	0.78 ± 0.00 [a]
Plasma adipokine			
Adiponectin (ng/mL)	0.26 ± 0.03 [a]	0.48 ± 0.03 [b]	0.71 ± 0.06 [c]
Leptin (ng/mL)	3.76 ± 0.27	3.32 ± 0.33	3.36 ± 0.26
Resistin (ng/mL)	32.55 ± 0.12 [c]	22.88 ± 1.43 [b]	18.25 ± 1.05 [a]
TNF-α (µg/mL)	9.58 ± 0.81 [c]	7.25 ± 0.58 [b]	4.51 ± 0.12 [a]
Hepatic glucose-regulating enzymes (µmol/min/mg protein)			
PEPCK	3.74 ± 0.87 [c]	2.98 ± 0.52 [b]	1.18 ± 0.41 [a]
GK	1.62 ± 0.13 [a]	2.89 ± 0.19 [b]	2.98 ± 0.22 [b]
G6pase	76.95 ± 1.32 [c]	68.33 ± 1.47 [b]	47.58 ± 1.51 [a]
GK/G6pase ratio	0.02 ± 0.00 [a]	0.04 ± 0.00 [b]	0.06 ± 0.00 [c]

[a–c] Values are means ± SE (*n* = 10). Means in the same row not sharing a common superscript are significantly different at $p < 0.05$. NC, normal control diet (AIN-93M); SH, normal diet + non-germinated Superhongmi rice; GSH, normal diet + germinated Superhongmi rice; HOMA-IR, homeostasis model of insulin resistance = (fasting insulin × fasting glucose)/22.5; TNF, tumor necrosis factor; PEPCK, phosphoenolpyruvate carboxynase; GK, glucokinase; G6pase, glucose-6-phosphatase.

3.3. Plasma Adipokine Level

The adiponectin level was highest in the GSH group (0.71 ng/mL) and lowest in the NC group (0.26 ng/mL) (Table 4). On the other hand, the levels of resistin and TNF-α were lowest in the GSH group and highest in the NC group. No significant difference was found in the leptin level among the animal groups.

3.4. Hepatic Glucose-Regulating Enzymes Activities

The hepatic PEPCK and G6pase activities were lowest in GSH rats and highest in the NC group (Table 4). Both the SH and GSH rats exhibited significantly higher GK activity (2.89–2.98 µmol/min/mg protein) than the control ones (1.62 µmol/min/mg protein). The GK to G6pase ratio was highest in the GSH group (0.06), followed by the SH group (0.04), then the NC group (0.02).

3.5. Biochemical Markers of Bone Metabolism

The GSH group showed significantly higher levels of 17-β-estradiol (0.87 ng/mL) and lower levels of intact PTH (18.05 pg/mL), NTx-1 (121.44 nmol/L), and CTx-1 (13.29 nmol/L) than the NC and SH groups (Table 5). No significant difference was found in the calcium and osteocalcin contents among the groups. The ALP level, on the other hand, was below 0.50 µg/L in all groups.

Table 5. Biochemical markers of bone metabolism in ovariectomized rats fed with germinated Superhongmi rice powder.

	NC	SH	GSH
17-β-estradiol (ng/mL)	0.47 ± 0.03 [a]	0.52 ± 0.02 [a]	0.87 ± 0.05 [b]
Intact PTH (pg/mL)	22.58 ± 0.63 [b]	21.22 ± 1.02 [b]	18.05 ± 0.57 [a]
Calcium (mg/dL)	9.65 ± 0.53	10.68 ± 0.43	10.58 ± 0.58
Osteocalcin (ng/mL)	13.55 ± 1.23	13.16 ± 0.73	12.57 ± 0.54
Alkaline phosphatase (µg/L)	<0.50 ± 0.00	<0.50 ± 0.00	<0.50 ± 0.00
NTx-1 (nmol/L)	181.58 ± 2.37 [c]	145.25 ± 1.23 [b]	121.44 ± 3.45 [a]
CTx-1 (nmol/mL)	23.71 ± 0.85 [c]	18.69 ± 0.65 [b]	13.29 ± 1.58 [a]

[a–c] Values are means ± SE ($n = 10$). Means in the same row not sharing a common superscript are significantly different at $p < 0.05$. NC, normal control diet (AIN-93M); SH, normal diet + non-germinated Superhongmi rice; GSH, normal diet + germinated Superhongmi rice; PTH, parathyroid hormone; NTx-1, N-terminal telopeptide of type 1 collagen; CTx-1, C-terminal telopeptide of type 1 collagen.

4. Discussion

Ovarian hormone deficiency resulting from menopause or ovariectomy increases the risk of diabetes, obesity, dyslipidemia, and osteoporosis [14,17,36]. The present study analyzed the effect of germinated Superhongmi rice, a reddish-brown pigmented cultivar, on the glucose and bone metabolisms in the postmenopausal-like model of ovariectomized rats. Results showed that diet supplementation of germinated and non-germinated Superhongmi rice powder significantly decreased the body weight gain, amount of body fat, blood glucose level, and plasma insulin concentrations and increased the hepatic glycogen level in ovariectomized rats. Both the SH and GSH animal groups also exhibited a markedly lower HOMA-IR index—an indicator of insulin resistance—than the control group, suggesting an increase in the insulin sensitivity in these animals. Studies in the past have also shown that pigmented rice could lower the body weight gain and improve the glucose metabolism in both laboratory animals and human subjects [12,13]. Between the two Superhongmi rice-fed groups, the GSH rats exhibited a greater body weight-lowering effect and hypoglycemic activity than the SH group. Germinated rice, especially pigmented cultivar, contains substantially higher amounts of bioactive compounds than non-germinated rice [4,5,19]. In the present study, γ-oryzanol, GABA, phytic acid, tocols, and policosanol were significantly higher in a germinated rice sample than that of the non-germinated one. γ-oryzanol, GABA, and phytic acid have hypolipidemic, hypoglycemic, and anti-obesity effects [4,7,37–39]. The tocols and policosanol possess antioxidative and antidiabetic property [4,40,41]. Hence, the strong hypoglycemic activity observed in GSH rats relative to the SH group is probably due to the increased amounts of bioactives in the germinated Superhongmi rice. This increase in the bioactive content is caused by the breaking down of the cell wall during germination, releasing the free and bound materials, and the activation of dormant enzymes associated with the synthesis of bioactive compounds [3].

The metabolism of glucose is influenced by adipokines and glucose-regulating enzymes. The ovariectomized rats fed with germinated Superhongmi rice powder showed the lowest resistin and TNF-α levels and highest adiponectin concentration. They also exhibited the lowest PEPCK and G6pase activities and highest GK activity and GK/G6pase ratio. The adipokines resistin and TNF-α regulate the lipid and glucose metabolisms and their elevated levels have been associated with the progression of obesity and diabetes [42–44]. The adiponectin, on the other hand, induces insulin-sensitizing effects and its enhanced expression has been shown to improve insulin sensitivity and glucose tolerance while its deficiency could induce insulin resistance [42]. An elevated level of adiponectin has also been reported to protect postmenopausal women against the development of diabetes [45]. The PEPCK, GK, and G6pase are major enzymes associated with glucose metabolism, wherein PEPCK and G6pase are involved in the regulation of gluconeogenesis and hepatic glucose output and an increase in their activities could result in an increased production of glucose [46,47]. The GK enzyme, on the other hand, is involved in glucose homeostasis and its enhanced activity has been associated with an increased glycogen level and reduced blood glucose content [48]. The GK/G6pase ratio, which reflects the balance between glucose uptake and output, was highest in GSH rats, indicating an enhanced glucose metabolism in these animals. Thus, the increase in adiponectin level and GK activity and the reduction in resistin and TNF-α concentrations and PEPCK and G6pase activities are possibly responsible for the improved glucose profile found in the rice-fed ovariectomized rats, particularly the GSH group.

Menopause and ovariectomy cause metabolic dysfunctions due to the rapid decrease of the estrogen hormone [14]. In the present study, the GSH rats showed significantly higher amount of 17-β-estradiol—the most potent form of estrogen—than the control group, suggesting that the germinated Superhongmi rice was able to inhibit the ovariectomy-induced reduction of estrogen level in these animals. Estrogen plays a central role in the regulation of bone metabolism, and administration of 17-β-estradiol has been reported to decrease the rate of bone turnover and prevent bone loss in postmenopausal women [49–51]. The ovariectomized rats fed with germinated Superhongmi rice also exhibited relatively low levels of intact PTH, NTx-1, and CTx-1, which are biochemical markers of bone resorption, indicating a reduced bone turnover in the GSH group. Increased bone resorption and imbalanced bone turnover are considered the main cause of the rapid rate of bone loss and enhanced risk of bone fracture in postmenopausal women [51,52]. Rice cultivars with colored pericarp, such as Superhongmi, are rich in antioxidant compounds such as anthocyanins, tocols, γ-oryzanol, and phytic acid [53] and germination could further increase the amount of these antioxidant compounds. Germinated Superhongmi rice has been previously reported to contain a substantial amount of antioxidant compounds and to have a strong antioxidant capacity [19]. Past investigations revealed that dietary antioxidants could prevent bone loss in postmenopausal women and ovariectomized animals and may be useful in the prevention and treatment of osteoporosis [54,55]. Since oxidative stress plays a central role in the pathogenesis of osteoporosis [56,57], the antioxidant compounds present in germinated Superhongmi rice may have been partly responsible for the improved bone metabolism observed in GSH rats.

5. Conclusions

The pigmented rice Superhongmi significantly reduced the body weight gain, glucose level, insulin concentration, and bone turnover in the postmenopausal-like model of ovariectomized rats through a mechanism involving the regulation of adipokine production and modulation of glucose-regulating enzyme activities. Germination for 72 h further enhanced the hypoglycemic effect and bone metabolism-improving action of this pigmented rice cultivar which may have been due to the increased amounts of various bioactive compounds such as GABA, γ-oryzanol, and tocols. Germinated Superhongmi rice may be beneficial as a functional food with therapeutic potential against menopause-induced hyperglycemia and bone turnover imbalance.

Acknowledgments: This research was supported by Basic Science Research Program through the National Research Foundation of Republic of Korea funded by the Ministry of Education (2014R1A1A2056797), and Next-Generation BioGreen21 Program (PJ011089).

Author Contributions: S.I.C. and M.Y.K. conceived and designed the experiments; S.N.R. offered rice samples, S.I.C. performed the experiments and analyzed the data; S.I.C. and M.Y.K. wrote the paper. All authors approved the final version of the manuscript.

Conflicts of Interest: The authors declare no conflict of interest.

References

1. Wu, F.; Yang, N.; Toure, A.; Jin, Z.; Xu, X. Germinated brown rice and its role in human health. *Crit. Rev. Food Sci. Nutr.* **2013**, *53*, 451–463. [CrossRef] [PubMed]
2. Patil, S.B.; Khan, M.K. Germinated brown rice as a value added rice product: A review. *J. Food Sci. Technol.* **2011**, *48*, 661–667. [CrossRef] [PubMed]
3. Moongngarm, A.; Saetung, N. Comparison of chemical compositions andbioactive compounds of germinated rough rice and brown rice. *Food Chem.* **2010**, *122*, 782–788. [CrossRef]
4. Cho, D.H.; Lim, S.T. Germinated brown rice and its bio-functional compounds. *Food Chem.* **2016**, *196*, 259–271. [CrossRef] [PubMed]
5. Ng, L.T.; Huang, S.H.; Chen, Y.T.; Su, C.H. Changes of tocopherols, tocotrienols, γ-oryzanol, and γ-aminobutyric acid levels in the germinated brown rice of pigmented and nonpigmented cultivars. *J. Agric. Food Chem.* **2013**, *61*, 12604–12611. [CrossRef] [PubMed]
6. Mohd, E.N.; Abdul, K.K.K.; Amom, Z.; Azlan, A. Antioxidant activity of white rice, brown rice and germinated brown rice (in vivo and in vitro) and the effects on lipid peroxidation and liver enzymes in hyperlipidaemic rabbits. *Food Chem.* **2013**, *141*, 1306–1312. [CrossRef] [PubMed]
7. Kang, M.Y.; Rico, C.W.; Bae, H.J.; Lee, S.C. Antioxidant capacity of newly developed pigmented rice cultivars in Korea. *Cereal Chem.* **2013**, *90*, 497–501. [CrossRef]
8. Min, B.; McClung, A.M.; Chen, M.H. Phytochemicals and antioxidant capacities in rice brans of different color. *J. Food Sci.* **2011**, *76*, C117–C126. [CrossRef] [PubMed]
9. Deng, G.F.; Xu, X.R.; Zhang, Y.; Li, D.; Gan, R.Y.; Li, H.B. Phenolic compounds and bioactivities of pigmented rice. *Crit. Rev. Food Sci. Nutr.* **2013**, *53*, 296–306. [CrossRef] [PubMed]
10. Frank, T.; Reichardt, B.; Shu, Q.; Engel, K.H. Metabolite profiling of colored rice (*Oryza sativa* L.) grains. *J. Cereal Sci.* **2012**, *55*, 112–119. [CrossRef]
11. Ling, W.H.; Cheng, Q.X.; Ma, J.; Wang, T. Red and black rice decrease atherosclerotic plaque formation and increase antioxidant status in rabbits. *J. Nutr.* **2001**, *131*, 1421–1426. [PubMed]
12. Bae, H.J.; Rico, C.W.; Ryu, S.N.; Kang, M.Y. Hypolipidemic, hypoglycemic and antioxidantive effects of a new pigmented rice cultivar "Superjami" in high fat-fed mice. *J. Korean Soc. Appl. Biol. Chem.* **2014**, *57*, 685–691. [CrossRef]
13. Shimoda, H.; Aitani, M.; Tanaka, J.; Hitoe, S. Purple rice extract exhibits preventive activities on experimental diabetes models and human subjects. *J. Rice Res.* **2015**, *3*, 137. [CrossRef]
14. Carr, M.C. The emergence of the metabolic syndrome with menopause. *J. Clin. Endocrinol. Metab.* **2003**, *88*, 2404–2411. [CrossRef] [PubMed]
15. Akahoshi, M.; Soda, M.; Nakashima, E.; Shimaoka, K.; Seto, S.; Yano, K. Effects of menopause on trends of serum cholesterol, blood pressure, and body mass index. *Circulation* **1996**, *94*, 61–66. [CrossRef] [PubMed]
16. Otsuki, M.; Kasayama, S.; Morita, S.; Asanuma, N.; Saito, H.; Mukai, M.; Koga, M. Menopause, but not age, is an independent risk factor for fasting plasma glucose levels in nondiabetic women. *Menopause* **2007**, *14*, 404–407. [CrossRef] [PubMed]
17. Ji, M.X.; Yu, Q. Primary osteoporosis in postmenopausal women. *Chronic Dis. Transl. Med.* **2015**, *1*, 9–13. [CrossRef]
18. Brinton, R.D. Minireview: Translational animal models of human menopause: Challenges and emerging opportunities. *Endocrinology* **2012**, *153*, 3571–3578. [CrossRef] [PubMed]
19. Chung, S.I.; Lo, L.M.P.; Kang, M.Y. Effect of germination on the antioxidant capacity of pigmented rice (*Oryza sativa* L. cv. Superjami and Superhongmi). *Food Sci. Technol. Res.* **2016**, *22*, 387–394. [CrossRef]
20. Lo, L.M.P.; Kang, M.Y.; Yi, S.J.; Chung, S.I. Dietary supplementation of germinated pigmented rice (*Oryza sativa* L.) lowers dyslipidemia risk in ovariectomized Sprague-Dawley rats. *Food Nutr. Res.* **2016**, *60*. [CrossRef] [PubMed]
21. Wu, F.; Chen, H.; Yang, N.; Wang, J.; Duan, X.; Jin, Z.; Xu, X. Effect on germination time on physicochemical properties of brown rice flour and starch from different rice cultivars. *J. Cereal Sci.* **2013**, *58*, 263–271. [CrossRef]
22. Chakuton, K.; Puangpronpitag, D.; Nakornriab, M. Phytochemical Content and Antioxidant Activity of Colored and Non-colored Thai Rice Cultivars. *Asian J. Plant Sci.* **2012**, *11*, 285–293.

23. Islam, M.A.; Becerra, J.X. Analysis of chemical components involved in germination process of rice variety Jhapra. *J. Sci. Res.* **2012**, *4*, 251–262. [CrossRef]
24. Jeng, T.L.; Shih, Y.J.; Ho, P.T.; Lai, C.C.; Lin, Y.W. γ -Oryzanol, tocol and mineral compositions in different grain fractions of giant embryo rice mutants. *J. Sci. Food Agric.* **2012**, *92*, 1468–1474. [CrossRef] [PubMed]
25. Kim, N.H.; Kwak, J.; Baik, J.Y.; Yoon, M.R.; Lee, J.S.; Yoon, S.W.; Kim, I.H. Changes in lipid substances in rice during grain development. *Phytochemistry* **2015**, *116*, 170–179. [CrossRef] [PubMed]
26. Konwachara, T.; Ahromrit, A. Effect of cooking on functional properties of germinated black glutinous rice (KKU-URL012). *Songklanakarin J. Sci. Technol.* **2014**, *36*, 283–290.
27. Association of Official Analytical Chemists Inc. *AOAC Official Methods of Analysis*; Association of Official Analytical Chemists Inc.: Arlington, VA, USA, 2003.
28. American Institute of Nutrition. Report of ad hoc committee on standards for nutritional studies. *J. Nutr.* **1977**, *107*, 1340–1347.
29. Seifter, S.; Dayton, S.; Navic, B.; Muntwyler, E. The estimation of glycogen with the anthrone reagent. *Arch. Biochem.* **1950**, *25*, 191–200. [PubMed]
30. Vogeser, M.; Konig, D.; Frey, I.; Predel, H.G.; Parhofer, K.G.; Berg, A. Fasting serum insulin and the homeostasis model of insulin resistance (HOMA-IR) in the monitoring of lifestyle interventions in obese persons. *Clin. Biochem.* **2007**, *40*, 964–968. [CrossRef] [PubMed]
31. Hulcher, F.H.; Oleson, W.H. Simplified spectrophotometric assay for microsomal 3-hydroxy-3-methylglutaryl CoA reductase by measurement of coenzyme A. *J. Lipid Res.* **1973**, *14*, 625–631. [PubMed]
32. Bradford, M.M. A rapid sensitive method for the quantitation of microgram quantities of protein utilizing the principle of protein-dye binding. *Anal. Biochem.* **1976**, *72*, 248–254. [CrossRef]
33. Bentle, L.A.; Lardy, H.A. Interaction of anions and divalent metal ions with phosphoenolpyruvate carboxykinase. *J. Biol. Chem.* **1976**, *251*, 2916–2921. [PubMed]
34. Davidson, A.L.; Arion, W.J. Factors underlying significant underestimations of glucokinase activity in crude liver extracts: Physiological implications of higher cellular activity. *Arch. Biochem. Biophys.* **1987**, *253*, 156–167. [CrossRef]
35. Alegre, M.; Ciudad, C.J.; Fillat, C.; Guinovart, J.J. Determination of glucose-6-phosphatase activity using the glucose dehydrogenase-coupled reaction. *Anal. Biochem.* **1988**, *173*, 185–189. [CrossRef]
36. Seidlova-Wuttke, D.; Nguyen, B.T.; Wuttke, W. Long-term effects of ovariectomy on osteoporosis and obesity in estrogen-receptor-β-deleted mice. *Comp. Med.* **2012**, *62*, 8–13. [PubMed]
37. Kim, S.M.; Rico, C.W.; Lee, S.C.; Kang, M.Y. Modulatory effect of rice bran and phytic acid on glucose metabolism in high fat-fed C57BL/6N mice. *J. Clin. Biochem. Nutr.* **2010**, *47*, 12–17. [CrossRef] [PubMed]
38. Son, M.J.; Rico, C.W.; Nam, S.H.; Kang, M.Y. Influence of oryzanol and ferulic acid on the lipid metabolism and antioxidative status in high fat-fed mice. *J. Clin. Biochem. Nutr.* **2010**, *46*, 150–156. [CrossRef] [PubMed]
39. Son, M.J.; Rico, C.W.; Nam, S.H.; Kang, M.Y. Effect of oryzanol and ferulic acid on the glucose metabolism of mice fed with high fat diet. *J. Food Sci.* **2011**, *76*, H7–H10. [CrossRef] [PubMed]
40. Chauhan, K.; Chauhan, B. Policosanol: Natural wax component with potent health benefits. *Int. J. Med. Pharm. Sci.* **2015**, *5*, 15–24.
41. Lee, J.Y.; Choi, H.Y.; Kang, Y.R.; Chang, H.B.; Chun, H.S.; Lee, M.S.; Kwon, Y.I. Effects of long-term supplementation of policosanol on blood cholesterol/glucose levels and 3-hydroxy-3methylglutaryl coenzyme a reductase activity in a rat model fed high cholesterol diets. *Food Sci. Biotechnol.* **2016**, *25*, 899–904. [CrossRef]
42. Jung, U.J.; Choi, M.S. Obesity and its metabolic complications: The role of adipokines and the relationship between obesity, inflammation, insulin resistance, dyslipidemia and nonalcoholic fatty lover disease. *Int. J. Mol. Sci.* **2014**, *15*, 6184–6223. [CrossRef] [PubMed]
43. Silha, J.V.; Weiler, H.A.; Murphy, L.J. Plasma adipokines and body composition in response to modest dietary manipulations in the mouse. *Obesity* **2006**, *14*, 1320–1329. [CrossRef] [PubMed]
44. Steppan, C.M.; Bailey, S.T.; Bhat, S.; Brown, E.J.; Banerjee, R.R.; Wright, C.M.; Patel, H.R.; Ahima, R.S.; Lazar, M.A. The hormone resistin links obesity to diabetes. *Nature* **2001**, *409*, 307–312. [CrossRef] [PubMed]
45. Darabi, H.; Raeisi, A.; Kalantarhormozi, M.R.; Ostovar, A.; Assadi, M.; Asadipooya, K.; Vahdat, K.; Dobaradaran, S.; Nabipour, I. Adiponectin as protective factor against progression toward type 2 diabetes mellitus in postmenopausal women. *Medicine* **2015**, *94*, e1347. [CrossRef] [PubMed]

46. She, P.; Shiota, M.; Shelton, K.D.; Chalkley, R.; Postic, C.; Magnuson, M.A. Phosphoenolpyruvate carboxykinase is necessary for the integration of hepatic energy metabolism. *Mol. Cell. Biol.* **2000**, *20*, 6508–6517. [CrossRef] [PubMed]
47. Schaftingen, E.V.; Gerin, I. The glucose-6-phosphatase system. *Biochem. J.* **2002**, *362*, 513–532. [CrossRef] [PubMed]
48. Coope, G.J.; Atkinson, A.M.; Allott, C.; McKerrecher, D.; Johnstone, C.; Pike, K.G. Predictive blood glucose lowering efficacy by glucokinase activators in high fat fed female zucker rats. *Br. J. Pharmacol.* **2003**, *149*, 328–335. [CrossRef] [PubMed]
49. Curran, M.P.; Wagstaff, A.J. Spotlight on estradiol and norgestimate as hormone therapy in postmenopausal women. *Treat. Endocrinol.* **2002**, *1*, 127–129. [CrossRef] [PubMed]
50. Ettinger, B. Use of low-dosage 17 beta-estradiol for the prevention of osteoporosis. *Clin. Ther.* **1993**, *15*, 950–962. [PubMed]
51. Vaananen, H.K.; Harkonen, P.L. Estrogen and bone metabolism. *Maturitas* **1996**, *23*, S65–S69. [CrossRef]
52. Seibel, M.J. Biochemical markers of bone turnover part II: Clinical applications in the management of osteoporosis. *Clin. Biochem. Rev.* **2006**, *27*, 123–138. [PubMed]
53. Goufo, P.; Trindade, H. Rice antioxidants: Phenolic acids, flavonoids, anthocyanins, proanthocyanidins, tocopherols, tocotrienols, γ-oryzanol, and phytic acid. *Food Sci. Nutr.* **2014**, *2*, 75–104. [CrossRef] [PubMed]
54. Franca, N.A.G.; Camargo, M.B.; Lazaretti-Castro, M.; Martini, L.A. Antioxidant intake and bone status in a cross-sectional study of Brazilian women with osteoporosis. *Nutr. Health* **2013**, *22*, 133–142. [CrossRef] [PubMed]
55. Muhammad, N.; Luke, D.A.; Shuid, A.N.; Mohamed, N.; Soelaiman, I.N. Tocotrienol supplementation in postmenopausal osteoporosis: Evidence from a laboratory study. *Clinics* **2013**, *68*, 1338–1343. [CrossRef]
56. Altindag, O.; Erel, O.; Soran, N.; Celik, H.; Selek, S. Total oxidative/anti-oxidative status and relation to bone mineral density in osteoporosis. *Rheumatol. Int.* **2008**, *28*, 317–321. [CrossRef] [PubMed]
57. Sendur, O.F.; Turan, Y.; Tastaban, E.; Serter, M. Antioxidant status in patients with osteoporosis: A controlled study. *Jt. Bone Spine* **2009**, *76*, 514–518. [CrossRef] [PubMed]

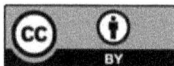

nutrients

MDPI

Review
Phytomedicine in Joint Disorders

Dorin Dragos [1,2], Marilena Gilca [3], Laura Gaman [3], Adelina Vlad [4], Liviu Iosif [5], Irina Stoian [3,5,]*
and Olivera Lupescu [6,7]

[1] Medical Semiology Department, Faculty of General Medicine, "Carol Davila" University of Medicine and Pharmacy, B-dul "Eroilor Sanitari" nr. 8, Sector 6, 76241 Bucharest, Romania; dordrag@drdorindragos.ro
[2] Nephrology Clinic, University Emergency Hospital Bucharest, 050098 Bucharest, Romania
[3] Biochemistry Department, Faculty of General Medicine, "Carol Davila" University of Medicine and Pharmacy, B-dul "Eroilor Sanitari" nr. 8, Sector 6, 76241 Bucharest, Romania; marilenagilca@gmail.com (M.G.); glauraelena@gmail.com (L.G.)
[4] Physiology Department, Faculty of General Medicine, "Carol Davila" University of Medicine and Pharmacy, B-dul "Eroilor Sanitari" nr. 8, Sector 6, 76241 Bucharest, Romania; adelina_munteanu@yahoo.com
[5] R&D IRIST LABMED SRL, Str. Miraslau, nr. 24, Sector 3, 031235 Bucharest, Romania; iristlabmed@gmail.com
[6] Orthopaedic and Trauma Clinic 2, Faculty of General Medicine, "Carol Davila" University of Medicine and Pharmacy, 020022 Bucharest, Romania; olivera_lupescu@yahoo.com
[7] Clinical Emergency Hospital Bucharest, 014461 Bucharest, Romania
* Correspondence: irina.stoian@umf.ro or irina_stoian64@yahoo.com; Tel.: +40-748-038-284

Received: 12 December 2016; Accepted: 12 January 2017; Published: 16 January 2017

Abstract: Chronic joint inflammatory disorders such as osteoarthritis and rheumatoid arthritis have in common an upsurge of inflammation, and oxidative stress, resulting in progressive histological alterations and disabling symptoms. Currently used conventional medication (ranging from pain-killers to biological agents) is potent, but frequently associated with serious, even life-threatening side effects. Used for millennia in traditional herbalism, medicinal plants are a promising alternative, with lower rate of adverse events and efficiency frequently comparable with that of conventional drugs. Nevertheless, their mechanism of action is in many cases elusive and/or uncertain. Even though many of them have been proven effective in studies done in vitro or on animal models, there is a scarcity of human clinical evidence. The purpose of this review is to summarize the available scientific information on the following joint-friendly medicinal plants, which have been tested in human studies: *Arnica montana*, *Boswellia* spp., *Curcuma* spp., *Equisetum arvense*, *Harpagophytum procumbens*, *Salix* spp., *Sesamum indicum*, *Symphytum officinalis*, *Zingiber officinalis*, *Panax notoginseng*, and *Whitania somnifera*.

Keywords: osteoarthritis; rheumatoid arthritis; medicinal plants; herbs

1. Introduction

Chronic joint inflammatory disorders such as osteoarthritis and rheumatoid arthritis have in common an upsurge of inflammation, and oxidative stress, resulting in progressive histological alterations and disabling symptoms.

Osteoarthritis, one of the most common musculoskeletal disorders, affecting approximately 15% of the population [1], is characterized by irreversible destruction of articular cartilage and bone erosion, induced by pro-inflammatory cytokines, e.g., interleukin 1 (IL-1), interleukin 6 (IL-6), and tumor necrosis factor α (TNF-α). These mediators increased the collagenase or matrix metaloproteinase (MMP) synthesis and the degradation of collagen type II, and decreased the synthesis of collagenase inhibitors, collagen and proteoglycans [2]. Degradation of collagen type II by collagenase-1 and collagenase-3 (also called MMP-13) represents one of the biochemical hallmarks of osteoarthritis [3].

Factors that increase the risk of OA are advanced age, sex, overweight, increased body mass index (BMI), genetics, ethnicity, diet, trauma, certain physical or occupational activities that imply biomechanical stress (e.g., pressure, load-bearing) across the joints [4–6]. Monitoring the OA evolution and therapy involves pain and physical function assessment for shorter studies, as well as joint imaging for longer studies (1 year or more). Pain is evaluated with visual analog scales (VAS), while the functional impairment with Western Ontario and McMaster Universities OA Index (WOMAC) [7]. Other useful assessment tools of functional impairment are Lequesne Functional Severity Index [8] and Karnofski Performance Scale Index [9].

Rheumatoid arthritis (RA) is a chronic progressive systemic autoimmune disease affecting 1% of the population and generating disability and increased risk for cardiovascular disease, lymphoma, and death [10], typically associated with high levels of oxidative stress and inflammatory mediators. RA is currently treated with a wide variety of medicines ranging from steroidal/nonsteroidal anti-inflammatory drugs (NSAID and pain killers), to potent biological agents targeting specific immune and inflammatory pathways, such as TNF-alpha (TNF-α) inhibitors and interleukin-1 receptor antagonists [11]. Among nonsteroidal anti-inflammatory drugs, acetaminophen is most frequently used in very high doses (4000 mg/day). Concerning the pain killers, tramadol is highly recommended, but also other opioids (e.g., morphine) [12]. Etanercept, infliximab and rituximab represent few examples of TNF-α inhibitors used for the treatment of severe RA [13,14]. Anakinra (an IL-1 receptor antagonist) [15] and methotrexat are other therapeutic choices for RA [16].

The biologic therapies have proven to be highly successful and effective in the majority of RA cases, including the severe ones.

Unfortunately, the use of standard drugs in arthropathies is accompanied by numerous and frequently serious side effects [17]: gastrointestinal ulcerations, hemorrhagic events, and nephrotoxicity induced by NSAID [18]; infusion hypersensitivity reactions, and auto-immune responses (e.g., lupus-like syndrome) triggered by TNFα inhibitors [19]; increased risk of severe infection, affecting mainly the respiratory tract, caused by biological drugs (anakinra, rituximab, or abatacept) [20]; fatal cytopenia induced by methotrexate [21]; etc.

Hence the renewed interest in medicines of botanical origin, which lack severe adverse effects and have a millennia-proven efficacy [22]. These remedies may be have a beneficial effect not only on the symptoms but also on the course of the disease [23].

The purpose of this review is to summarize the available scientific information obtained from medical databases and literature on medicinal plants that have been reported to have anti-arthritic activity in vitro, in animal models and also in human clinical studies.

A literature search was performed using the following phrases "medicinal plants or herb and osteoarthritis or arthritis or rheumatoid arthritis", "*specific herb Latin name* or *specific herb English name* and osteoarthritis or arthritis or rheumatoid arthritis" (e.g., *Curcuma longa* or turmeric and osteoarthritis or arthritis or rheumatoid arthritis), in PubMed database. Only medicinal plants studied in human clinical studies were selected, and presented in alphabetical order of their Latin names. For all the plants included in the paper, we have analyzed in vitro studies, animal studies, and human clinical studies using herbal extracts, and potentially active phytochemicals. The corresponding papers were retrieved and evaluated in terms of the relevance for the present paper topic. Supplementary information was also obtained by a manual search in various books, including books of traditional medicine.

Several herbal extracts presented in the present paper (see Table 1) showed benefits in terms of pain and physical mobility, with low risk of side effects in arthritic subjects. These results warranting further investigation.

2. Anti-Arthritic Medicinal Plants

2.1. Arnica montana, family (fam.) Asteraceae

Traditional knowledge. This plant has been used for centuries in traditional herbalism as a remedy for trauma-, strain- and/or inflammation-related conditions of the locomotor system [24], and is one of the natural remedies most often used for rheumatologic conditions [25].

Animal studies. An orally administered *Arnica* extract was shown (on the collagen induced arthritis rat model) to alleviate both the histological and radiological changes in the affected joints, in parallel with a decrease in NO, TNF-α, IL-1β, IL-6, and IL-12 concentrations, anti-type II collagen antibodies level, and an improvement of the oxidative status (higher antioxidant levels and milder peroxidative injury) [24].

Human clinical studies. In an open multicenter trial, a gel prepared form *Arnica montana* fresh plant was tested in knee OA and proven to alleviate symptoms, improve functionality, and to be well tolerated. Rare adverse events were reported. Allergy might be a concern, as is fitting for a true Asteraceae herb [26]. A double-blind study on 204 patients comparing *Arnica montana* with ibuprofen in topical applications for hand OA found no difference in terms of efficiency and side effects (less frequent for *Arnica*) [27], a result corroborated by another study [28]. The equipotency of *Arnica* with NSAID in the local treatment of hand OA was acknowledged also by a Cochrane review [29].

Active phytochemicals. The anti-arthritic efficiency is attributed by some authors to a synergism of phenolic and flavonoid compounds, the dominant active principles, detected in a methanol extract, which was found efficient on a collagen-induced arthritis (CIA) rat model [24].

2.2. Boswellia spp., fam. Burseraceae

Traditional knowledge. Used for centuries in Ayurveda medicine (where it is called sallaki) *Boswellia serrata* (BS) yields a gum resin, known as frankincense, efficacious in the treatment of inflammatory disorders [30], particularly arthritis. Nowadays, many anti-arthritic combinations contain BS.

In vitro studies. A BS preparation enriched in active principles was able to hinder cartilage breakdown by metalloproteinase-3 (MMP-3) and to block Intercellular Adhesion Molecule 1 (ICAM-1) and thereby the inflammatory reaction [31]. In another study, a *B. frereana* preparation decreased the synthesis/ activation of several inflammation-related mediators and enzymes (MMP-9 and MMP-13, cycloxygenase-2, nitric oxide, prostaglandin E2), thus thwarting collagen and cartilage dissolution [32].

A poly-herbal formulation containing *Zingiber officinale* root, *Tinospora cordifolia* stem, *Phyllanthus emblica* fruit and oleoresin of BS has been shown to halt cartilage degradation in the knee (decreased release of glycosaminoglycans and aggrecan) associated with anti-inflammatory activity (as assessed by lower levels of nitric oxide) [33].

Another combination including three herbs (*Uncaria tomentosa*, *Boswellia* spp., and *Lepidium meyenii*) and an amino acid (L-leucine) has been shown to hamper inflammation and protect the articular cartilage. Tested on OA chondrocytes, it blocked the IL-1β-triggered activation of NF-κB and consequently abrogated the activity of inflammation-related enzymes (iNOS, MMP-9 and MMP-13), leading to a decreased rate of NO production and of cartilage matrix deterioration (less glycosaminoglycans-GAGs-released); simultaneously, enhanced production of structural proteins (including aggrecan and type II collagen) was detected [23].

Animal studies. Using the rat model of collagen induced arthritis, an extract of BS was able to suppress pro-inflammatory mediators and to improve the antioxidant status, as reflected by lactoperoxidase, myeloperoxidase, catalase, superoxide dismutase (SOD), glutathione (GSH), nitric oxide (NO) [22]. A mixture of *Withania somnifera*, BS, *Zingiber officinale* and *Curcuma longa* was tested on a rat model of adjuvant induced arthritis and proven to relieve inflammation and arthritis, and also to diminish the production of TNF-α and NO [34].

Human clinical studies. A Cochrane systematic review concluded that preparations from BS "show trends of benefits" (when used for the treatment of OA) coupled with a low burden of side effects, citing two high-quality and two moderate-quality studies demonstrating superiority compared to placebo in reducing pain and increasing functionality, and a moderate-quality study indicating a favorable adverse events profile [35]. Indeed, a couple of double-blind, randomized, placebo-controlled studies done on patients with knee OA demonstrated that phytopreparations from BS gum resin are able to reduce pain and increase functionality after only a few days (a week or so at most) with no serious adverse effects [31,36]. A phytosomal *Boswellia* preparation has been shown to be beneficial in the treatment of knee OA when added to the standard management of this condition (ameliorating the functional status (higher Karnofski Scale Index) and the symptoms (lower WOMAC (Western Ontario and McMaster Universities questionnaire) Score) [37]). It also hasten functional recovery and diminished pain and objective physical and humoral signs of inflammations in persons with arthritis of the hand induced by work-related overstraining [38]. A combination of *Curcuma longa* and BS was proven to be safe and efficient in patients with osteoarthritis, alleviating symptoms and objective signs, even better than celecoxib (a selective COX-2 inhibitor) and being practically devoid of side effects [39]. However other studies failed to confirm the efficiency of BS in the treatment of active RA [40].

Active phytochemicals. The role of bioactive principles is revendicated by the boswellic acids [41,42], a family of pentacyclic triterpenes, among which the main contenders were, initially, 11-keto-β-boswellic acid and acetyl-11-keto-β-boswellic acid. Oral or local administration of boswellic acids in a bovine serum albumin-induced arthritis model ameliorated the electrophoretic pattern of the synovial fluid proteins and decreased the infiltration of leucocytes into the knee joint [43]. These compounds were considered until recently to inhibit leukotriene synthesis by suppressing lipoxygenase-5 (LOX-5) in vitro and in animal models [30,44]. Other mechanisms were also invoked such as suppression of NF-κB activation, reduction of the production of pro-inflammatory cytokines (TNF-α, IL-1, IL-2, IL-4, IL-6 and IFN-γ), and reduced cleavage of C3 into the active components C3a and C3b, hampering the activation of the classic path of the complement [45]. These were showed in various in vivo experiments, with various arthritic or non-arthritic inflammation models (e.g., hypersensitivity reaction in mice) [46]. More recently, concerns were raised regarding both the action intensity of 11-keto-β-boswellic acid and acetyl-11-keto-β-boswellic acid, and their bioavailability, the latter being too poor to provide concentrations high enough for bioactivity [47]. Nonetheless, another member of the family was proposed as active principle, namely β-boswellic acid, able to reach much higher levels in plasma, enough to efficiently exert its inhibitory action on microsomal prostaglandin E synthase-1 and on the serine protease cathepsin G, which might be the substrate of the inflammation-suppressing aptitude of BS preparations [17].

2.3. *Curcuma spp., fam. Zingiberaceae*

Traditional knowledge. Several members of the *Curcuma* genus are used in traditional medicine, most important being *Curcuma longa* (CL), turmeric. Its rhizome has a centuries-long use as a dietary spice as well as an Ayurveda herb prized for its anti-inflammatory properties, hence its utility in arthritic conditions including RA [48].

Animal studies. In an animal arthritis model a preparation from CL lacking essential oil strongly suppressed joint inflammation and periarticular damage in correlation with decreased activation of NF-κB and of the ensuing cascade of events (involving mediators of inflammation and injury such as chemokines, cyclooxygenase 2, and receptor activator of nuclear factor kappa-B ligand (RANKL)) [49]. The ability to prevent the destructive changes in joints and periarticular bone seems to be comparable to that of betamethasone [50,51]. Liposomal encapsulation may help overcome the poor bioavailability problem generated by the low water-solubility [52]. The osteoclast-osteoblast balance is tipped in favor of bone building, while halting the OA progression [52]. In a rat-model of experimentally induced arthritis, a combination of ginger and turmeric rhizomes was superior to indomethacin (a potent NSAID) regarding the ability to alleviate both joint histopathological changes, and the extra-articular manifestations, including systemic inflammation (leukocytosis, thrombocytosis, and hyperglobulinemia), malnutrition (decreased body weight gain, and hypoalbuminemia), and iron deficiency anemia, with no prejudice to kidney function and reduced risk of cardiovascular disease (favorable lipid and oxidative profile) [53].

Human clinical studies. A mixture of *Curcuma longa* and *Boswellia serrata* has been shown to be more efficient than a standard dose of celecoxib (a selective COX-2 inhibitor) in the treatment of osteoarthritis, improving both objectively and subjectively the condition of the patients, with no toxicity detectable by clinical examination and laboratory tests (hemogram, liver and renal function tests) [39]. *Curcuma domestica* extracts have been shown to be useful in knee osteoarthritis, reducing the pain and preserving functionality with an efficiency equivalent to ibuprofen, but with fewer gastrointestinal side effects [54]. A recent meta-analysis found relevant scientific evidence for the efficacy of turmeric as a therapeutic option in arthritis, but concluded that more studies are necessary in order to definitively pin it down [55].

Active phytochemicals. The active ingredient is diferuloylmethane, a yellow phenolic pigment commonly known as curcumin, which has a multifaceted beneficial action in various fields of pathology (diabetes, cancer, inflammation, oxidative stress) due to its ability to favorably influence a variety of signaling pathways and mediators [56]. In a rat model of arthritis, it has been shown to ameliorate the joint inflammation (evaluated by the neutrophil infiltrate density), in the first six hours after the arthritis-inducing event (zymosan infiltration) being even more effective than a low dose of prednisone [57].

The reduction of the systemic oxidative stress as reflected by enhanced serum SOD activity, increased GSH level, and decreased malondialdehyde level was considered part of the mechanism of action [58]. The blockage of glial activation resulting in decreased synthesis and secretion of inflammatory mediators in the spinal cord, corroborated by similar results in studies on cultures of astrocytes and microglia can be responsible for arthritic pain reduction [59].

β-Elemene, found in *Curcuma Wenyujin*, an herb used in Traditional Chinese Medicine for the treatment of rheumatoid arthritis, may be another phytochemical active in arthropathies. This compound antiproliferative activity (useful in neoplastic diseases) may explain the suppressive effect on accumulation of fibroblast-like synoviocytes. One in vitro study showed that the underlying mechanism may be represented by the apoptosis induction via increased production of reactive oxygen species and activation of p38 mitogen-activated protein kinase (MAPK) [60].

2.4. Equisetum arvense, fam. Equisetaceae

Traditional knowledge. *Equisetum arvense*, also known as horsetail, has a long history of use in European ethnomedicine as an anti-inflammatory remedy [61].

Animal studies. An animal model of arthritis induced through an antigen challenge was used to prove the downregulating effects of *Equisetum giganteum* on lymphocyte proliferation. B and T lymphocytes are both affected by the immunomodulatory action of this plant, which is nevertheless free of cytotoxicity [62].

Human clinical studies. The beneficial effect of horsetail in RA was substantiated by a study that pointed out the decrease in TNF-α as one of the contributing mechanisms [63].

Active phytochemicals. Kynurenic acid was proposed as a putative mediator of the anti-inflammatory and antalgic effect of several herbs beneficial in RA, horsetail among them [64]. The anti-inflammatory potential of kynurenic acid was showed until now only in non-arthritic animal models (e.g., acute experimental colitis in rat) [65]. Kynurenic acid is also an endogenous oxidative metabolite of tryptophan, with glutamate-receptor antagonist activity, which may explain partially its analgesic properties. One in vitro study showed that kynurenic acid is able to inhibit the proliferation of synoviocytes [66]. Its level was significantly lower in human subjects with RA than that in those with OA [67], fact which suggests the beneficial potential of kynurenic acid supplementation in RA patients.

2.5. Harpagophytum procumbens, fam. Pedaliaceae

Traditional knowledge. Harpagophytum procumbens (HP), also known as devil's claw, a medicinal plant native to Africa, is a "celebrity" among anti-osteoarthritis natural remedies, being approved by German Commission E for the treatment of degenerative diseases of the musculoskeletal system [68].

In vitro studies. HP extracts showed chondroprotective activity, several mechanisms being potentially responsible for this: decreased synthesis of inflammatory mediators (e.g., TNF-α, and interleukin-1β), and inhibition of matrix metalloproteinases and elastase [69].

Animal studies. A dried aqueous extract of HP has been shown to have a significant dose-dependent analgesic and anti-inflammatory activity in rats at 5 and 10 mg/kg. Nevertheless, carrageenan-induced paw edema was not affected by the isolated harpagoside constituent. This signifies that harpagoside may not have an anti-inflammatory effect, at least in the dosage used in this study [70,71]. This suggests that other HP constituents may be responsible for the anti-inflammatory effect.

Human clinical studies. Several human clinical studies showed that various HP tuber extracts (equivalent to 50–60 mg harpagoside daily, administered for a variable period between 8 and 16 weeks, depending on the study) significantly improved the clinical picture of subjects with knee and hip osteoarthritis in terms of pain, movement limitation, and joint crepitus [72–74]. The severity of pain and other symptoms was assessed by the WOMAC questionnaire, VAS, Lequesne Index, physician exam and/or pain-relieving medication dose.

Active phytochemicals. The major phytochemicals responsible for the anti-osteoarthritis effect are the iridoid glycosides (harpagoside, harpagide, and procumbide), which are found in a higher amount in tubers and root. Although, it is worthy to mention that the whole-plant extracts seem to have a better therapeutic effect than those obtained from isolated parts [75]. Harpagoside inhibited in vitro the synthesis of various pro-inflammatory mediators via suppression of iNOS and COX-2 expression through inhibition of NF-κB activation [76], but showed no anti-inflammatory activity in one animal model of inflammation (carrageenan-induced paw edema) [70]. The scientists suggested that other phytochemicals than harpagoside may be contributors to the anti-inflammatory effect of HP [70,77].

2.6. Panax notoginseng, fam. Araliaceae

Traditional knowledge. Panax notoginseng (PN), known as sanqi in Chinese, has a long history of clinical use for the treatment of traumatic injuries, swellings and pains [78].

In vitro studies. An n-butanol extract of PN inhibited the synthesis of pro-inflammatory mediators (TNF-alpha, IL-1, inducible NOS, and MMP-13) in vitro [79].

Animal studies. PN in combination with other two herbs (*Rehmannia glutinosa* and *Eleutherococcus senticosus*), had a suppressive effect on collagen-induced arthritis in mice, through inhibition of TNF-alpha, IL-1, iNOS, and MMP-13 synthesis [80].

Human clinical studies. The same combination of PN with *Rehmannia glutinosa* and *Eleutherococcus senticosus*, administered as capsules, 4 capsules of 400 mg daily for six weeks (containing ginsenoside Rb1, 19.49 ± 3.89 mg/g, stachyose 0.87 ± 0.17 mg/g and eleutheroside E 0.07 ± 0.014 mg/g) improved the physical function and pain according to the Korean version of WOMAC questionnaire in 57 patients with knee OA, and was considered effective for symptomatic relief [2].

Active phytochemicals. Saponins are considered the main osteo-active phytochemicals from PN. PN saponins promoted the autograft tendon healing in bone tunnel [81], and amplified the effect of routine therapy (diclofenac sodium, Leflunomide and prednisone) in terms of joint swelling, tenderness, and pain index, as well as time of morning stiffness, VAS and immunological parameters, in patients with RA [82].

2.7. Salix spp., fam. Salicaceae

Traditional knowledge. Various species from the genus *Salix*, or willow, were already in common use for pain relief in antiquity [83,84], being first mentioned in the Ebers papyrus (about 1550 BC) [85], and afterwards by all the great masters of medicine in antiquity, middle ages, and modern times [86].

In vitro studies. The inflammation-suppressing effect of willow bark extract (WBE) relies, at least partially, on its ability to antagonize the activated monocytes, by blocking the activity of pro-inflammatory cytokines (TNFα), enzymes (COX-2), and mediators (NF-κB) [87].

Animal studies. The mechanism of the anti-inflammatory action of WBE was examined on two animal models of arthritis, an acute and a chronic one. WBE decreased the inflammatory infiltrate and exudate and blocked the cytokine surge with a potency at least equivalent to that of acetylsalicylic acid (ASA), was better than ASA in reducing leukotrienes levels and in inhibiting COX-2, and as good as ASA in decreasing prostaglandins levels. WBE influenced favorably the oxidative stress increasing GSH and decreasing malondialdehyde levels more efficiently than ASA or celecoxib (a selective COX-2 inhibitor). Despite being more potent than ASA, on a molar basis, the salicin amount in WBE is much less than the salicylate content of ASA, suggesting that active principles other than salicin might play a role in the anti-inflammatory and antioxidative action of WBE, the polyphenols being among the candidates, at least regarding the protection against free radicals [88]. The ability to mitigate pro-inflammatory cytokines and oxidative stress was corroborated by still another study on the collagen induced arthritis animal model [89].

Human clinical studies. The first clinical trial of aspirin, albeit uncontrolled and non-randomized, was conducted in the 18th century by the English Reverend Edward Stone—the good fellow, struck by the quinine-like bitterness of aspirin, surmised an antifebrile activity and, indeed, was able to cure fever in 50 patients [86]. A two-week, double-blind, randomized, placebo-controlled trial demonstrated the ability of willow bark extract (in a dose equivalent to 240 mg salicin/day) to control the symptoms of patients with OA, especially to reduce pain, although with rather subdued efficiency [90]. The same dose of willow bark extract was used in two other six-week, randomized, controlled, double-blind trials in patients with OA and RA, respectively, the herbal preparation being compared with a potent NSAID (diclofenac) and with placebo. The two trials yielded sobering results, as in neither was willow bark extract significantly better than placebo in pain relief [91]. In a six-week, open, multicentric observational study with reference treatment, WBE was evaluated as better as conventional therapy by physicians and patients alike, in terms of both therapeutic efficiency and side effects, when used for hip and knee degenerative disease [92].

A systematic review concluded that there is moderate evidence for the efficiency of WBE in low back pain, but insufficient data for OA and RA, suggesting that higher doses should be tested [84].

In a longer (six months) observational study on 436 patients with OA and back pain, WBE significantly decreased pain and was well tolerated [93].

Active phytochemicals. Although traditionally salicin was considered as the active principle, there are opinions that this substance cannot explain the whole range of effects of WBE, and that other phytochemicals might be involved, such as polyphenols and flavonoids, which showed inhibitory activity on COX-2 and decreased synthesis of pro-inflammatory mediators in vitro, in human monocytes and differentiated macrophages [87,88,94–96].

2.8. Sesamum indicum, fam. Pedaliaceae

Traditional knowledge. Sesame oil (SO) extracted from *Sesamum indicum* (SI) has been used in various Asian traditional medicines to alleviate pain in inflammatory conditions of the joints, teeth, skin, etc. [97].

Animal studies. SO was tested in a rat model of adjuvant (Freund's adjuvant)-induced arthritis and was able to dampen the biochemical consequences of oxidative stress: lower plasmatic levels of thiobarbituric acid reactive substances and reduced gamma-glutamyltransferase activity in the joints and spleen [98]. In a rat model of acute gout-like arthritis, SO strongly hindered the inflammatory reaction, thinning the inflammatory infiltrate, lowering the levels of inflammatory mediators (TNF-α, IL-1β, IL-6), impeding the activity of nuclear factor-κB (NF-κB) (at least in the mast cells) and complement system activation [97]. In another rat model of OA, SO alleviated joint pain by inhibiting oxidative aggression (decline in the peroxidation of lipids and in the production of superoxide anion and peroxynitrite, and a surge in glutathione and glutathione peroxidase levels) in the muscles associated with nuclear factor erythroid-2-related factor [1]. SO is active in experimentally induced arthritis through its minor constituents (devoid of these minor constituents it is inactive), decreasing not only the clinically visible joint inflammation, but also its serum markers (oxidative stress related molecules, RA markers, inflammatory eicosanoids and cytokines) and the activity of hydrolytic enzymes; additionally, bone loss was also diminished [99].

Human clinical studies. In a study on patients with knee OA, oral administration of sesame together with standard therapy produced better outcomes in terms of objective and subjective manifestations compared to standard therapy alone [100]. In a placebo controlled trial on patients with knee OA, sesame seed administration was associated with a statistically significant drop in serum levels of malondialdehyde and of high-sensitivity C-reactive protein (hs-CRP) after two months of treatment. and significantly lowered levels of IL-6 after treatment [101].

Active phytochemicals. The ability of SI to protect from the dire consequences of inflammation and oxidative stress (aging, cancer, cardiovascular disease, to name only a few) seems to be due to the lignans. It contains sesamin and its hydroxylated counterpart, sesamolin. Similar biological activity has a phenolic compound, sesamol (3,4-methylene-dioxy-phenol) which results from the degradation of sesamolin [102]. Sesamol has been proven to mitigate joint inflammation, cartilage degradation, and periarticular bone resorbtion in adjuvant-induced arthritis animal model. This action was paralleled by a drop in the level of pro-inflammatory cytokines and in the activity of tissue-destructive enzymes [103]. In addition, a restoration of the oxidant homeostasis reflected in decreased oxidative stress markers and a boost in the activity of protective enzymes were noticed [103]. The hydroperoxides-scavenging capacity of sesamol makes it able to arrest the oxidation state of iron and consequently the conversion of inactive LOX (Fe^{2+}) to active LOX (Fe^{3+}), which leads to the inhibition of this inflammation-promoting enzyme [102].

In a study done on porcine cartilage explant exposed to the pro-inflammatory action of TNF-α and oncostatin M (as an animal RA model), sesamin has been proven to preclude the cytokine-induced cartilage degeneration by slowing down the degradation of constitutive glycosaminoglycans and collagen [104].

2.9. Symphytum officinalis, fam. Boraginaceae

Traditional knowledge. Symphytum officinalis, also known as comfrey, is a medicinal plant traditionally used in Europe for the treatment of inflammatory disorders [105,106].

In vitro studies. An extract of comfrey significantly inhibited the respiratory burst of polymorphonuclear leukocytes, suggesting an anti-inflammatory potential [107].

Animal studies. Comfrey extracts showed anti-inflammatory activity, by *inhibiting carrageenan-induced* rat paw oedema [108,109].

Human clinical studies. A study on people aged 50–80 with OA of the knee proved that topically applied comfrey preparation decreased pain, although was unable to decrease the burden of inflammatory molecules or the rate of cartilage breakdown, the only noticeable adverse effect being local rash [110].

Similar results yielded another study on a similar population of years-long sufferers from OA of the knee: a comfrey-containing ointment improved the quality of life by decreasing pain and increasing knee-mobility [111].

Active phytochemicals. Phenolic acids (e.g., rosmarinic acid), glycopeptides and amino acids are considered to be, at least in part, responsible for the anti-inflammatory potential of comfrey root extracts, in various vitro models [108,112]. Rosmarinic acid inhibited prostaglandin synthesis, and carrageenan- and gelatine-induced erythrocyte aggregation [113].

2.10. Zingiber officinalis, fam. Zingiberaceae

Traditional knowledge. *Zingiber officinalis* (ZO), also known as ginger, is a common spice used in Asian cuisine, and a traditional remedy for joint diseases in ethnomedicine [48].

In vitro studies. ZO is thought to have anti-inflammatory effects, possibly by inhibiting COX-1, COX-2 and LOX [114–116]. Nevertheless, the squeezed ginger extract paradoxically increased the synthesis of pro-inflammatory cytokines (TNF-α, IL-6, and monocyte chemotactic protein-1) in RAW 264 cell culture [117].

Animal studies. The oral administration of the squeezed ginger extract had a dual effect on TNF-α synthesis in mice, in peritoneal cells: ZO extract initially augmented it, but after repeated administrations decreased it [117]. In addition, it augmented the serum corticosterone level, and this may contribute to the anti-inflammatory effect of ZO.

Human clinical studies. A recent study found that ZO powder supplementation (1 g/day) for three months can reduce the serum level of nitric oxide and high-sensitivity reactive protein hs-CRP in patients with knee OA. The inflammatory markers started to decrease after three weeks of treatment [118]. Several other studies showed clinical improvement in OA patients with ZO extract, as evaluated by the pain score with VAS, reduction in intake of rescue medication, having mostly mild gastrointestinal adverse events, and similar or even better efficacy and satisfaction score than the standard treatment prescribed by the orthopedic specialist [119–121].

Another study found that the oral daily administration of one ZO preparation (340 mg EV.EXT 35 *Zingiber officinalis* extract) and glucosamine (1000 mg) for four weeks, in 21 patients with confirmed knee and hip OA, significantly reduced the arthritic pain on standing and moving, according to VAS scale evaluation. Moreover, this treatment had a similar efficacy as diclofenac (100 mg/day) plus glucosamine (1000 mg/day), but a higher safety, due to the decrease of gastrointestinal pain and increase of gastroprotective prostaglandin (PGE1, PGE2, and PGF2α) levels in the stomach mucosa [122]. However, one cross-over study (a wash-out period of one week followed by three treatment periods of three weeks duration each) found no significant difference between placebo and ginger extract in OA patients [123].

Active phytochemicals. Pungent constituents of ZO were thought to contribute to the anti-inflammatory activity of this medicinal plant. For instance, 1-dehydro-[10]-gingerdione inhibited κB kinase β activity required for NF-κB activation and suppressed NF-κB-regulated expression of inflammatory genes in lipopolysaccharide S-activated macrophage [124]. 6-Dehydrogingerdione attenuated iNOS, COX-2, IL-1β, IL-6, and TNF-α gene expression in vitro, in RAW 264.7 macrophages. [114]. Other compounds from ZO (10-gingerol, 8-shogaol and 10-shogaol) showed the capacity to decrease COX-2 activity in vitro [115].

2.11. Whitania somnifera, fam. Solanaceae

Withania somnifera (WS), also known as ashwagandha, is a potent anti-osteoarthritic and anti-inflammatory plant used in Ayurveda [125].

In vitro. One study showed that the WS extract inhibited liposaccharyde S induced synthesis of pro-inflammatory cytokines (TNF-alpha, IL-1beta and IL-12) in peripheral and synovial fluid mononuclear cells from rheumatoid arthritis subjects in vitro, but had no effect on IL-6 synthesis [126]. The WS extract also showed inhibitory effects on collagenase activity against the degradation of the bovine Achilles tendon type I collagen, that may be useful in joint disease treatment [127].

Animal studies. WS root powder had protective effect on bone collagen in experimental induced arthritis model in rats [128].

Human clinical studies. A randomized, double blind placebo controlled study showed that the aqueous extract of WS produced significant reduction of scores for pain, stiffness and disability in human subjects with knee joint pain [129].

Active phytochemicals. Withaferin A, belonging to the steroid class of phytochemicals, is thought to be one of contributor compounds to the beneficial effects of WS in OA subjects [126]. Whitaferin A reverted to near normal levels the increase in paw volume, lysosomal enzymes, lipid peroxidation, and TNFα in an monosodium urate crystal-induced arthritis in mice [130]. Withaferin A supressess NF-κB activation by targeting a crucial cysteine 179 in IκB kinase β, and by inhibition of the NF-κB Essential Modulator/ IκB kinase β association complex formation, according to molecular docking and molecular dynamics simulations studies [131,132].

Table 1. Medicinal plants with therapeutic potential in ostheoarthritis and rheumatoid arthritis (Legend: AM, animal model; CAT, catalase; COX, cyclooxygenase; GPx, glutathione peroxidase; GSH, glutathione; GST, glutathione-S-transferase; HS, human study; IL, interleukine; iNOS, inducible nitric oxide synthase; LOX, lipooxygenase; PGE1-S, prostaglandin E2 synthase; ROS, reactive oxygen species; SOD, superoxide dismutase; MAPK, mitogen-activated protein kinase; MCP-1, monocyte chemoattractant protein-1; MIP-1α, monocyte inflammatory protein-1; MMP, matrix metaloproteinase; NO, nitric oxide; TNF, tumoral necrosis factor; (−), decreased synthesis/decreased activation/inhibition of various mediators, enzymes, transcription factors, and processes; (+), increased synthesis/increased activation of various mediators, enzymes, transcription factors, and processes). Note: References in the table correspond only to the mechanism of action.

Plant	Active Phytochemicals	Mechanism of Action	References
Arnica montana	phenols, flavonoids	(−) NO, TNF-α, IL-1β, IL-6, IL-12, anti-type II collagen antibodies, (+) antioxidants (AM)	[24]
Boswelia spp.	boswelic acids	(−) PGE1-S, cathepsin G, LOX-5, MMP-9, MMP-13, COX-2, NO, PGE1, TNF-α, IL-1, IL-2, IL-4, IL-6, IFN-γ (in vitro, AM)	[17,30,31,41]
		(−) leukocyte infiltration in knee (AM)	[43]
Curcuma spp.	curcuminoids	(+) SOD, GSH, (−) MDA (HS)	[58]
		(−) neutrophil infiltrate in knee, (AM), (−) IL-1β, TNFα, MCP-1, and MIP-1α (in vitro, AM)	[57,59]
	β-elemene	(+) p38 MAPK (in vitro)	[60]
Equisetum arvense	kynurenic acid	(−) synoviocyte proliferation (in vitro)	[64,66]
Harpagophytum procumbens	iridoid glycosides	(−) iNOS and COX-2 (in vitro)	[76]
Panax notoginseng	saponins	(−) TNF-alpha, IL-1, iNOS, MMP-13 (AM)	[79,80]
Salix spp.	salicin, polyphenols, flavonoids	(−) TNFα, COX-2, IL-1, IL-6 (in vitro)	[87,95]
Sesamum indicum	sesamin, sesamol, sesamolin	(−) thiobarbituric acid reactive substances, LOX (in vitro), TNF-α, IL-1β, IL-6, hyaluronidase, MMP-13, MMP-3, MMP-9, exoglycosidases, cathepsin D, phosphatases, COX-2, PGE2, ROS, H2O2, MDA (AM), IL-6 (HS)	[1,97,98,101–103]
		(+) GSH, GPx (AM)	
Symphitum officinalis	rosmarinic acids, glycopeptides, amino acids	(−) PG (in vitro)	[108,112,113]
Zingiber officinalis	gingerdione derivatives, 10-gingerol, 8,10-shogaol	(−) COX-1, COX-2, LOX, iNOS, TNF-α, IL-1β, IL-6, MCP-1, κB kinase β (in vitro, AM), NO (HS)	[114,115,117,118,124]
		(+) cortisone (AM)	
Whitania somnifera	whitaferin A	(−)TNF-alpha, IL-1β, IL-12, collagenase (in vitro), NF kB (docking studies)	[126,127,131,132]

3. Concluding Remarks

Several medicinal plant extracts showed trends of clinical and biochemical benefits with low risk of side effects in arthritic patients that warrant further investigation, including imagistic and histological evaluation. The search for effective herbal supplements as a complementary therapy of degenerative arthropathies is a complex issue and implies a long process, in the end of which the conclusions are difficult to be drawn, due to the differences in terms of study design and protocols [133]. The available studies did not evaluate the effect of plant extracts on disease progression, or whether it halts the aggravation of arthropathies. For this purpose, studies of longer duration should be performed.

Almost no studies confirmed in humans the biological mechanisms of herbal extracts found in vitro or in animal studies, the majority of the available ones being focused only on the evaluation of the symptomatic relief induced by the herbal treatment.

Despite their advantages, herbal treatments raise several concerns, such as drug–herbal interactions, low bioavailability, lack of standardization, insufficient regulatory guidelines at national and international levels, and therefore possibility of adulteration [134–137].

More evidence of medicinal plant efficacy, safety and mechanisms of action are needed before herbal treatment can gain a place in therapeutic guidelines of OA and RA.

Author Contributions: Dorin Dragos and Marilena Gilca equally contributed to this work as first authors. All the authors have contributed to all of the following steps: (1) the conception of the study, search of literature, and acquisition of data; (2) analysis and interpretation of data retrieved from the literature; and (3) writing the draft of the manuscript and revision of the article. All authors have read and approved the final manuscript.

Conflicts of Interest: The authors declare no conflict of interest.

References

1. Hsu, D.-Z.; Chu, P.-Y.; Jou, I.-M. Daily sesame oil supplement attenuates joint pain by inhibiting muscular oxidative stress in osteoarthritis rat model. *J. Nutr. Biochem.* **2016**, *29*, 36–40. [CrossRef] [PubMed]
2. Park, S.-H.; Kim, S.-K.; Shin, I.-H.; Kim, H.-G.; Choe, J.-Y. Effects of AIF on Knee Osteoarthritis Patients: Double-blind, Randomized Placebo-controlled Study. *Korean J. Physiol. Pharmacol.* **2009**, *13*, 33–37. [CrossRef] [PubMed]
3. Peat, G.; McCarney, R.; Croft, P. Knee pain and osteoarthritis in older adults: A review of community burden and current use of primary health care. *Ann. Rheum. Dis.* **2001**, *60*, 91–97. [CrossRef] [PubMed]
4. McWilliams, D.F.; Leeb, B.F.; Muthuri, S.G.; Doherty, M.; Zhang, W. Occupational risk factors for osteoarthritis of the knee: A meta-analysis. *Osteoarthr. Cartil.* **2011**, *19*, 829–839. [CrossRef]
5. Smith, R.L.; Carter, D.R.; Schurman, D.J. Pressure and shear differentially alter human articular chondrocyte metabolism: A review. *Clin. Orthop. Relat. Res.* **2004**, *427*, S89–S95.
6. Murphy, N.J.; Eyles, J.P.; Hunter, D.J. Hip Osteoarthritis: Etiopathogenesis and Implications for Management. *Adv. Ther.* **2016**, *33*, 1921–1946. [CrossRef]
7. Dougados, M. Monitoring osteoarthritis progression and therapy. *Osteoarthr. Cartil.* **2004**, *12* (Suppl. A), S55–S60. [CrossRef] [PubMed]
8. Lequesne, M.G.; Mery, C.; Samson, M.; Gerard, P. Indexes of severity for osteoarthritis of the hip and knee. Validation—Value in comparison with other assessment tests. *Scand. J. Rheumatol. Suppl.* **1987**, *65*, 85–89. [CrossRef] [PubMed]
9. Johnson, M.J.; Bland, J.M.; Davidson, P.M.; Newton, P.J.; Oxberry, S.G.; Abernethy, A.P.; Currow, D.C. The relationship between two performance scales: New York Heart Association Classification and Karnofsky Performance Status Scale. *J. Pain Symptom Manag.* **2014**, *47*, 652–658. [CrossRef] [PubMed]
10. Yang, C.L.H.; Or, T.C.T.; Ho, M.H.K.; Lau, A.S.Y. Scientific Basis of Botanical Medicine as Alternative Remedies for Rheumatoid Arthritis. *Clin. Rev. Allergy Immunol.* **2013**, *44*, 284–300. [CrossRef] [PubMed]
11. Smolen, J.S.; Landewe, R.; Breedveld, F.C.; Buch, M.; Burmester, G.; Dougados, M.; Emery, P.; Gaujoux-Viala, C.; Gossec, L.; Nam, J.; et al. EULAR recommendations for the management of rheumatoid arthritis with synthetic and biological disease-modifying antirheumatic drugs: 2013 update. *Ann. Rheum. Dis.* **2014**, *73*, 492–509. [CrossRef] [PubMed]
12. Hochberg, M.C.; Altman, R.D.; April, K.T.; Benkhalti, M.; Guyatt, G.; McGowan, J.; Towheed, T.; Welch, V.; Wells, G.; Tugwell, P. American College of Rheumatology 2012 recommendations for the use of nonpharmacologic and pharmacologic therapies in osteoarthritis of the hand, hip, and knee. *Arthritis Care Res.* **2012**, *64*, 465–474. [CrossRef]

13. Hyrich, K.L.; Watson, K.D.; Silman, A.J.; Symmons, D.P.M. Predictors of response to anti-TNF-alpha therapy among patients with rheumatoid arthritis: Results from the British Society for Rheumatology Biologics Register. *Rheumatology* **2006**, *45*, 1558–1565. [CrossRef] [PubMed]

14. Soliman, M.M.; Hyrich, K.L.; Lunt, M.; Watson, K.D.; Symmons, D.P.M.; Ashcroft, D.M. Effectiveness of rituximab in patients with rheumatoid arthritis: Observational study from the British Society for Rheumatology Biologics Register. *J. Rheumatol.* **2012**, *39*, 240–246. [CrossRef] [PubMed]

15. Cavalli, G.; Dinarello, C.A. Treating rheumatological diseases and co-morbidities with interleukin-1 blocking therapies. *Rheumatology* **2015**, *54*, 2134–2144. [CrossRef] [PubMed]

16. Nishina, N.; Kaneko, Y.; Kameda, H.; Kuwana, M.; Takeuchi, T. Reduction of plasma IL-6 but not TNF-alpha by methotrexate in patients with early rheumatoid arthritis: A potential biomarker for radiographic progression. *Clin. Rheumatol.* **2013**, *32*, 1661–1666. [CrossRef] [PubMed]

17. Abdel-Tawab, M.; Werz, O.; Schubert-Zsilavecz, M. *Boswellia serrata*: An overall assessment of in vitro, preclinical, pharmacokinetic and clinical data. *Clin. Pharmacokinet.* **2011**, *50*, 349–369. [CrossRef] [PubMed]

18. McAlindon, T.E.; Bannuru, R.R.; Sullivan, M.C.; Arden, N.K.; Berenbaum, F.; Bierma-Zeinstra, S.M.; Hawker, G.A.; Henrotin, Y.; Hunter, D.J.; Kawaguchi, H.; et al. OARSI guidelines for the non-surgical management of knee osteoarthritis. *Osteoarthr. Cartil.* **2014**, *22*, 363–388. [CrossRef] [PubMed]

19. Matucci, A.; Cammelli, D.; Cantini, F.; Goletti, D.; Marino, V.; Milano, G.M.; Scarpa, R.; Tocci, G.; Maggi, E.; Vultaggio, A. Influence of anti-TNF immunogenicity on safety in rheumatic disease: A narrative review. *Expert Opin. Drug Saf.* **2016**, *15*, 3–10. [CrossRef] [PubMed]

20. Cabral, V.P.; Andrade, C.A.; Passos, S.R.; Martins, M.F.; Hökerberg, Y.H. Severe infection in patients with rheumatoid arthritis taking anakinra, rituximab, or abatacept: A systematic review of observational studies. *Rev. Bras. Reumatol.* **2016**, *56*, 543–550. [CrossRef] [PubMed]

21. Mameli, A.; Barcellona, D.; Marongiu, F. Fatal Cytopenia Induced by Low-Dose Methotrexate in Elderly With Rheumatoid Arthritis. Identification of Risk Factors. *Am. J. Ther.* **2017**, *24*, e106–e107. [CrossRef]

22. Umar, S.; Umar, K.; Sarwar, A.H.M.G.; Khan, A.; Ahmad, N.; Ahmad, S.; Katiyar, C.K.; Husain, S.A.; Khan, H.A. *Boswellia serrata* extract attenuates inflammatory mediators and oxidative stress in collagen induced arthritis. *Phytomedicine* **2014**, *21*, 847–856. [CrossRef]

23. Akhtar, N.; Miller, M.J.; Haqqi, T.M. Effect of a Herbal-Leucine mix on the IL-1β-induced cartilage degradation and inflammatory gene expression in human chondrocytes. *BMC Complement. Altern. Med.* **2011**, *11*, 66. [CrossRef] [PubMed]

24. Sharma, S.; Arif, M.; Nirala, R.K.; Gupta, R.; Thakur, S.C. Cumulative therapeutic effects of phytochemicals in *Arnica montana* flower extract alleviated collagen-induced arthritis: Inhibition of both pro-inflammatory mediators and oxidative stress. *J. Sci. Food Agric.* **2016**, *96*, 1500–1510. [CrossRef] [PubMed]

25. Álvarez-Hernández, E.; César Casasola-Vargas, J.; Lino-Pérez, L.; Burgos-Vargas, R.; Vázquez-Mellado, J. Frecuencia de uso de medicinas complementarias y alternativas en sujetos que acuden por primera vez al servicio de reumatología. Análisis de 800 casos. *Reumatol. Clín.* **2006**, *2*, 183–189. [CrossRef]

26. Knuesel, O.; Weber, M.; Suter, A. *Arnica montana* gel in osteoarthritis of the knee: An open, multicenter clinical trial. *Adv. Ther.* **2002**, *19*, 209–218. [CrossRef] [PubMed]

27. Widrig, R.; Suter, A.; Saller, R.; Melzer, J. Choosing between NSAID and *Arnica* for topical treatment of hand osteoarthritis in a randomised, double-blind study. *Rheumatol. Int.* **2007**, *27*, 585–591. [CrossRef]

28. Ross, S.M. Osteoarthritis. *Holist. Nurs. Pract.* **2008**, *22*, 237–239. [CrossRef] [PubMed]

29. Cameron, M.; Chrubasik, S. Topical herbal therapies for treating osteoarthritis. *CDSR* **2013**, *2013*, CD010538. [CrossRef]

30. Ammon, H.P.T. Boswellic acids (components of frankincense) as the active principle in treatment of chronic inflammatory diseases. *Wien. Med. Wochenschr.* **2002**, *152*, 373–378. (In German) [CrossRef] [PubMed]

31. Sengupta, K.; Krishnaraju, A.V.; Vishal, A.A.; Mishra, A.; Trimurtulu, G.; Sarma, K.V.S.; Raychaudhuri, S.K.; Raychaudhuri, S.P. Comparative efficacy and tolerability of 5-Loxin and AflapinAgainst osteoarthritis of the knee: A double blind, randomized, placebo controlled clinical study. *Int. J. Med. Sci.* **2010**, *7*, 366–377. [CrossRef] [PubMed]

32. Blain, E.J.; Ali, A.Y.; Duance, V.C. *Boswellia frereana* (frankincense) suppresses cytokine-induced matrix metalloproteinase expression and production of pro-inflammatory molecules in articular cartilage. *Phyther. Res.* **2009**, *24*, 905–912. [CrossRef] [PubMed]

33. Sumantran, V.N.; Joshi, A.K.; Boddul, S.; Koppikar, S.J.; Warude, D.; Patwardhan, B.; Chopra, A.; Chandwaskar, R.; Wagh, U.V. Antiarthritic Activity of a Standardized, Multiherbal, Ayurvedic Formulation containing *Boswellia serrata*: In Vitro Studies on Knee Cartilage from Osteoarthritis Patients. *Phyther. Res.* **2011**, *25*, 1375–1380. [CrossRef] [PubMed]

34. Dey, D.; Chaskar, S.; Athavale, N.; Chitre, D. Inhibition of LPS-Induced TNF-α and NO Production in Mouse Macrophage and Inflammatory Response in Rat Animal Models by a Novel Ayurvedic Formulation, BV-9238. *Phyther. Res.* **2014**, *28*, 1479–1485. [CrossRef]

35. Cameron, M.; Chrubasik, S. Oral herbal therapies for treating osteoarthritis. *CDSR* **2014**, *2014*, CD002947. [CrossRef]

36. Vishal, A.A.; Mishra, A.; Raychaudhuri, S.P. A double blind, randomized, placebo controlled clinical study evaluates the early efficacy of aflapin in subjects with osteoarthritis of knee. *Int. J. Med. Sci.* **2011**, *8*, 615–622. [CrossRef] [PubMed]

37. Belcaro, G.; Dugall, M.; Luzzi, R.; Ledda, A.; Pellegrini, L.; Cesarone, M.R.; Hosoi, M.; Errichi, M.; Francis, S.; Cornelli, U. FlexiQule (*Boswellia* extract) in the supplementary management of osteoarthritis: A supplement registry. *Minerva Med.* **2014**, *105*, 9–16.

38. Belcaro, G.; Feragalli, B.; Cornelli, U.; Dugall, M. Hand "stress" arthritis in young subjects: Effects of Flexique (pharma-standard *Boswellia* extract). A preliminary case report. *Minerva Gastroenterol. Dietol.* **2015**, in press.

39. Kizhakkedath, R. Clinical evaluation of a formulation containing *Curcuma longa* and *Boswellia serrata* extracts in the management of knee osteoarthritis. *Mol. Med. Rep.* **2013**, *8*, 1542–1548. [CrossRef] [PubMed]

40. Sander, O.; Herborn, G.; Rau, R. Is H15 (resin extract of *Boswellia serrata*, "incense") a useful supplement to established drug therapy of chronic polyarthritis? Results of a double-blind pilot study. *Z. Rheumatol.* **1998**, *57*, 11–16. [CrossRef] [PubMed]

41. Wang, H.; Zhang, C.; Wu, Y.; Ai, Y.; Lee, D.Y.-W.; Dai, R. Comparative pharmacokinetic study of two boswellic acids in normal and arthritic rat plasma after oral administration of *Boswellia serrata* extract or Huo Luo Xiao Ling Dan by LC-MS. *Biomed. Chromatogr.* **2014**, *28*, 1402–1408. [CrossRef] [PubMed]

42. Hamidpour, R.; Hamidpour, S.; Hamidpour, M.; Shahlari, M. Frankincense (Rǔ Xiāng; *Boswellia* Species): From the Selection of Traditional Applications to the Novel Phytotherapy for the Prevention and Treatment of Serious Diseases. *J. Tradit. Complement. Med.* **2013**, *3*, 221–226. [CrossRef] [PubMed]

43. Sharma, M.L.; Bani, S.; Singh, G.B. Anti-arthritic activity of boswellic acids in bovine serum albumin (BSA)-induced arthritis. *Int. J. Immunopharmacol.* **1989**, *11*, 647–652. [CrossRef]

44. Singh, S.; Khajuria, A.; Taneja, S.C.; Johri, R.K.; Singh, J.; Qazi, G.N. Boswellic acids: A leukotriene inhibitor also effective through topical application in inflammatory disorders. *Phytomedicine* **2008**, *15*, 400–407. [CrossRef] [PubMed]

45. Ammon, H.P.T. Modulation of the immune system by *Boswellia serrata* extracts and boswellic acids. *Phytomedicine* **2010**, *17*, 862–867. [CrossRef] [PubMed]

46. Khajuria, A.; Gupta, A.; Suden, P.; Singh, S.; Malik, F.; Singh, J.; Gupta, B.D.; Suri, K.A.; Srinivas, V.K.; Ella, K.; et al. Immunomodulatory activity of biopolymeric fraction BOS 2000 from *Boswellia serrata*. *Phyther. Res.* **2008**, *22*, 340–348. [CrossRef] [PubMed]

47. Sengupta, K.; Kolla, J.N.; Krishnaraju, A.V.; Yalamanchili, N.; Rao, C.V.; Golakoti, T.; Raychaudhuri, S.; Raychaudhuri, S.P. Cellular and molecular mechanisms of anti-inflammatory effect of Aflapin: A novel *Boswellia serrata* extract. *Mol. Cell. Biochem.* **2011**, *354*, 189–197. [CrossRef] [PubMed]

48. Sharma, R.; Dash, B. *Caraka Samhita*, 2006th ed.; Chowkhamba Sanskrit Series Office: Varanasi, India, 2006.

49. Funk, J.L.; Frye, J.B.; Oyarzo, J.N.; Kuscuoglu, N.; Wilson, J.; McCaffrey, G.; Stafford, G.; Chen, G.; Lantz, R.C.; Jolad, S.D.; et al. Efficacy and mechanism of action of turmeric supplements in the treatment of experimental arthritis. *Arthritis Rheum.* **2006**, *54*, 3452–3464. [CrossRef] [PubMed]

50. Taty Anna, K.; Elvy Suhana, M.R.; Das, S.; Faizah, O.; Hamzaini, A.H. Anti-inflammatory effect of *Curcuma longa* (turmeric) on collagen-induced arthritis: An anatomico-radiological study. *Clin. Ter.* **2011**, *162*, 201–207. [PubMed]

51. Kamarudin, T.A.; Othman, F.; Mohd Ramli, E.S.; Md Isa, N.; Das, S. Protective effect of curcumin on experimentally induced arthritic rats: Detailed histopathological study of the joints and white blood cell count. *EXCLI J.* **2012**, *11*, 226–236. [PubMed]

52. Chang, H.-I.; Su, Y.-H.; Lin, Y.-J.; Chen, P.-J.; Shi, C.-S.; Chen, C.-N.; Yeh, C.-C. Evaluation of the protective effects of curcuminoid (curcumin and bisdemethoxycurcumin)-loaded liposomes against bone turnover in a cell-based model of osteoarthritis. *Drug Des. Dev. Ther.* **2015**, *9*, 2285–2300. [CrossRef] [PubMed]

53. Ramadan, G.; El-Menshawy, O. Protective effects of ginger-turmeric rhizomes mixture on joint inflammation, atherogenesis, kidney dysfunction and other complications in a rat model of human rheumatoid arthritis. *Int. J. Rheum. Dis.* **2013**, *16*, 219–229. [CrossRef] [PubMed]

54. Kuptniratsaikul, V.; Dajpratham, P.; Taechaarpornkul, W.; Buntragulpoontawee, M.; Lukkanapichonchut, P.; Chootip, C.; Saengsuwan, J.; Tantayakom, K.; Laongpech, S. Efficacy and safety of *Curcuma* domestica extracts compared with ibuprofen in patients with knee osteoarthritis: A multicenter study. *Clin. Interv. Aging* **2014**, *9*, 451–458. [CrossRef] [PubMed]

55. Daily, J.W.; Yang, M.; Park, S. Efficacy of Turmeric Extracts and Curcumin for Alleviating the Symptoms of Joint Arthritis: A Systematic Review and Meta-Analysis of Randomized Clinical Trials. *J. Med. Food* **2016**, *19*, 717–729. [CrossRef] [PubMed]

56. Ghosh, S.; Banerjee, S.; Sil, P.C. The beneficial role of curcumin on inflammation, diabetes and neurodegenerative disease: A recent update. *Food Chem. Toxicol.* **2015**, *83*, 111–124. [CrossRef] [PubMed]

57. Nonose, N.; Pereira, J.A.; Machado, P.R.M.; Rodrigues, M.R.; Sato, D.T.; Martinez, C.A.R. Oral administration of curcumin (*Curcuma longa*) can attenuate the neutrophil inflammatory response in zymosan-induced arthritis in rats. *Acta Cir. Bras.* **2014**, *29*, 727–734. [CrossRef] [PubMed]

58. Panahi, Y.; Alishiri, G.H.; Parvin, S.; Sahebkar, A. Mitigation of Systemic Oxidative Stress by Curcuminoids in Osteoarthritis: Results of a Randomized Controlled Trial. *J. Diet. Suppl.* **2016**, *13*, 209–220. [CrossRef] [PubMed]

59. Chen, J.-J.; Dai, L.; Zhao, L.-X.; Zhu, X.; Cao, S.; Gao, Y.-J. Intrathecal curcumin attenuates pain hypersensitivity and decreases spinal neuroinflammation in rat model of monoarthritis. *Sci. Rep.* **2015**, *5*, 10278. [CrossRef]

60. Zou, S.; Wang, C.; Cui, Z.; Guo, P.; Meng, Q.; Shi, X.; Gao, Y.; Yang, G.; Han, Z. β-Elemene induces apoptosis of human rheumatoid arthritis fibroblast-like synoviocytes via reactive oxygen species-dependent activation of p38 mitogen-activated protein kinase. *Pharmacol. Rep.* **2016**, *68*, 7–11. [CrossRef]

61. Gründemann, C.; Lengen, K.; Sauer, B.; Garcia-Käufer, M.; Zehl, M.; Huber, R. *Equisetum arvense* (common horsetail) modulates the function of inflammatory immunocompetent cells. *BMC Complement. Altern. Med.* **2014**, *14*, 283. [CrossRef]

62. Farinon, M.; Lora, P.S.; Francescato, L.N.; Bassani, V.L.; Henriques, A.T.; Xavier, R.M.; de Oliveira, P.G. Effect of Aqueous Extract of Giant Horsetail (*Equisetum giganteum* L.) in Antigen-Induced Arthritis. *Open Rheumatol. J.* **2013**, *7*, 129–133. [CrossRef] [PubMed]

63. Jiang, X.; Qu, Q.; Li, M.; Miao, S.; Li, X.; Cai, W. Horsetail mixture on rheumatoid arthritis and its regulation on TNF-α and IL-10. *Pak. J. Pharm. Sci.* **2014**, *27*, 2019–2023. [PubMed]

64. Zgrajka, W.; Turska, M.; Rajtar, G.; Majdan, M.; Parada-Turska, J. Kynurenic acid content in anti-rheumatic herbs. *Ann. Agric. Environ. Med.* **2013**, *20*, 800–802. [PubMed]

65. Varga, G.; Erces, D.; Fazekas, B.; Fulop, M.; Kovacs, T.; Kaszaki, J.; Fulop, F.; Vecsei, L.; Boros, M. N-Methyl-D-aspartate receptor antagonism decreases motility and inflammatory activation in the early phase of acute experimental colitis in the rat. *Neurogastroenterol. Motil.* **2010**, *22*, 217–225. [CrossRef] [PubMed]

66. Parada-Turska, J.; Rzeski, W.; Zgrajka, W.; Majdan, M.; Kandefer-Szerszen, M.; Turski, W. Kynurenic acid, an endogenous constituent of rheumatoid arthritis synovial fluid, inhibits proliferation of synoviocytes in vitro. *Rheumatol. Int.* **2006**, *26*, 422–426. [CrossRef]

67. Parada-Turska, J.; Zgrajka, W.; Majdan, M. Kynurenic acid in synovial fluid and serum of patients with rheumatoid arthritis, spondyloarthropathy, and osteoarthritis. *J. Rheumatol.* **2013**, *40*, 903–909. [CrossRef] [PubMed]

68. Blumenthal, M.; Busse, W.R. *The Complete German Commission E Monographs*; American Botanical Council: Austin, TX, USA, 1998.

69. Fiebich, B.; Heinrich, M.; Hiller, K.; Kammerer, N. Inhibition of TNF-α synthesis in LPS-stimulated primary human monocytes by *Harpagophytum* extract SteiHap 69. *Phytomedicine* **2001**, *8*, 28–30. [CrossRef]

70. Lanhers, M.; Fleurentin, J.; Mortier, F.; Al, E. Antiinflammatory and analgesic effects of an aqueous extract of *Harpagophytum procumbens*. *Planta Med.* **1992**, *58*, 117–123. [CrossRef] [PubMed]

71. Akhtar, N.; Haqqi, T.M. Current nutraceuticals in the management of osteoarthritis: A review. *Ther. Adv. Musculoskelet. Dis.* **2012**, *4*, 181–207. [CrossRef] [PubMed]

72. Wegener, T.; Lupke, N. Treatment of patients with arthrosis of hip or knee with an aqueous extract of devil's claw (*Harpagophytum procumbens* DC.). *Phytother. Res.* **2003**, *17*, 1165–1172. [CrossRef] [PubMed]

73. Chantre, P.; Cappelaere, A.; Leblan, D.; Al, E. Efficacy and tolerance of *Harpagophytum procumbens* versus diacerhein in treatment of osteoarthritis. *Phytomedicine* **2000**, *7*, 177–183. [CrossRef]

74. Chrubasik, S.; Thanner, J.; Kunzel, O.; Al, E. Comparison of outcome measures during treatment with the proprietary *Harpagophytum* extract Doloteffin in patients with pain in the lower back, knee, or hip. *Phytomedicine* **2002**, *9*, 181–194. [CrossRef] [PubMed]

75. *Harpagophytum procumbens* (devil's claw). Monograph. *Altern. Med. Rev.* **2008**, *13*, 248–252.

76. Huang, T.H.-W.; Tran, V.H.; Duke, R.K.; Tan, S.; Chrubasik, S.; Roufogalis, B.D.; Duke, C.C. Harpagoside suppresses lipopolysaccharide-induced iNOS and COX-2 expression through inhibition of NF-κB activation. *J. Ethnopharmacol.* **2006**, *104*, 149–155. [CrossRef] [PubMed]

77. Kaszkin, M.; Beck, K.; Koch, E.; Al, E. Downregulation of iNOS expression in rat mesangial cells by special extracts of *Harpagophytum procumbens* derives from harpagoside-dependent and independent effects. *Phytomedicine* **2004**, *11*, 585–595. [CrossRef]

78. Liu, Z.; Liu, L. *Essentials of Chinese Medicine*; Liu, Z., Liu, L., Eds.; Springer: London, UK, 2009.

79. Chang, S.-H.; Choi, Y.; Park, J.-A.; Jung, D.-S.; Shin, J.; Yang, J.-H.; Ko, S.-Y.; Kim, S.-W.; Kim, J.-K. Anti-inflammatory effects of BT-201, an *n*-butanol extract of *Panax notoginseng*, observed in vitro and in a collagen-induced arthritis model. *Clin. Nutr.* **2007**, *26*, 785–791. [CrossRef] [PubMed]

80. Chang, S.-H.; Sung, H.-C.; Choi, Y.; Ko, S.-Y.; Lee, B.-E.; Baek, D.-H.; Kim, S.-W.; Kim, J.-K. Suppressive effect of AIF, a water extract from three herbs, on collagen-induced arthritis in mice. *Int. Immunopharmacol.* **2005**, *5*, 1365–1372. [CrossRef] [PubMed]

81. Zhang, L.; Li, Z.; Sun, J.; Ma, J.; Zhang, S.; Liu, J.; Zhu, J. Effect of *Panax Notoginseng* Saponins on autograft tendon healing in bone tunnel: Interface histological characteristics. *Zhongguo Gu Shang* **2011**, *24*, 132–136. [PubMed]

82. Zhang, J.; Wang, J.; Wang, H. Clinical study on effect of total *Panax notoginseng* saponins on immune related inner environment imbalance in rheumatoid arthritis patients. *Zhongguo Zhong Xi Yi Jie He Za Zhi/Chin. J. Integr. Tradit. West. Med.* **2007**, *27*, 589–592.

83. Appelboom, T. Arthropathy in art and the history of pain management—Through the centuries to cyclooxygenase-2 inhibitors. *Rheumatology* **2002**, *41* (Suppl. 1), 28–34. [CrossRef] [PubMed]

84. Vlachojannis, J.E.; Cameron, M.; Chrubasik, S. A systematic review on the effectiveness of willow bark for musculoskeletal pain. *Phyther. Res.* **2009**, *23*, 897–900. [CrossRef] [PubMed]

85. Mackowiak, P.A. Brief History of Antipyretic Therapy. *Clin. Infect. Dis.* **2000**, *31*, S154–S156. [CrossRef]

86. Vane, J.R. The fight against rheumatism: From willow bark to COX-1 sparing drugs. *J. Physiol. Pharmacol.* **2000**, *51*, 573–586. [PubMed]

87. Bonaterra, G.A.; Heinrich, E.U.; Kelber, O.; Weiser, D.; Metz, J.; Kinscherf, R. Anti-inflammatory effects of the willow bark extract STW 33-I (Proaktiv®) in LPS-activated human monocytes and differentiated macrophages. *Phytomedicine* **2010**, *17*, 1106–1113. [CrossRef] [PubMed]

88. Khayyal, M.; El-Ghazaly, M.; Abdallah, D.; Okpanyi, S.; Kelber, O.; Weiser, D. Mechanisms Involved in the Anti-inflammatory Effect of a Standardized Willow Bark Extract. *Arzneimittelforschung* **2011**, *55*, 677–687. [CrossRef] [PubMed]

89. Sharma, S.; Sahu, D.; Das, H.R.; Sharma, D. Amelioration of collagen-induced arthritis by *Salix nigra* bark extract via suppression of pro-inflammatory cytokines and oxidative stress. *Food Chem. Toxicol.* **2011**, *49*, 3395–3406. [CrossRef] [PubMed]

90. Schmid, B.; Lüdtke, R.; Selbmann, H.K.; Kötter, I.; Tschirdewahn, B.; Schaffner, W.; Heide, L. Efficacy and tolerability of a standardized willow bark extract in patients with osteoarthritis: Randomized placebo-controlled, double blind clinical trial. *Phytother. Res.* **2001**, *15*, 344–350. [CrossRef] [PubMed]

91. Biegert, C.; Wagner, I.; Lüdtke, R.; Kötter, I.; Lohmüller, C.; Günaydin, I.; Taxis, K.; Heide, L. Efficacy and safety of willow bark extract in the treatment of osteoarthritis and rheumatoid arthritis: Results of 2 randomized double-blind controlled trials. *J. Rheumatol.* **2004**, *31*, 2121–2130.

92. Beer, A.-M.; Wegener, T. Willow bark extract (*Salicis cortex*) for gonarthrosis and coxarthrosis—Results of a cohort study with a control group. *Phytomedicine* **2008**, *15*, 907–913. [CrossRef] [PubMed]

93. Uehleke, B.; Müller, J.; Stange, R.; Kelber, O.; Melzer, J. Willow bark extract STW 33-I in the long-term treatment of outpatients with rheumatic pain mainly osteoarthritis or back pain. *Phytomedicine* **2013**, *20*, 980–984. [CrossRef] [PubMed]

94. Nahrstedt, A.; Schmidt, M.; Jäggi, R.; Metz, J.; Khayyal, M.T. Willow bark extract: The contribution of polyphenols to the overall effect. *Wien. Med. Wochenschr.* **2007**, *157*, 348–351. [CrossRef] [PubMed]

95. Drummond, E.M.; Harbourne, N.; Marete, E.; Martyn, D.; Jacquier, J.; O'Riordan, D.; Gibney, E.R. Inhibition of Proinflammatory Biomarkers in THP1 Macrophages by Polyphenols Derived From Chamomile, Meadowsweet and Willow bark. *Phyther. Res.* **2013**, *27*, 588–594. [CrossRef] [PubMed]

96. Shara, M.; Stohs, S.J. Efficacy and Safety of White Willow Bark (*Salix alba*) Extracts. *Phyther. Res.* **2015**, *29*, 1112–1116. [CrossRef] [PubMed]

97. Hsu, D.-Z.; Chen, S.-J.; Chu, P.-Y.; Liu, M.-Y. Therapeutic effects of sesame oil on monosodium urate crystal-induced acute inflammatory response in rats. *Springerplus* **2013**, *2*, 659. [CrossRef] [PubMed]

98. Sotnikova, R.; Ponist, S.; Navarova, J.; Mihalova, D.; Tomekova, V.; Strosova, M.; Bauerova, K. Effects of sesame oil in the model of adjuvant arthritis. *Neuro Endocrinol. Lett.* **2009**, *30* (Suppl. 1), 22–24.

99. Yadav, N.V.; Sadashivaiah; Ramaiyan, B.; Acharya, P.; Belur, L.; Talahalli, R.R. Sesame Oil and Rice Bran Oil Ameliorates Adjuvant-Induced Arthritis in Rats: Distinguishing the Role of Minor Components and Fatty Acids. *Lipids* **2016**, *51*, 1385–1395. [CrossRef] [PubMed]

100. Eftekhar Sadat, B.; Khadem Haghighian, M.; Alipoor, B.; Malek Mahdavi, A.; Asghari Jafarabadi, M.; Moghaddam, A. Effects of sesame seed supplementation on clinical signs and symptoms in patients with knee osteoarthritis. *Int. J. Rheum. Dis.* **2013**, *16*, 578–582. [CrossRef] [PubMed]

101. Khadem Haghighian, M.; Alipoor, B.; Malek Mahdavi, A.; Eftekhar Sadat, B.; Asghari Jafarabadi, M.; Moghaddam, A. Effects of sesame seed supplementation on inflammatory factors and oxidative stress biomarkers in patients with knee osteoarthritis. *Acta Med. Iran.* **2015**, *53*, 207–213. [PubMed]

102. Yashaswini, P.S.; Rao, A.G.A.; Singh, S.A. Inhibition of lipoxygenase by sesamol corroborates its potential anti-inflammatory activity. *Int. J. Biol. Macromol.* **2017**, *94*, 781–787. [CrossRef] [PubMed]

103. Hemshekhar, M.; Thushara, R.M.; Jnaneshwari, S.; Devaraja, S.; Kemparaju, K.; Girish, K.S. Attenuation of adjuvant-induced arthritis by dietary sesamol via modulation of inflammatory mediators, extracellular matrix degrading enzymes and antioxidant status. *Eur. J. Nutr.* **2013**, *52*, 1787–1799. [CrossRef] [PubMed]

104. Khansai, M.; Boonmaleerat, K.; Pothacharoen, P.; Phitak, T.; Kongtawelert, P. Ex vivo model exhibits protective effects of sesamin against destruction of cartilage induced with a combination of tumor necrosis factor-alpha and oncostatin M. *BMC Complement. Altern. Med.* **2016**, *16*. [CrossRef] [PubMed]

105. Cavero, R.Y.; Calvo, M.I. Medicinal plants used for musculoskeletal disorders in Navarra and their pharmacological validation. *J. Ethnopharmacol.* **2015**, *168*, 255–259. [CrossRef] [PubMed]

106. Di Lorenzo, C.; Dell'Agli, M.; Badea, M.; Dima, L.; Colombo, E.; Sangiovanni, E.; Restani, P.; Bosisio, E. Plant food supplements with anti-inflammatory properties: A systematic review (II). *Crit. Rev. Food Sci. Nutr.* **2013**, *53*, 507–516. [CrossRef] [PubMed]

107. Gilca, M.; Gaman, L.; Lixandru, D.; Stoian, I. Estimating the yin-yang nature of Western herbs: A potential tool based on antioxidation-oxidation theory. *Afr. J. Tradit. Complement. Altern. Med.* **2014**, *11*, 210–216. [CrossRef] [PubMed]

108. Hiermann, A.; Writzel, M. Antiphlogistic glycopeptide from the roots of *Symphytum officinale*. *Pharm. Pharmacol. Lett.* **1998**, *8*, 154–157.

109. Mascolo, N.; Autore, G.; Capasso, F.; Menghini, A.; Fasulo, M.P. Biological screening of Italian medicinal plants for anti-inflammatory activity. *Phyther. Res.* **1987**, *1*, 28–31. [CrossRef]

110. Laslett, L.L.; Quinn, S.J.; Darian-Smith, E.; Kwok, M.; Fedorova, T.; Körner, H.; Steels, E.; March, L.; Jones, G. Treatment with 4Jointz reduces knee pain over 12 weeks of treatment in patients with clinical knee osteoarthritis: A randomised controlled trial. *Osteoarthr. Cartil.* **2012**, *20*, 1209–1216. [CrossRef] [PubMed]

111. Grube, B.; Grünwald, J.; Krug, L.; Staiger, C. Efficacy of a comfrey root (*Symphyti offic. radix*) extract ointment in the treatment of patients with painful osteoarthritis of the knee: Results of a double-blind, randomised, bicenter, placebo-controlled trial. *Phytomedicine* **2007**, *14*, 2–10. [CrossRef] [PubMed]

112. Gracza, L.; Koch, H.; Loffler, E. Biochemical-pharmacologic studies of medicinal plants. 1. Isolation of rosmarinic acid from *Symphytum officinale* L. and its anti-inflammatory activity in an in vitro model. *Arch. Pharm.* **1985**, *318*, 1090–1095. [CrossRef]

113. Gracza, L. Prüfung der membranabdichtenden Wirkung eines Phytopharmakons und dessen Wirkstoffe. *Z. Phytother.* **1987**, *8*, 78–81.

114. Huang, S.-H.; Lee, C.-H.; Wang, H.-M.; Chang, Y.-W.; Lin, C.-Y.; Chen, C.-Y.; Chen, Y.-H. 6-Dehydrogingerdione restrains lipopolysaccharide-induced inflammatory responses in RAW 264.7 macrophages. *J. Agric. Food Chem.* **2014**, *62*, 9171–9179. [CrossRef] [PubMed]

115. Van Breemen, R.B.; Tao, Y.; Li, W. Cyclooxygenase-2 inhibitors in ginger (*Zingiber officinale*). *Fitoterapia* **2011**, *82*, 38–43. [CrossRef] [PubMed]

116. Grzanna, R.; Lindmark, L.; Frondoza, C.G. Ginger—An herbal medicinal product with broad anti-inflammatory actions. *J. Med. Food* **2005**, *8*, 125–132. [CrossRef] [PubMed]

117. Ueda, H.; Ippoushi, K.; Takeuchi, A. Repeated oral administration of a squeezed ginger (*Zingiber officinale*) extract augmented the serum corticosterone level and had anti-inflammatory properties. *Biosci. Biotechnol. Biochem.* **2010**, *74*, 2248–2252. [CrossRef] [PubMed]

118. Naderi, Z.; Mozaffari-Khosravi, H.; Dehghan, A.; Nadjarzadeh, A.; Huseini, H.F. Effect of ginger powder supplementation on nitric oxide and C-reactive protein in elderly knee osteoarthritis patients: A 12-week double-blind randomized placebo-controlled clinical trial. *J. Tradit. Complement. Med.* **2016**, *6*, 199–203. [CrossRef]

119. Altman, R.D.; Marcussen, K.C. Effects of a ginger extract on knee pain in patients with osteoarthritis. *Arthritis Rheum.* **2001**, *44*, 2531–2538. [CrossRef]

120. Alipour, Z.; Asadizaker, M.; Fayazi, S.; Yegane, N.; Kochak, M.; Haghighi Zadeh, M.H. The Effect of Ginger on Pain and Satisfaction of Patients with Knee Osteoarthritis. *Jundishapur J. Chronic Dis. Care* **2016**, *6*, e34798. [CrossRef]

121. Haghighi, M.; Khalvat, A.; Toliat, T.; Jallaei, S. Comparing the effects of ginger extract and ibuprofen in patients with osteoporosis. *Arch. Iran. Med.* **2005**, *8*, 267–271.

122. Drozdov, V.N.; Kim, V.A.; Tkachenko, E.V.; Varvanina, G.G. Influence of a specific ginger combination on gastropathy conditions in patients with osteoarthritis of the knee or hip. *J. Altern. Complement. Med.* **2012**, *18*, 583–588. [CrossRef] [PubMed]

123. Bliddal, H.; Rosetzsky, A.; Schlichting, P.; Weidner, M.S.; Andersen, L.A.; Ibfelt, H.H.; Christensen, K.; Jensen, O.N.; Barslev, J. A randomized, placebo-controlled, cross-over study of ginger extracts and ibuprofen in osteoarthritis. *Osteoarthr. Cartil.* **2000**, *8*, 9–12. [CrossRef] [PubMed]

124. Lee, H.Y.; Park, S.H.; Lee, M.; Kim, H.-J.; Ryu, S.Y.; Kim, N.D.; Hwang, B.Y.; Hong, J.T.; Han, S.-B.; Kim, Y. 1-Dehydro-[10]-gingerdione from ginger inhibits IKKβ activity for NF-κB activation and suppresses NF-κB-regulated expression of inflammatory genes. *Br. J. Pharmacol.* **2012**, *167*, 128–140. [CrossRef] [PubMed]

125. Singh, N.; Bhalla, M.; de Jager, P.; Gilca, M. An overview on Ashwagandha: A Rasayana (Rejuvenator) of Ayurveda. *Afr. J. Tradit. Complement. Altern. Med.* **2011**, *8*, 208–213. [CrossRef] [PubMed]

126. Singh, D.; Aggarwal, A.; Maurya, R.; Naik, S. Withania somnifera inhibits NF-κB and AP-1 transcription factors in human peripheral blood and synovial fluid mononuclear cells. *Phytother. Res.* **2007**, *21*, 905–913. [CrossRef] [PubMed]

127. Ganesan, K.; Sehgal, P.K.; Mandal, A.B.; Sayeed, S. Protective effect of Withania somnifera and Cardiospermum halicacabum extracts against collagenolytic degradation of collagen. *Appl. Biochem. Biotechnol.* **2011**, *165*, 1075–1091. [CrossRef] [PubMed]

128. Rasool, M.; Varalakshmi, P. Protective effect of Withania somnifera root powder in relation to lipid peroxidation, antioxidant status, glycoproteins and bone collagen on adjuvant-induced arthritis in rats. *Fundam. Clin. Pharmacol.* **2007**, *21*, 157–164. [CrossRef] [PubMed]

129. Ramakanth, G.S.H.; Uday Kumar, C.; Kishan, P.V.; Usharani, P. A randomized, double blind placebo controlled study of efficacy and tolerability of Withaina somnifera extracts in knee joint pain. *J. Ayurveda Integr. Med.* **2016**, *7*, 151–157. [CrossRef] [PubMed]

130. Sabina, E.P.; Chandal, S.; Rasool, M.K. Inhibition of monosodium urate crystal-induced inflammation by withaferin A. *J. Pharm. Pharm. Sci.* **2008**, *11*, 46–55. [PubMed]

131. Grover, A.; Shandilya, A.; Punetha, A.; Bisaria, V.S.; Sundar, D. Inhibition of the NEMO/IKKβ association complex formation, a novel mechanism associated with the NF-κB activation suppression by Withania somnifera's key metabolite withaferin A. *BMC Genom.* **2010**, *11* (Suppl. 4), S25. [CrossRef] [PubMed]

132. Heyninck, K.; Lahtela-Kakkonen, M.; van der Veken, P.; Haegeman, G.; Vanden Berghe, W. Withaferin A inhibits NF-κB activation by targeting cysteine 179 in IKKβ. *Biochem. Pharmacol.* **2014**, *91*, 501–509. [CrossRef] [PubMed]

133. Bee, T.A.; Liew, A.; Hons, P. Dietary Supplements Used in Osteoarthritis. *Proc. Singap. Healthc.* **2010**, *19*, 237–247. [CrossRef]

134. Posadzki, P.; Watson, L.; Ernst, E. Contamination and adulteration of herbal medicinal products (HMPs): An overview of systematic reviews. *Eur. J. Clin. Pharmacol.* **2013**, *69*, 295–307. [CrossRef] [PubMed]

135. Ernst, E. Risks of herbal medicinal products. *Pharmacoepidemiol. Drug Saf.* **2004**, *13*, 767–771. [CrossRef] [PubMed]

136. Posadzki, P.; Watson, L.; Ernst, E. Herb-drug interactions: An overview of systematic reviews. *Br. J. Clin. Pharmacol.* **2013**, *75*, 603–618. [CrossRef] [PubMed]

137. Bhattaram, V.A.; Graefe, U.; Kohlert, C.; Veit, M.; Derendorf, H. Pharmacokinetics and bioavailability of herbal medicinal products. *Phytomedicine* **2002**, *9* (Suppl. 3), 1–33. [CrossRef] [PubMed]

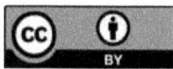

nutrients

MDPI

Article

The Effects of Tocotrienol and Lovastatin Co-Supplementation on Bone Dynamic Histomorphometry and Bone Morphogenetic Protein-2 Expression in Rats with Estrogen Deficiency

Kok-Yong Chin [1], Saif Abdul-Majeed [2], Norazlina Mohamed [1] and Soelaiman Ima-Nirwana [1,*]

[1] Department of Pharmacology, Universiti Kebangsaan Malaysia Medical Centre, Cheras 56000, Malaysia; chinkokyong@ppukm.ukm.edu.my (K.-Y.C.); azlina@ppukm.ukm.edu.my (N.M.)
[2] Department of Anatomy and Cell Biology, University of Pennsylvania, PA 19104, USA; saif_saad83@yahoo.com
* Correspondence: imasoel@ppukm.ukm.edu.my; Tel.: +60-3-9145-5002

Received: 17 January 2017; Accepted: 13 February 2017; Published: 15 February 2017

Abstract: Both tocotrienol and statins are suppressors of the mevalonate pathway. Supplementation of tocotrienol among statin users could potentially protect them against osteoporosis. This study aimed to compare the effects of tocotrienol and lovastatin co-supplementation with individual treatments on bone dynamic histomorphometric indices and bone morphogenetic protein-2 (BMP-2) gene expression in ovariectomized rats. Forty-eight female Sprague-Dawley rats were randomized equally into six groups. The baseline was sacrificed upon receipt. All other groups were ovariectomized, except for the sham group. The ovariectomized groups were administered orally daily with (1) lovastatin 11 mg/kg/day alone; (2) tocotrienol derived from annatto bean (annatto tocotrienol) 60 mg/kg/day alone; (3) lovastatin 11 mg/kg/day, and annatto tocotrienol 60 mg/kg/day. The sham and ovariectomized control groups were treated with equal volume of vehicle. After eight weeks of treatment, the rats were sacrificed. Their bones were harvested for bone dynamic histomorphometry and BMP-2 gene expression. Rats supplemented with annatto tocotrienol and lovastatin concurrently demonstrated significantly lower single-labeled surface, but increased double-labeled surface, mineralizing surface, mineral apposition rate and bone formation rate compared to individual treatments ($p < 0.05$). There was a parallel increase in BMP-2 gene expression in the rats receiving combined treatment ($p < 0.05$). The combination of annatto tocotrienol and lovastatin exerted either additively or synergistically on selected bone parameters. In conclusion, tocotrienol can augment the bone formation and mineralization in rats receiving low-dose statins. Supplementation of tocotrienol in statin users can potentially protect them from osteoporosis.

Keywords: calcium; mineralization; menopause; mevalonate; osteopenia; osteoporosis; vitamin E

1. Introduction

Hypercholesterolemia is a prevalent condition among middle-aged and elderly populations worldwide [1–3]. Statins are the most commonly prescribed medication for the treatment of this condition to prevent cardiovascular disease [4]. The middle-aged and elderly populations are also susceptible to osteoporosis. It is a condition characterized by degeneration of bone mass and deterioration of skeletal microarchitecture, leading to decreased bone strength and increased risk of fracture [5]. Post-menopausal women are particularly susceptible to osteoporosis because rapid bone loss occurs after the cessation of ovarian estrogen production [6].

Meta-analyses have concluded that statins could increase bone mineral density of its users and protect them from osteoporosis [7–9]. This pleiotropic effect of statins on bone is mediated through the suppression of the mevalonate pathway, which plays an integral part in both cholesterol synthesis and bone metabolism. The inhibition of 3-hydroxy-3-methyl-glutaryl-coenzyme A reductase (HMGCR) and the subsequent reduction in isoprenoid synthesis tilt the bone remodeling process in favor of formation over resorption [10]. However, most animal studies indicated that statins at doses higher than the clinical hypocholesterolemia regimen are required to exploit its bone-protective potential [11,12]. High-dose statins are often accompanied by adverse side-effects, such as myopathy, rhabdomyolysis, increased circulating transaminase level and risk of diabetes mellitus [13]. Thus, it is not a safe osteoporosis treatment option.

Tocotrienol, a member of vitamin E family in addition to tocopherol, has been shown to exhibit bone protective action in various animal bone loss models [14–16]. Homologues of tocotrienol, namely alpha-, beta-, gamma-, and delta-tocotrienol, are available in mixtures derived from plant sources [17,18]. Oil derived from palm kernel, annatto seed and rice bran is rich in tocotrienol [19–21]. The skeletal protective actions of palm tocotrienol mixtures in post-menopausal animal model have been studied extensively [22–25]. Recent evidence also suggested that annatto tocotrienol supplementation at 60 mg/kg/day for eight weeks could prevent post-menopausal bone loss in rats by preserving the integrity of trabecular structure, increasing the number of osteoblast (bone forming cells), decreasing the number of osteoclast (bone resorbing cells) and maintaining bone biomechanical strength [26,27]. Annatto tocotrienol at 60 mg/kg/day also exerted strong skeletal anabolic effects in rats with testosterone deficiency by increasing the expression of bone formation genes coding for alkaline phosphatase (ALPL), beta-catenin (CTNNB1), collagen type I alpha 1 (COL1A1) and osteopontin (SPP1) [28]. A study by Deng et al. suggested that the bone protective activity of tocotrienol was mediated by the mevalonate pathway [29].

Taking all evidence into consideration, tocotrienol can potentially enhance the bone protective effects of statins among its users. Two previous reports indicated that concurrent supplementation of lovastatin at normal hypocholesterolemic dosage (11 mg/kg/day) and annatto tocotrienol at 60 mg/kg/day body weight prevented the degeneration of trabecular structure and bone strength in ovariectomized rats [26,27]. Lovastatin, alone, failed to do the same within the same treatment period [26,27]. However, the effects of lovastatin and annatto tocotrienol co-supplementation on bone formation and mineralization activity, as indicated by dynamic histomorphometric parameters, in ovariectomized rats have not been explored. The dynamic histomorphometry utilizes fluorescent labeling agents to visualize mineral deposition and formation activity in bone [30]. There is also no literature on the effects of the combined treatment on BMP-2, an integral bone formation signal that bridges mevalonate pathway and osteoblastic differentiation [31].

This study is a continuation of our previous studies [26,27] and aimed to compare the effects of lovastatin, annatto tocotrienol and the combination of both agents on bone dynamic parameters and skeletal BMP-2 mRNA expression in ovariectomized rats. We hypothesized that the combined treatment would result in better bone mineralization and formation in rats compared to individual treatments. This would be brought about by an increased skeletal BMP-2 expression. This study will complement our earlier attempts and establish tocotrienol as a bone protective agent for post-menopausal women at risk of both osteoporosis and hypercholesterolemia.

2. Materials and Methods

2.1. Preparation of Annatto Tocotrienol and Lovastatin

Annatto tocotrienol containing 90% delta-tocotrienol and 10% gamma-tocotrienol was a gift from American River Nutrition (Hadley, MA, USA). This mixture was chosen because previous studies showed that tocotrienol mixture with less alpha-tocopherol was more effective in suppressing the activity of HMGCR [32]. In addition, gamma- and delta-tocotrienol were shown to be more effective compared to other isomers in lowering cholesterol level [33]. It was diluted 10 times in olive oil (Bartolini Emilio, Arrone Terni, Italy). Mevacor tablets (Merck, NJ, USA) containing 40 mg lovastatin was grounded and suspended in 0.5% carboxymethycellulose (Sigma-Aldrich, St. Louis, MO, USA).

2.2. Animal Treatment

The study protocol was reviewed and approved by Universiti Kebangsaan Malaysia Animal Ethics Committee. A total of 48 three-month-old Sprague-Dawley female rats weighing 200–250 g were obtained from the Laboratory Animal Resource Unit, Universiti Kebangsaan Malaysia (Kuala Lumpur, Malaysia). They were housed in the animal laboratory of the Department of Pharmacology, Universiti Kebangsaan Malaysia Medical Centre (Kuala Lumpur, Malaysia) under standard conditions (27 °C; ambient humidity; natural dark light cycle; standard rat chow, and tap water ad libitum). After one week of acclimatization, they were randomly divided into six groups: baseline (BL), sham (SH), ovariectomized control (OVX), ovariectomized and treated with lovastatin (OVX+LOV), ovariectomized and treated with annatto tocotrienol (OVX+AnTT), ovariectomized and treated with lovastatin and annatto tocotrienol (OVX+LOV+AnTT). The BL group was sacrificed upon receipt. All groups except the SH underwent bilateral ovariectomy. The SH group was subjected to similar surgical stress but the ovaries were not removed. Treatment was initiated one week after ovariectomy to allow the rats to recuperate. The OVX+LOV and OVX+LOV+AnTT group received daily oral administration of lovastation (11 mg/kg/day) while the other groups received equal volume of 0.5% carboxymethylcellulose as vehicle. Annatto tocotrienol at 60 mg/kg body weight was administered daily orally to the OVX+AnTT and OVX+LOV+AnTT group while the other groups was given equal volume of olive oil as vehicle. All treatments regimens were administered using an 18 gauge oral gavage needle with round end when the animals were restrained. The rats were sacrificed after eight weeks of treatment by anesthetic overdose. Left and right femoral and tibial bones were harvested for analysis.

2.3. Preparation of Bone Sample

The rats were administered calcein (Sigma-Aldrich, St. Louis, MO, USA) at 20 mg/kg body weight nine days and two days prior to euthanasia. Calcein is a fluorescent chromophore, which binds specifically to the skeleton, allowing direct visualization of mineralization. The left femurs was harvested, sectioned into halves sagittally, and fixed using alcohol. Next, the undecalcified bone was infiltrated and embedded using methyl methacrylate resin (Osteo-bed bone embedding kit, Polyscience, Warrington, PA, USA). The resin block was sectioned at thickness of 8 μm using a microtome (Leica, Wetzlar, Germany).

2.4. Assessment of Dynamic Histomorphometric Indices

The unstained slides were observed using a fluorescence microscope (Nikon Eclipse 80i, Tokyo, Japan). The secondary spongiosa in the metaphyseal region located 3–7 mm from the lowest point of growth plate and 1 mm from the cortical wall was sampled. The calcein-labeled surface of trabecular bone was measured manually using a Weibel grid with the aid of an image analyzer (MediaCybernetics Image Pro-Plus, Rockville, MD, USA). The dynamic histomorphometric parameters measured included single- (sLS/BS) and double-labeled surface (dLS/BS), mineralizing surface (MS/BS; extent of bone surface actively mineralizing), mineral apposition rate (MAR; distance between two labels in a double-labelled surface divided by the time between two calcein injections) and bone formation rate (BFR; the product of MAR multiplied by the fraction of labelled bone surface).

2.5. Determination of Bone Morphogenetics Protein-2 (BMP-2) Expression in Bone

Approximately 40 g of bone tissue sampled from proximal tibial metaphyseal region was homogenized and RNA was extracted using RNeasy Lipid Tissue Mini Kit (QIAGEN, Venlo, The Netherlands). Concentration and purity of RNA was determined using the Nanodrop

2000 device (Thermo Fisher Scientific, Waltham, MA, USA). The real-time PCR reaction mixture was prepared using iScript One-Step RT-PCR reagent with SYBR Green (Bio-Rad, Hercules, CA, USA). GADPH was used as the internal control. The forward and reverse sequence of primers for GAPDH and BMP-2 are shown in Table 1. Real-time PCR and data analysis were performed using iQ5 Real Time PCR Detection System (Bio-Rad, Hercules, CA, USA). The cycling conditions were as the following: cDNA synthesis for 10 min at 50 °C; reverse transcription inactivation for 5 min at 95 °C; PCR amplification for 45 cycles with 10 s at 95 °C and 30 s at 60 °C. Melt curve analysis was performed as the following: 1 min at 95 °C, 1 minute at 55 °C and 80 cycles of 10 s at 55–95 °C. Expression of BMP-2 will be normalized to GADPH and $2 - \Delta Ct$ values will be calculated.

Table 1. Primers for GADPH and BMP-2.

Gene	Accession Number	Primer Sequence	Base Pairs
GAPDH	NM 017008	F: 5′-GTGGACCTCATGGCCTACAT-3′ R: 5′-TGTGAGGGAGATGCTCAGTG-3′	129
BMP-2	NM 017178	F: 5′-TGAACACAGCTGGTCTCAGG-3′ R: 5′-TTAAGACGCTTCCGCTGTTT-3′	120

2.6. Statistical Analysis

Statistical analysis was performed using Statistical Package for Social Sciences version 20.0 (IBM, Armonk, NY, USA). Normality of the data was assessed using Shapiro-Wilks test. All data were normally distributed. Comparison of mean among the study groups were performed using one-way analysis of variance (ANOVA) with suitable post-hoc test. Additionally, the data were analyzed using factorial ANOVA considering the effects of lovastatin and annatto tocotrienol separately and together on each parameter. Statistical significance was defined as $p < 0.05$. The data were presented as mean ± standard error of mean.

3. Results

From the fluorescent micrographs, trabecular bone of the ovariectomized rats treated with annatto tocotrienol alone or lovastatin and annatto tocotrienol together showed more calcein double-labelled surface compared to untreated rats and rats treated with lovastatin alone (Figure 1). Quantification using a Weibel grid revealed that the sLS/BS was significantly higher ($p < 0.001$), but dLS/BS ($p < 0.001$), MS/BS ($p = 0.006$), MAR ($p < 0.001$), BFR ($p < 0.001$) were significant lower in the OVX group compared to the SH group. These parameters were not significantly different in OVX+LOV group compared to OVX group ($p > 0.05$). In contrast, OVX+AnTT and OVX+LOV+AnTT group possessed significantly lower sLS/BS, but higher dLS dLS/BS, MS/BS, MAR, and BFR compared to the OVX group ($p < 0.001$ for all comparisons). The sLS/BS ($p = 0.935$), MS/BS ($p = 0.127$), MAR ($p = 0.458$), and BFR ($p = 0.175$) between ovariectomized rats receiving combined treatment of annatto tocotrienol and lovastatin and those receiving annatto tocotrienol alone were not significantly different. Only the dLS/BS was significantly different between the two groups ($p = 0.002$) (Figure 2A–E).

The relative expression of BMP-2 mRNA was significantly lower in the OVX group compared to the SH group ($p < 0.001$). Treatment with lovastatin did not elevate the expression of BMP-2 mRNA significantly compared to the OVX group ($p = 0.409$). Annatto alone ($p < 0.001$) or in combination with lovastatin ($p < 0.001$) significantly increased the expression of BMP-2 mRNA compared to the OVX group. The increase was significantly higher in the OVX+LOV+AnTT group compared to the OVX+AnTT group ($p = 0.006$) (Figure 3).

The data were analyzed again using factorial ANOVA to determine the individual and combined effects of lovastatin and annatto tocotrienol on each parameter. The main effect of lovastatin was significant for dLS/BS ($p < 0.001$), MAR ($p = 0.006$), BFR ($p = 0.003$), and BMP-2 ($p < 0.001$). The main effect of annatto tocotrienol was significant for all parameters studied (p for all parameters < 0.001).

Significant interaction (lovastatin × annatto tocotrienol) was observed for dLS/BS ($p < 0.001$) and BFR ($p = 0.037$). These results indicated that the effects of annatto tocotrienol and lovastatin on MAR and BMP-2 could be additive, and on dLS/BS and BFR could be synergistic.

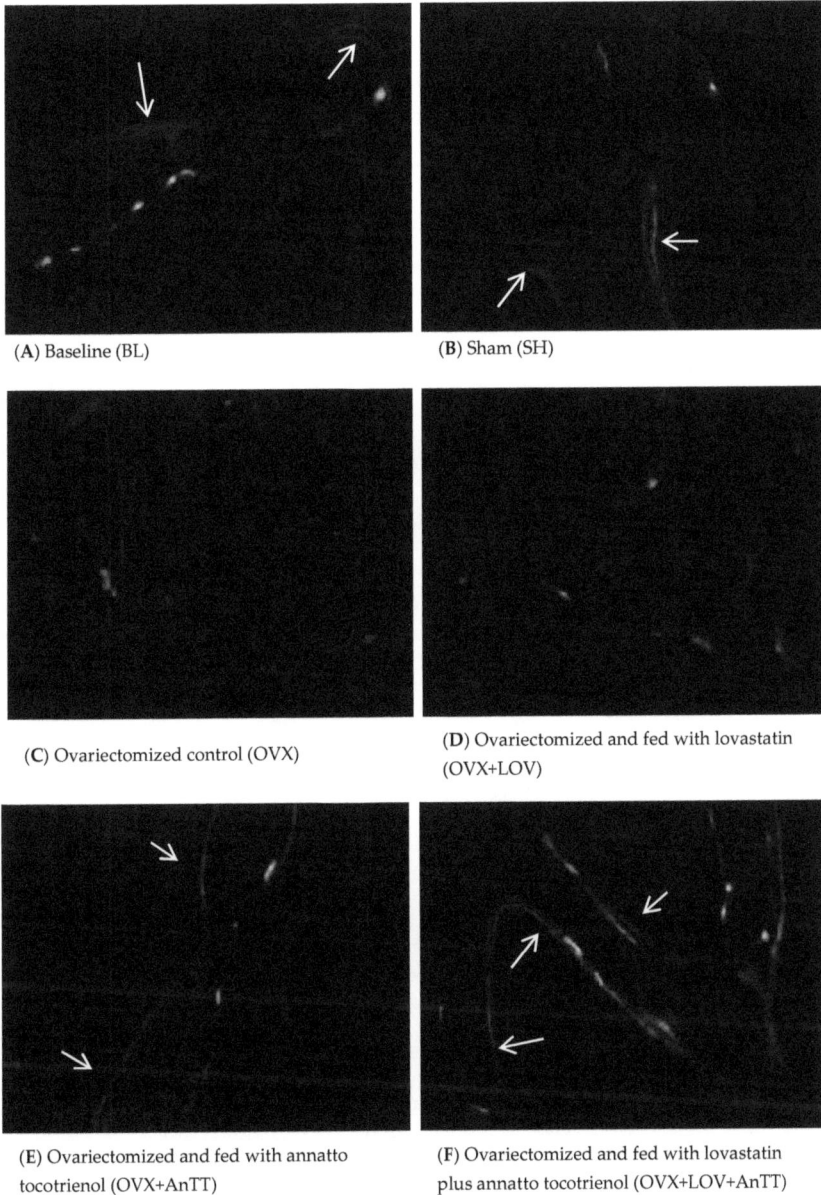

(A) Baseline (BL)

(B) Sham (SH)

(C) Ovariectomized control (OVX)

(D) Ovariectomized and fed with lovastatin (OVX+LOV)

(E) Ovariectomized and fed with annatto tocotrienol (OVX+AnTT)

(F) Ovariectomized and fed with lovastatin plus annatto tocotrienol (OVX+LOV+AnTT)

Figure 1. Micrograph of calcein-labeled trabecular bone. Rats treated with annatto tocotrienol alone or in combination with statin showed more calcein double-labeled surface. The white arrows show double-labeled surface.

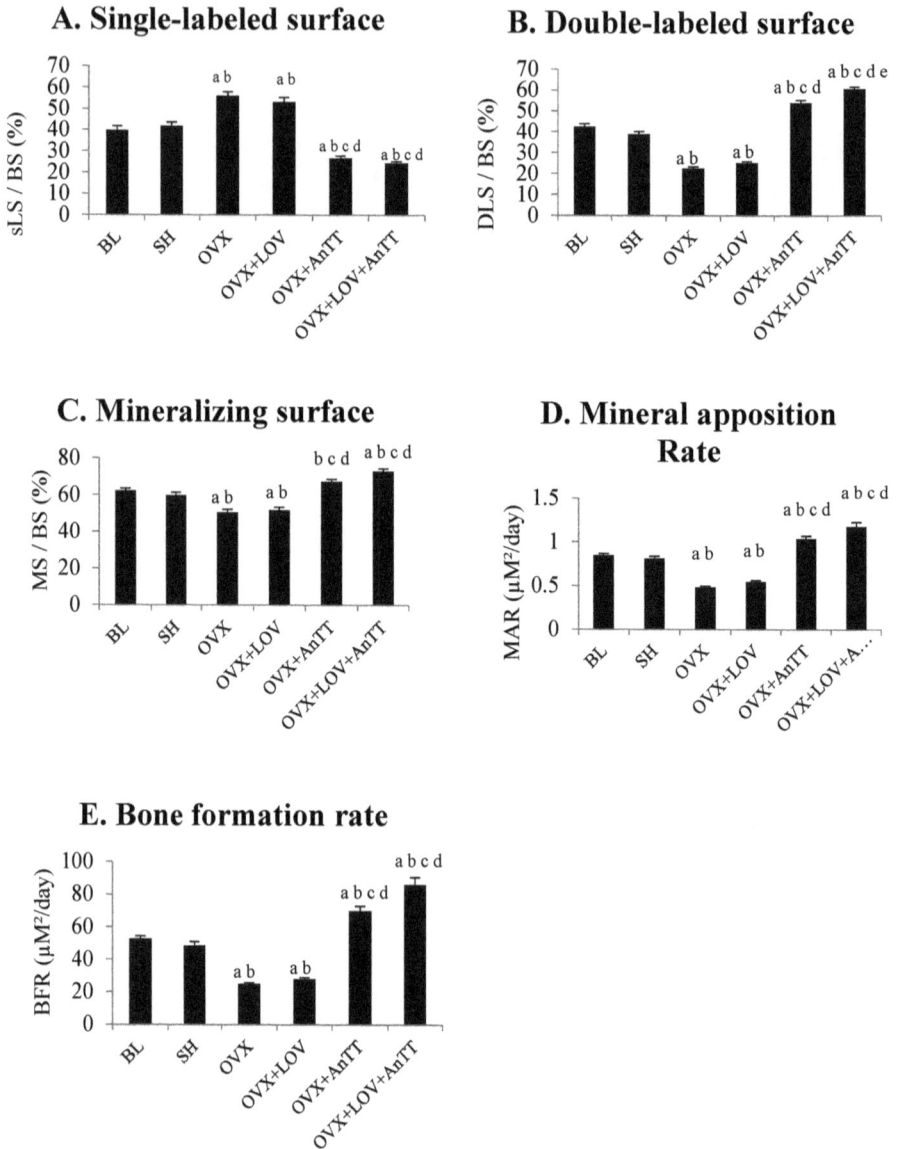

Figure 2. Bone dynamic histomorphometric parameters among the study group. Legend: Letters indicates significant difference between the marked group and 'a' BL; 'b' SH; 'c' OVX+LOV'; 'd' OVX+AnTT or 'e' OVX+LOV+AnTT. Abbreviation: BL = baseline; SH = sham-operated; OVX = ovariectomized; OVX+LOV = ovariectomized and supplemented with lovastatin (11 mg/day); OVX+AnTT = ovariectomized and supplemented with annatto tocotrienol (60 mg/kg/day); OVX+LOVAnTT = ovariectomized and supplemented with lovastatin (11 mg/day) and annatto tocotrienol (60 mg/kg/day).

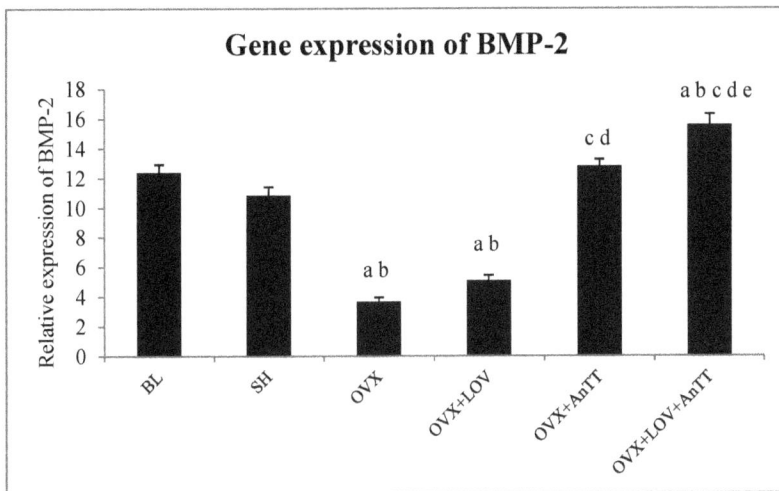

Figure 3. Gene expression of BMP-2 among the study groups. Legend: Letters indicates significant difference between the marked group and 'a' BL; 'b' SH; 'c' OVX+LOV'; 'd' OVX+AnTT or 'e' OVX+LOV+AnTT. Abbreviation: BL = baseline; SH = sham-operated; OVX = ovariectomized; OVX+LOV = ovariectomized and supplemented with lovastatin (11 mg/day); OVX+AnTT = ovariectomized and supplemented with annatto tocotrienol (60 mg/kg/day); OVX+LOVAnTT = ovariectomized and supplemented with lovastatin (11 mg/day) and annatto tocotrienol (60 mg/kg/day).

4. Discussion

The current study showed that co-supplementation of lovastatin and annatto tocotrienol was superior to lovastatin or tocotrienol alone in improving bone formation and mineralization activity in rats with estrogen deficiency, indicated by lower sLS/BS, but higher dLS/BS, MS/BS, MAR, and BFR compared to the untreated group. Annatto tocotrienol at 60 mg/kg body weight was able to improve bone dynamic histomorphometry of the ovariectomized rats. The combined treatment was more efficacious than annatto tocotrienol alone in increasing dLS/BS and BMP-2 expression. Lovastatin at the usual hypocholesterolemic dose in rats failed to augment the bone dynamic histomorphometry in ovariectomized rats within eight weeks. The skeletal anabolic effects of the aforementioned treatment regimens corresponded well to the increase in skeletal expression of BMP-2 of the rats (OVX+LOV+AnTT > OVX+AnTT = SH > OVX+LOV = OVX). The effects of annatto tocotrienol and lovastatin could be additive for MAR and BMP-2, and synergistic for dLS/BS and BFR.

Considering the higher metabolic rate of rats, 10 mg/kg/day of statins to rats was equivalent to 70 mg/day in humans [34]. The dose of lovastatin administrated to rats in this study was 11 mg/kg/day, which was equivalent to 77 mg/day to human. Oral administration of lovastatin as low as 10 mg/kg was shown to reduce the serum cholesterol level in ovariectomized rats [35]. The lovastatin dose used in this study does not exceed the recommended statin dose for high-intensity hypocholesterolemic effects in humans (80 mg/day) [36]. Monteiro et al. showed that oral supplementation of very-high-dose simvastatin (20 mg/kg/day, equivalent to 140 mg/day in humans) improved the bone microstructure of ovariectomized rats in 14 days [37]. Similar effects were not observed with a lower dose within the same treatment period [37]. Thus, it is reasonable that lovastatin at the dose used in the current study produced no effects on bone dynamic histormorphometric parameters in ovariectomized rats. Similarly, a study showed that simvastatin at 10 mg/kg/day for five weeks did not exert bone anabolic effects in normal female rats [38]. Our previous studies also showed that lovastatin at 11 mg/kg did not improve bone microstructure and mechanical strength in ovariectomized rats [26,27]. Another study showed that simvastatin at 10 mg/kg/day could not reverse established osteoporosis in ovariectomized rats [39]. The lack of improvement in bone formation and mineralization in rats supplemented by statins at hypocholesterolemic dose, as illustrated in this study, provided an explanation for the aforementioned studies. Deposition of statins in skeletal tissue after oral administration of statins is very low [35], thus a lower dosage and short treatment period prevents statins from achieving their bone protective potential.

Tocotrienol has been shown to promote bone mineralization and formation process in various animal studies [23,28,40,41]. Despite the difference in composition of tocotrienol homologues, bone dynamic histomorphometric changes caused by palm tocotrienol in ovariectomized rats were comparable with alterations induced by annatto tocotrienol observed in this study [23,40]. They were marked by a reduction in sLS/BS, and an increment in dLS/BS, MS/BS, MAR, and BFR in the supplemented ovariectomized rats compared to the untreated group [23,40]. The improvement in bone dynamic histomorphometry caused by palm tocotrienol was greater than estrogen treated group in a study by Aktifanus et al. [40]. In orchidectomized rats, annatto tocotrienol at 60 mg/kg/day for eight weeks caused a decrease in sLS/BS and an increase in dLS/BS, but the changes in MS/BS, MAR and BFR were not significant [28]. This might indicate that annatto tocotrienol works better in a female bone loss model. The rise in bone formation and mineralization caused by annatto tocotrienol could be explained by increased osteoblastic activity, marked by increased circulating bone formation markers and increased gene expression of osteoblastic differentiation markers [26,28,42]. It also corresponded to the previous findings that osteoblast number, osteoid surface, osteoid volume were inflated in ovariectomized rats supplemented with annatto or palm tocotrienol [22,26,42]. The dose of tocotrienol used in this study (60 mg/kg/day) is well below the toxic dose detected in previous animal studies [43].

The combination of tocotrienol and lovastatin was found to increase the dLS/BS and BMP-2 expression better than individual treatments. In addition, there were potential additive effects (MAR and BMP-2) and synergistic effects (dLS/BS and BFR) between annatto tocotrienol and lovastatin. This indicates that statin users could experience bone protection without increasing the dose of medication beyond the current recommendation. Previous studies have demonstrated that the combined treatment of tocotrienol and lovastatin enhanced the bone microstructure, increased osteoblast number and osteoid production, and decreased osteoclast number and bone erosion in ovariectomized rats better than both agents alone [26,27]. The rats treated with both agents concurrently also had significantly higher bone biomechanical strength compared to rats receiving single treatment of either agent [27]. Both tocotrienol and lovastatin are suppressors of the mevalonate pathway important for isoprenoid synthesis by inhibiting the rate-determining HMGCR enzyme via modulation of sterol regulatory element-binding proteins (SREBPs) [10,44]. These isoprenoids are materials for cholesterol synthesis or prenylation with GTPases to produce prenylated proteins, which act as negative regulators for bone formation [10,44]. Gamma- and delta-tocotrienol, the constituents of annatto tocotrienol mixture, modulate HMGCR in slightly different ways. Delta-tocotrienol enhances the ubiquitination of HMGCR and inhibits SREBP processing [45]. Gamma-tocotrienol is more selective in HMGCR degradation than blocking SREBPs [45]. Structurally, tocotrienols with their long carbon chain with double bonds are similar to farnesyl, a compound preceding geranyl-pyrophosphate that will enter isoprenoid synthesis [46]. The presence of tocotrienol stimulates the farnesol production instead of farnesyl, thus reducing the input for isoprenoid synthesis pathway [46]. On the other hand, statins are competitive inhibitor of HMGCR because they are structurally similar with HMGCo-A, the substrate for HMGCR [47]. The benefits of tocotrienol and statins co-treatment extend beyond bone health, and have been proven in anticancer studies [48,49].

Bone morphogenetic protein-2 plays an important role in the differentiation of osteoblasts. Through Smad signaling pathway, BMP-2 activates runt-related factor-2 (RUNX2), the master transcription factor for osteoblastic gene expression [50]. It can also activate osterix, an essential transcription factor for the differentiation of osteoblasts directly via distal-less homeobox 5 or indirectly via RUNX2 [50]. The expression of BMP-2 is influenced by the mevalonate pathway. Simvastatin treatment was shown to increase the expression of BMP-2 in preosteoblasts, decrease post-translation modification of Ras, regulate intracellular protein associated to Ras, and subsequently increase osteoblast differentiation [51]. Results of the current study showed that hypocholesterolemic dose of lovastatin could not upregulate the expression of BMP-2 in bone probably due to poor deposition of the compound in the skeleton. On the other hand, tocotrienol alone or in combination with lovastatin increased the expression of skeletal BMP-2. The extent of improvement was greater in the latter compared with the former, partly due to the additive effect of both agents. Previous studies have established that tocotrienol was able to preserve BMP-2, RUNX2, and OSX expression in nicotine-treated osteoporotic rats [52]. Tocotrienol was also shown to increase gene expression of osteoblast markers, such as ALPL, COL1A1, SPP1, and CTNNB1 in orchidectomized rats [28]. The current study showed that these changes could be a result of BMP-2 up-regulation since they are all downstream genes of BMP-2 signaling.

Several limitations should be considered in this study. Only gene expression of BMP-2 was determined. Its expression level was not validated by protein expression assay. Tocotrienol has similar cholesterol-lowering effects as statins [53,54]. However, this study did not investigate whether concurrent treatment with tocotrienol would potentiate the hypocholesterolemic effects of statins. Despite strong evidence from previous studies, we could not validate the involvement of the mevalonate pathway in the bone protective action of both agents directly. This is because we did not quantify the inhibition of HMGCR and level of prenylated proteins in the bone. In spite of these limitations, this study successfully showed that tocotrienol could aggrandize the bone protective actions of low-dose statins by increasing bone mineralization and formation. This could protect middle-aged and elderly populations already taking statins for hypercholesteremia against osteoporosis.

5. Conclusions

Tocotrienol alone or in combination with low-dose lovastatin can augment bone formation and mineralization in a rat model of bone loss due to estrogen deficiency. The enhanced protection can be contributed by the additive or synergistic effects between lovastatin and annatto tocotrienol on bone. The bone protective action of both regimens is mediated by an increased skeletal BMP-2 expression. This provides a justification to conduct a clinical trial supplementing tocotrienol in statins users to protect them against osteoporosis.

Acknowledgments: We thank Universiti Kebangsaan Malaysia for funding this study via grants GGPM-2015-036 and DIP-2014-040. We express our gratitude to American River Nutrition for providing the annatto tocotrienol. We also thank the following persons from the Department of Pharmacology, Universiti Kebangsaan Malaysia Medical Centre for their technical assistance: Fadlullah Zuhair Japar Sidik, Juliana Abdul Hamid, Nurul Hafizah Abas, Sabariah Adnan, and Nur Farhana Mohd Fozi.

Author Contributions: K.-Y.C. analyzed the data and wrote the manuscript; S.A.-M. analyzed the data and performed the experiments; S.I.-M. and N.M. conceived and designed the experiments, as well as supervised the project; S.I.-M. obtained funding for the project, provided critical review and final approval for this manuscript.

Conflicts of Interest: The authors declare no conflict of interest. The sponsors had no role in the design of the study; in the collection, analyses, or interpretation of data; in the writing of the manuscript, and in the decision to publish the results.

References

1. Basulaiman, M.; El Bcheraoui, C.; Tuffaha, M.; Robinson, M.; Daoud, F.; Jaber, S.; Mikhitarian, S.; Wilson, S.; Memish, Z.A.; Al Saeedi, M.; et al. Hypercholesterolemia and its associated risk factors-Kingdom of Saudi Arabia, 2013. *Ann. Epidemiol.* **2014**, *24*, 801–808. [CrossRef] [PubMed]
2. Guallar-Castillon, P.; Gil-Montero, M.; Leon-Munoz, L.M.; Graciani, A.; Bayan-Bravo, A.; Taboada, J.M.; Banegas, J.R.; Rodriguez-Artalejo, F. Magnitude and management of hypercholesterolemia in the adult population of Spain, 2008–2010: The Enrica Study. *Rev. Esp. Cardiol.* **2012**, *65*, 551–558. [CrossRef] [PubMed]

3. Kim, H.J.; Kim, Y.; Cho, Y.; Jun, B.; Oh, K.W. Trends in the prevalence of major cardiovascular disease risk factors among Korean adults: Results from the Korea National Health and Nutrition Examination Survey, 1998–2012. *Int. J. Cardiol.* **2014**, *174*, 64–72. [CrossRef] [PubMed]

4. Stone, N.J.; Robinson, J.G.; Lichtenstein, A.H.; Bairey Merz, C.N.; Blum, C.B.; Eckel, R.H.; Goldberg, A.C.; Gordon, D.; Levy, D.; Lloyd-Jones, D.M.; et al. 2013 acc/aha guideline on the treatment of blood cholesterol to reduce atherosclerotic cardiovascular risk in adults: A report of the American college of cardiology/american heart association task force on practice guidelines. *J. Am. Coll. Cardiol.* **2014**, *63*, 2889–2934. [CrossRef] [PubMed]

5. Edwards, M.H.; Dennison, E.M.; Aihie Sayer, A.; Fielding, R.; Cooper, C. Osteoporosis and sarcopenia in older age. *Bone* **2015**, *80*, 126–130. [CrossRef] [PubMed]

6. Cauley, J.A. Estrogen and bone health in men and women. *Steroids* **2015**, *99*, 11–15. [CrossRef] [PubMed]

7. Liu, J.; Zhu, L.P.; Yang, X.L.; Huang, H.L.; Ye, D.Q. Hmg-coa reductase inhibitors (statins) and bone mineral density: A meta-analysis. *Bone* **2013**, *54*, 151–156. [CrossRef] [PubMed]

8. Uzzan, B.; Cohen, R.; Nicolas, P.; Cucherat, M.; Perret, G.Y. Effects of statins on bone mineral density: A meta-analysis of clinical studies. *Bone* **2007**, *40*, 1581–1587. [CrossRef] [PubMed]

9. Wang, Z.; Li, Y.; Zhou, F.; Piao, Z.; Hao, J. Effects of statins on bone mineral density and fracture risk: A prisma-compliant systematic review and meta-analysis. *Medicine (Baltimore)* **2016**, *95*, e3042. [CrossRef] [PubMed]

10. Mo, H.; Yeganehjoo, H.; Shah, A.; Mo, W.K.; Soelaiman, I.N.; Shen, C.L. Mevalonate-suppressive dietary isoprenoids for bone health. *J. Nutr. Biochem.* **2012**, *23*, 1543–1551. [CrossRef] [PubMed]

11. Maritz, F.J.; Conradie, M.M.; Hulley, P.A.; Gopal, R.; Hough, S. Effect of statins on bone mineral density and bone histomorphometry in rodents. *Arterioscler. Thromb. Vasc. Biol.* **2001**, *21*, 1636–1641. [CrossRef] [PubMed]

12. Soares, E.A.; Novaes, R.D.; Nakagaki, W.R.; Fernandes, G.J.; Garcia, J.A.; Camilli, J.A. Metabolic and structural bone disturbances induced by hyperlipidic diet in mice treated with simvastatin. *Int. J. Exp. Pathol.* **2015**, *96*, 261–268. [CrossRef] [PubMed]

13. Simic, I.; Reiner, Z. Adverse effects of statins—Myths and reality. *Curr. Pharm. Des.* **2015**, *21*, 1220–1226. [CrossRef] [PubMed]

14. Chin, K.Y.; Ima-Nirwana, S. The biological effects of tocotrienol on bone: A review on evidence from rodent models. *Drug Des. Devel. Ther.* **2015**, *9*, 2049–2061. [CrossRef] [PubMed]

15. Chin, K.-Y.; Ima-Nirwana, S. Vitamin E as an antiosteoporotic agent via receptor activator of nuclear factor kappa-B ligand signaling disruption: Current evidence and other potential research areas. *Evid. Based Complement. Altern. Med.* **2012**, *2012*, 747020. [CrossRef] [PubMed]

16. Chin, K.-Y.; Mo, H.; Soelaiman, I.-N. A review of the possible mechanisms of action of tocotrienol–A potential antiosteoporotic agent. *Curr. Drug Targets* **2013**, *14*, 1533–1541. [CrossRef] [PubMed]

17. Chin, K.Y.; Pang, K.L.; Soelaiman, I.N. Tocotrienol and its role in chronic diseases. *Adv. Exp. Med. Biol.* **2016**, *928*, 97–130. [PubMed]

18. Aggarwal, B.; Sundaram, C.; Prasad, S.; Kannappan, R. Tocotrienols, the vitamin E of the 21st century: It's potential against cancer and other chronic diseases. *Biochem. Pharmacol.* **2010**, *80*, 1613–1631. [CrossRef] [PubMed]

19. Frega, N.; Mozzon, M.; Bocci, F. Identification and estimation of tocotrienols in the annatto lipid fraction by gas chromatography-mass spectrometry. *J. Am. Oil Chem. Soc.* **1998**, *75*, 1723–1727. [CrossRef]

20. Ng, M.; Choo, Y.; Ma, A.; Chuah, C.; Hashim, M. Separation of vitamin E (tocopherol, tocotrienol, and tocomonoenol) in palm oil. *Lipids* **2004**, *39*, 1031–1035. [CrossRef] [PubMed]

21. Chen, M.H.; Bergman, C.J. A rapid procedure for analysing rice bran tocopherol, tocotrienol and γ-oryzanol contents. *J. Food Compost. Anal.* **2005**, *18*, 139–151. [CrossRef]

22. Muhammad, N.; Luke, D.A.; Shuid, A.N.; Mohamed, N.; Soelaiman, I.N. Two different isomers of vitamin E prevent bone loss in postmenopausal osteoporosis rat model. *Evid. Based Complement. Altern. Med.* **2012**, *2012*, 161527. [CrossRef] [PubMed]

23. Soelaiman, I.N.; Ming, W.; Abu Bakar, R.; Hashnan, N.A.; Mohd Ali, H.; Mohamed, N.; Muhammad, N.; Shuid, A.N. Palm tocotrienol supplementation enhanced bone formation in oestrogen-deficient rats. *Int. J. Endocrinol.* **2012**, *2012*, 532862. [CrossRef] [PubMed]

24. Nazrun, A.; Khairunnur, A.; Norliza, M.; Norazlina, M.; Ima Nirwana, S. Effects of palm tocotrienol on oxidative stress and bone strength in ovariectomised rats. *Med. Health* **2008**, *3*, 83–90.

25. Muhammad, N.; Razali, S.; Shuid, A.N.; Mohamed, N.; Soelaiman, I.N. Membandingkan kesan antara fraksi-kaya tokotrienol, kalsium dan estrogen terhadap metabolisme tulang tikus terovariektomi. *Sains Malays.* **2013**, *42*, 1591–1597.

26. Abdul-Majeed, S.; Mohamed, N.; Soelaiman, I.-N. Effects of tocotrienol and lovastatin combination on osteoblast and osteoclast activity in estrogen-deficient osteoporosis. *Evid. Based Complement. Altern. Med.* **2012**, *2012*, 960742. [CrossRef] [PubMed]

27. Abdul-Majeed, S.; Mohamed, N.; Soelaiman, I.N. The use of delta-tocotrienol and lovastatin for anti-osteoporotic therapy. *Life Sci.* **2015**, *125*, 42–48. [CrossRef] [PubMed]

28. Chin, K.Y.; Ima Nirwana, S. The effects of annatto-derived tocotrienol supplementation in osteoporosis induced by testosterone deficiency in rats. *Clin. Interv. Aging* **2014**, *9*, 1247–1259. [CrossRef] [PubMed]

29. Deng, L.; Ding, Y.; Peng, Y.; Wu, Y.; Fan, J.; Li, W.; Yang, R.; Yang, M.; Fu, Q. γ-Tocotrienol protects against ovariectomy-induced bone loss via mevalonate pathway as HMG-CoA reductase inhibitor. *Bone* **2014**, *67*, 200–207. [CrossRef] [PubMed]

30. Vedi, S.; Compston, J. Bone histomorphometry. *Methods Mol. Med.* **2003**, *80*, 283–298. [PubMed]

31. Kanazawa, I.; Yamaguchi, T.; Yano, S.; Hayashi, K.; Yamauchi, M.; Sugimoto, T. Inhibition of the mevalonate pathway rescues the dexamethasone-induced suppression of the mineralization in osteoblasts via enhancing bone morphogenetic protein-2 signal. *Horm. Metab. Res.* **2009**, *41*, 612–616. [CrossRef] [PubMed]

32. Khor, H.T.; Ng, T.T. Effects of administration of alpha-tocopherol and tocotrienols on serum lipids and liver HMG CoA reductase activity. *Int. J. Food Sci. Nutr.* **2000**, *51*, S3–S11. [CrossRef] [PubMed]

33. Yu, S.G.; Thomas, A.M.; Gapor, A.; Tan, B.; Qureshi, N.; Qureshi, A.A. Dose-response impact of various tocotrienols on serum lipid parameters in 5-week-old female chickens. *Lipids* **2006**, *41*, 453–461. [CrossRef] [PubMed]

34. Park, J.B. The use of simvastatin in bone regeneration. *Med. Oral Patol. Oral Cir. Bucal.* **2009**, *14*, e485–e488. [PubMed]

35. Jadhav, S.B.; Narayana Murthy, P.S.; Singh, M.M.; Jain, G.K. Distribution of lovastatin to bone and its effect on bone turnover in rats. *J. Pharm. Pharmacol.* **2006**, *58*, 1451–1458. [CrossRef] [PubMed]

36. US Preventive Services Task Force. Statin use for the primary prevention of cardiovascular disease in adults: US preventive services task force recommendation statement. *JAMA* **2016**, *316*, 1997–2007.

37. Monteiro, L.O.; Macedo, A.P.; Shimano, R.C.; Shimano, A.C.; Yanagihara, G.R.; Ramos, J.; Paulini, M.R.; Tocchini de Figueiredo, F.A.; Gonzaga, M.G.; Issa, J.P. Effect of treatment with simvastatin on bone microarchitecture of the femoral head in an osteoporosis animal model. *Microsc. Res. Tech.* **2016**, *79*, 684–690. [CrossRef] [PubMed]

38. Starnes, J.W.; Neidre, D.B.; Nyman, J.S.; Roy, A.; Nelson, M.J.; Gutierrez, G.; Wang, X. Synergistic effect of exercise and statins on femoral strength in rats. *Exp. Gerontol.* **2013**, *48*, 751–755. [CrossRef] [PubMed]

39. Yao, W.; Farmer, R.; Cooper, R.; Chmielewski, P.A.; Tian, X.Y.; Setterberg, R.B.; Jee, W.S.; Lundy, M.W. Simvastatin did not prevent nor restore ovariectomy-induced bone loss in adult rats. *J. Musculoskelet. Neuron. Interact.* **2006**, *6*, 277–283.

40. Aktifanus, A.T.; Shuid, A.N.; Rashid, N.H.A.; Tam, H.L.; Chua, Y.L.; Saat, N.M.; Muhammad, N.; Mohamed, N.; Ima Nirwana, S. Comparison of the effects of tocotrienol and estrogen on the bone markers and dynamic changes in postmenopausal osteoporosis rat model. *Asian J. Anim. Vet. Adv.* **2012**, *7*, 225–234.

41. Hermizi, H.; Faizah, O.; Ima-Nirwana, S.; Ahmad Nazrun, S.; Norazlina, M. Beneficial effects of tocotrienol and tocopherol on bone histomorphometric parameters in sprague–dawley male rats after nicotine cessation. *Calcif. Tissue Int.* **2009**, *84*, 65–74. [CrossRef] [PubMed]

42. Chin, K.Y.; Abdul-Majeed, S.; Fozi, N.F.; Ima-Nirwana, S. Annatto tocotrienol improves indices of bone static histomorphometry in osteoporosis due to testosterone deficiency in rats. *Nutrients* **2014**, *6*, 4974–4983. [CrossRef] [PubMed]

43. Ima-Nirwana, S.; Nurshazwani, Y.; Nazrun, A.S.; Norliza, M.; Norazlina, M. Subacute and subchronic toxicity studies of palm vitamin E in mice. *J. Pharmacol. Toxicol.* **2011**, *6*, 166–173. [CrossRef]

44. Abdul-Majeed, S.; Mohamed, N.; Soelaiman, I. A review on the use of statins and tocotrienols, individually or in combination for the treatment of osteoporosis. *Curr. Drug Targets* **2013**, *14*, 1579–1590. [CrossRef] [PubMed]

45. Song, B.L.; DeBose-Boyd, R.A. Insig-dependent ubiquitination and degradation of 3-hydroxy-3-methylglutaryl coenzyme a reductase stimulated by delta- and gamma-tocotrienols. *J. Biol. Chem.* **2006**, *281*, 25054–25061. [CrossRef] [PubMed]

46. Parker, R.A.; Pearce, B.C.; Clark, R.W.; Gordon, D.A.; Wright, J.J. Tocotrienols regulate cholesterol production in mammalian cells by post-transcriptional suppression of 3-hydroxy-3-methylglutaryl-coenzyme a reductase. *J. Biol. Chem.* **1993**, *268*, 11230–11238. [PubMed]

47. Tiwari, V.; Khokhar, M. Mechanism of action of anti-hypercholesterolemia drugs and their resistance. *Eur. J. Pharmacol.* **2014**, *741*, 156–170. [CrossRef] [PubMed]

48. McAnally, J.A.; Gupta, J.; Sodhani, S.; Bravo, L.; Mo, H. Tocotrienols potentiate lovastatin-mediated growth suppression in vitro and in vivo. *Exp. Biol. Med.* **2007**, *232*, 523–531.

49. Wali, V.B.; Sylvester, P.W. Synergistic antiproliferative effects of gamma-tocotrienol and statin treatment on mammary tumor cells. *Lipids* **2007**, *42*, 1113–1123. [CrossRef] [PubMed]

50. Chen, G.; Deng, C.; Li, Y.P. TGF-beta and bmp signaling in osteoblast differentiation and bone formation. *Int. J. Biol. Sci.* **2012**, *8*, 272–288. [CrossRef] [PubMed]

51. Chen, P.Y.; Sun, J.S.; Tsuang, Y.H.; Chen, M.H.; Weng, P.W.; Lin, F.H. Simvastatin promotes osteoblast viability and differentiation via ras/smad/erk/bmp-2 signaling pathway. *Nutr. Res.* **2010**, *30*, 191–199. [CrossRef] [PubMed]

52. Abukhadir, S.S.A.; Mohamed, N.; Makpol, S.; Muhammad, N. Effects of palm vitamin E on bone-formation-related gene expression in nicotine-treated rats. *Evid. Based Complement. Altern. Med.* **2012**, *2012*, 656025. [CrossRef] [PubMed]

53. Salman Khan, M.; Akhtar, S.; Al-Sagair, O.A.; Arif, J.M. Protective effect of dietary tocotrienols against infection and inflammation-induced hyperlipidemia: An in vivo and in silico study. *Phytother. Res.* **2011**, *25*, 1586–1595. [CrossRef] [PubMed]

54. Qureshi, A.A.; Reis, J.C.; Qureshi, N.; Papasian, C.J.; Morrison, D.C.; Schaefer, D.M. Delta-tocotrienol and quercetin reduce serum levels of nitric oxide and lipid parameters in female chickens. *Lipids Health Dis.* **2011**, *10*, 39. [CrossRef] [PubMed]

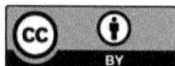

nutrients

MDPI

Article

Antiosteoporotic Activity of Genistein Aglycone in Postmenopausal Women: Evidence from a Post-Hoc Analysis of a Multicenter Randomized Controlled Trial

Vincenzo Arcoraci [1,†], Marco Atteritano [1,*,†], Francesco Squadrito [1], Rosario D'Anna [2],
Herbert Marini [1], Domenico Santoro [1], Letteria Minutoli [1], Sonia Messina [2], Domenica Altavilla [3]
and Alessandra Bitto [1]

[1] Department of Clinical and Experimental Medicine, University of Messina, 98100 Messina, Italy;
    varcoraci@unime.it (V.A.); fsquadrito@unime.it (F.S.); hrmarini@unime.it (H.M.); santisi@hotmail.com (D.S.);
    lminutoli@unime.it (L.M.); abitto@unime.it (A.B.)
[2] Department of Neurosciences and Nemo Sud Clinical Center, University of Messina, 98100 Messina, Italy;
    rdannna@unime.it (R.D.); smessina@unime.it (S.M.)
[3] Department of Paediatric, Gynaecological, Microbiological and Biomedical Sciences, University of Messina,
    98100 Messina, Italy; daltavilla@unime.it
*   Correspondence: matteritano@unime.it; Tel.: +39-90-2212388
†   These authors contributed equally to this work.

Received: 20 December 2016; Accepted: 20 February 2017; Published: 22 February 2017

Abstract: Genistein has a preventive role against bone mass loss during menopause. However, experimental data in animal models of osteoporosis suggest an anti-osteoporotic potential for this isoflavone. We performed a post-hoc analysis of a previously published trial investigating the effects of genistein in postmenopausal women with low bone mineral density. The parent study was a randomized, double-blind, placebo-controlled trial involving postmenopausal women with a femoral neck (FN) density <0.795 g/cm^2. A cohort of the enrolled women was, in fact, identified at the baseline as osteoporotic ($n = 121$) on the basis of their T-score and analyzed thereafter for the 24 months' treatment with either 1000 mg of calcium and 800 IU vitamin D3 (placebo; $n = 59$); or calcium, vitamin D3, and Genistein aglycone (54 mg/day; genistein; $n = 62$). According to the femoral neck T-scores, 31.3% of the genistein and 30.9% of the placebo recipients were osteoporotic at baseline. In the placebo and genistein groups, the 10-year hip fracture probability risk assessed by Fracture Risk Assessment tool (FRAX) was 4.1 ± 1.9 (SD) and 4.2 ± 2.1 (SD), respectively. Mean bone mineral density (BMD) at the femoral neck increased from 0.62 g/cm^2 at baseline to 0.68 g/cm^2 at 1 year and 0.70 g/cm^2 at 2 years in genistein recipients, and decreased from 0.61 g/cm^2 at baseline to 0.60 g/cm^2 at 1 year and 0.57 g/cm^2 at 2 years in placebo recipients. At the end of the study only 18 postmenopausal women had osteoporosis in the genistein group with a prevalence of 12%, whereas in the placebo group the number of postmenopausal women with osteoporosis was unchanged, after 24 months. This post-hoc analysis is a proof-of concept study suggesting that genistein may be useful not only in postmenopausal osteopenia but also in osteoporosis. However, this proof-of concept study needs to be confirmed by a large, well designed, and appropriately focused randomized clinical trial in a population at high risk of fractures.

Keywords: bone mineral density; genistein; postemenopausal osteoporosis

1. Introduction

Estrogen deficiency is a major cause of osteoporosis worldwide. Hormone Replacement Therapy (HRT) increases the bone mineral density (BMD) and decreases the fracture risk, but the adverse effects limit its use in a large cohort of subjects [1–3]. In the last few years, many researchers have focused their attention on natural alternatives to HRT, such as phytoestrogen. Epidemiological data indicate that women consuming high amounts of phytoestrogens, in the form of soy-derived dietary products, have less menopausal symptoms than those on Western diets, and consequently, it was assumed that bone mineral density may be favorably influenced by phytoestrogens [4,5]. A major phytoestrogen is genistein, which prevents bone mass loss and improves quality of life without the harmful estrogenic activity on reproductive tissues, or genotoxic effects in postmenopausal women, at least at the dose of 54 mg/day [6–12]. We have studied the effects of pure genistein (in its aglycone form) on BMD and bone metabolism in a large cohort of postmenopausal women [6], showing that a long-term intake of genistein produced a positive effect on bone metabolism with no clinically significant adverse effects on the breast and uterus [7–9]. Overall, these results agree with previous intervention trials in which >40 mg/day of genistein equivalents yielded the most positive effects on bone mineral density and bone markers when compared to other trials with lower amounts of genistein [13–16]. Animal studies suggest that genistein has an antiosteoporotic activity, improving bone morphology parameters in osteoporotic ovarictomized mice [17] and preventing bone fragility in rats with glucocorticoid-induced osteoporosis [18]. To date, no data are available on osteoporotic subjects, however a re-analysis of the 389 postmenopausal women enrolled in our previous trial, evaluating the efficacy of genistein in osteopenic women, revealed that a significant number was actually osteoporotic, according to the T-score. The aim of this study was to perform a post-hoc analysis to evaluate the efficacy of genistein aglycone on bone mineral density in women with osteoporosis.

2. Materials and Methods

2.1. Design Overview, Setting, Participants

A post-hoc analysis was carried out using data from the main multicenter randomized controlled trial "Effects of the phytoestrogen genistein on bone metabolism in osteopenic postmenopausal women". The study subjects and methods are described in detail elsewhere [6–8]. The protocol is consistent with the principles of the Declaration of Helsinki, was approved by the Ethics Committee of Palermo University (RODA-12254) and the participants gave their written informed consent. The trial included 389 postmenopausal women, randomly assigned to receive the isoflavone genistein (n = 198), or placebo (n = 191). Placebo and genistein (54 mg/day) tablets were identical in appearance and taste. The purity of genistein was >98%. All patients were co-prescribed with 1000 mg calcium carbonate and 800 IU vitamin D3, in two tablets. The bone mineral density was assumed as the primary outcome. The femoral neck (FN), lumbar spine (LN), and total hip (TH) bone mineral density, were measured by Dual-Energy X-ray Absorptiometry (DXA; Hologic QDR 4500 W, Technologic Srl, Turin, Italy) at baseline and after 12 and 24 months of treatment as previously published [6–8]. In addition, the ten-year fracture probability was assessed with the Fracture Risk Assessment (FRAX) tool, as a secondary outcome.

2.2. Study Population

This primary analysis included all postmenopausal women with osteoporosis at the femoral neck. A cohort of the enrolled postmenopausal women was identified at the baseline as osteoporotic (n = 121) on the basis of their T-score on the femoral neck and were analyzed thereafter for the 24 months' treatment with either placebo (n = 59) or genistein (n = 62). Data from postmenopausal women with osteopenia are also shown to assess whether these patients had similar beneficial effects on BMD and incidence of adverse events.

2.3. Assessment of Fracture Risk

The ten-year fracture probability was assessed with the FRAX tool (version 2.0; University of Sheffield, South Yorkshire, England) in osteoporotic and osteopenic patients. FRAX is a computer-based algorithm [19] that provides models for the assessment of fracture probability in men and women. In this analysis, FN BMD was included since fracture risk prediction is enhanced with the input of BMD.

The probability of fracture is calculated in women according to age, body mass index, and dichotomized risk variables that comprise: a prior fragility fracture, parental history of hip fracture, current tobacco smoking, ever long-term use of oral glucocorticoids, rheumatoid arthritis, other causes of secondary osteoporosis, and alcohol consumption of three or more units daily [20].

2.4. Statistical Analysis

Descriptive statistical analyses were performed to evaluate basal demographic and clinical characteristics. All results were expressed as mean with standard deviation (SD) for continuous variables, and absolute and percentage frequencies for categorical variables. All variables were evaluated at basal time and after 12 and 24 months of treatment and absolute values were evaluated in both genistein and placebo patients to verify differences between the groups. The primary efficacy data on BMD were analyzed as already described [6–8]. The significance of differences in mean values between placebo and genistein groups at year 1 and 2 was assessed by two-way analysis of variance (2-way ANOVA). A *p* value of 0.05 or less was considered statistically significant and 95% confidence intervals were calculated wherever possible. Statistical analysis was performed by using SAS software, version 9.1 (SAS Institute, Inc., Cary, NC, USA).

3. Results

Of the 389 postmenopausal women who were enrolled in the main study, 121 (31.1%) were osteoporotic and were included in this analysis. The baseline characteristics of the osteoporotic and osteopenic women are shown in Table 1. The number of osteoporotic women was similar in both groups: 59 (30.9%) in the placebo group and 62 (31.3%) in the genistein group.

Table 1. Baseline characteristics of postmenopausal women with osteoporosis and osteopenia in both groups.

Variable	Osteoporotic		Osteopenic	
	Placebo (59)	Genistein (62)	Placebo (132)	Genistein (136)
Mean age (SD), year	54.3 (2.4)	54.5 (2.9)	54.6 (2.7)	54.8 (2.2)
Mean body mass index (SD), Kg/m^2	25.2 (3.0)	25.5 (2.8)	25.4 (3.9)	24.8 (3.7)
Mean time since menopause (SD), m	69.4 (44.7)	68.3 (39.2)	69.1 (35.9)	66.4 (38.3)
Mean BMD Femoral neck (SD), g/cm^2	0.61 (0.07)	0.62 (0.05)	0.79 (0.04)	0.78 (0.05)
Mean BMD Lumbar Spine (SD), g/cm^2	0.81 (0.10)	0.82 (0.08)	0.85 (0.10	0.85 (0.08)
Mean BMD Total hip (SD), g/cm^2	0.72 (0.08)	0.73 (0.06)	0.93 (0.04)	0.92 (0.05)
B-ALP (µg/L)	10.8 (1.79)	10.0 (2.21)	10.0 (1.87)	10.6 (2.09)
D-Pyr (pmol/µmol of urinary creatinine)	22.0 (6.92)	22.7 (7.86)	20.6 (5.19)	21.2 (3.97)
FRAX index				
Major fractures (SD)	6.5 (2.8)	6.6 (2.4)	3.3 (0.5)	3.4 (0.5)
Femur fractures (SD)	4.1 (1.9)	4.2 (2.1)	0.7 (0.1)	0.7 (0.1)

BMD: Mean bone mineral density.

Mean bone mineral density (BMD) at the femoral neck increased from 0.62 g/cm^2 ± 0.05 (SD) at baseline to 0.68 g/cm^2 ± 0.06 (SD) at 1 year and to 0.70 g/cm^2 ± 0.07 (SD) at 2 years in the genistein recipients. Conversely, in the placebo group, BMD decreased from 0.61 g/cm^2 ± 0.07 (SD) at baseline to 0.60 g/cm^2 ± 0.06 (SD) at 1 year and to 0.57 g/cm^2 ± 0.07 (SD) at 2 years. Over time the BMD significantly improved in the genistein group compared to the placebo group (*p* = 0.0046).

Moreover, a significant time effect ($p = 0.0068$) and treatment-time interaction ($p = 0.0073$) were also observed. Similar trends, on bone mineral density at the femoral neck, were observed in osteopenic patients when considering treatment ($p = 0.0130$) and treatment-time interaction ($p = 0.0241$), while no significance was found for the time effect ($p = 0.4929$) (Figure 1). In genistein-treated osteoporotic patients, a significant increase of BMD at the lumbar spine (from 0.82 ± 0.08 at baseline to 0.85 ± 0.09 at 1 year and to 0.88 ± 0.08 at 2 years) and total hip (from 0.73 ± 0.06 at baseline to 0.80 ± 0.07 at 1 year and to 0.82 ± 0.08 at 2 years) was observed.

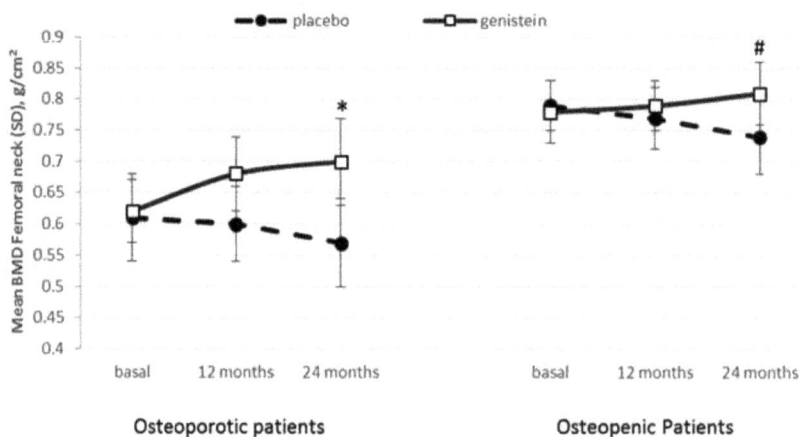

Figure 1. Femoral Neck Bone mineral density changes in absolute values over time in placebo and genistein group. (**left**) Femoral neck Bone Mineral Density changes in osteoporotic postmenopausal women groups; (**right**) Femoral neck Bone Mineral Density changes in osteopenic postmenopausal women groups. 2-way ANOVA: Over time, genistein vs. placebo: * Treatment $p = 0.0046$; # Treatment $p = 0.0130$; * Time $p = 0.0068$; # Time $p = 0.4929$; * Interaction $p = 0.0073$; # Interaction $p = 0.0241$.

Treatment also affected the bone turnover rate. Indeed, in genistein-treated osteoporotic women, B-ALP increased from 10.0 ± 2.2 at baseline to 13.8 ± 2.3 after 1 year and to 14.6 ± 2.2 at 2 years, while no differences were observed in the placebo group (basal: 10.8 ± 1.8; 1 year 10.3 ± 1.6; 2 year 10.4 ± 1.6).

Over time a significant treatment effect ($p < 0.01$), time effect ($p < 0.01$), and treatment-time interaction ($p < 0.01$) were observed using the 2-way ANOVA. Similar results were observed in osteopenic women. D-Pyr excretion in osteoporotic patients was affected only by time ($p = 0.002$).

According to the World Health Organization (WHO) classification criteria, at baseline, the number of postmenopausal women with osteoporosis was 62 in the genistein group and 59 in the placebo group. At the end of the study only 18 (29%) genistein-treated subjects were osteoporotic, while no changes were observed in the placebo group.

Gastrointestinal side effects were the most common reason for dropout, possibly because of the presence of calcium. There were no significant changes in routine biochemistry, liver function, or hematology results. The daily administration of 54 mg of genistein did not cause any significant change in the endometrial thickness.

4. Discussion

In a cohort of postmenopausal osteoporotic subjects, we confirmed the protective effects of genistein treatment on bone loss, as previously observed in osteopenic women. Postmenopausal osteoporosis significantly increases the risk of fractures and requires adequate prevention and appropriate medical treatment [21]. Since the lack of estrogen is the main etiopathogenetic element of postmenopausal bone loss, as a result, estrogen replacement therapy represents an established treatment for the prevention of osteoporosis [22]. However, the possibility of side-effects related to the estrogenic treatment requires therapeutic alternatives [23].

We previously showed that a daily administration of genistein aglycone produced a net gain in bone mass after 2 years of therapy in postmenopausal women with low bone mineral density and low fracture risk [6,7]. Although BMD and the bone markers previously assessed in our clinical trial are considered good surrogates of bone strength and bone quality, they may not correlate perfectly with a reduction in fracture risk. Fracture risk can be assessed more accurately by considering more variables than BMD alone, by using the FRAX tool. In this post-hoc analysis, our population had a medium-high fracture risk according to the FRAX scores; in fact, at baseline a 10-year fracture probability at the femur was 4.1 (1.9) in the placebo group and 4.2 (2.1) in the genistein group. This post-hoc comparison was made between the two treatment groups, showing for the first time that genistein aglycone (54 mg/day) plus calcium and vitamin D3 compared to only calcium and vitamin D3 supplementation significantly reduced the rate of osteoporosis, increasing BMD in postmenopausal women with medium-high 10-year fracture risk at the femur site. This analysis shows novel and additional findings distinct from those previously published [6–8]. More specifically, it appears that genistein has possible implications for the reduction of fracture risk in postmenopausal women with osteoporosis.

We believe that these data are particularly intriguing: in fact, this surrogate result on fractures overcomes one of the main limitations of our previous study, which was the lack of data on this major outcome. Additionally, the possibility to include, through the FRAX calculation, different risk factors in every patient enrolled in our clinical trial represents a strong advantage in terms of analysis for therapeutic efficacy.

Women enrolled in the parent trial were osteopenic rather than osteoporotic and this might represent a limitation for the current analysis; nevertheless, our study [6] remains, to date, the largest double-blind, placebo-controlled trial on genistein aglycone in the literature. To fill this gap, additional trials involving osteoporotic women are needed to further confirm the present results.

5. Conclusions

In conclusion, genistein plus calcium and vitamin D3 treatment demonstrated similar effects in terms of BMD increase at the femur versus placebo over 2 years in the subgroup of patients with osteoporosis. Collectively, these data confirm the positive and unique role of genistein aglycone, suggesting that it may be the most active isoflavone for treating postmenopausal bone loss, with a time-dependent effect, and suggesting that a long-term intake of genistein produces ongoing effects on bone health. This post-hoc analysis represents a proof-of concept study: it points out that genistein may counteract osteoporosis in postmenopausal women. However, this proof-of concept study needs to be confirmed by a large, well designed, and appropriately focused randomized clinical trial in a population at high risk of fractures. Currently, a clinical trial is investigating the effects of genistein on the fracture rate in glucocorticoid-induced osteoporosis and the final results are expected to be released in late 2018. These results will definitely clarify whether genistein may be useful not only in osteopenia but also in osteoporosis.

Acknowledgments: The authors are thankful to Bruce Burnett for his support in performing the analysis. Funding sources: Grant of the Italian Ministry of Education, University and Research, Code: 20073XZSR3; liberal donation from Primus Pharmaceuticals, Inc., Scottsdale, AZ, USA.

Author Contributions: V.A., M.A., F.S. and A.B. conceived and designed the experiments; M.A., R.D., H.M., D.S., L.M., S.M., D.A. performed the experiments; V.A., M.A., F.S. and A.B. analyzed the data; F.S., R.D., H.M., D.S., L.M., S.M., D.A. contributed reagents/materials/analysis tools; V.A., M.A., F.S., A.B. wrote the paper. All authors approved the final version of the manuscript.

Conflicts of Interest: The authors declare no conflict of interest.

References

1. Writing Group for the Women's Health Initiative Investigators. Risks and benefits of estrogen plus progestin in healthy postmenopausal women: Principal results from the Women's Health Initiative randomized controlled trial. *JAMA* **2002**, *288*, 321–333.
2. Collaborative group on Hormonal Factors in Breast Cancer. Breast Cancer and hormone replacement therapy: Collaborative reanalysis of data from 51 epidemiological studies of 52,705 women with breast cancer and 108,411 women without breast cancer. *Lancet* **1997**, *350*, 1047–1059.
3. Beral, V.; Million Women Study Collaborators. Breast cancer and hormone replacement therapy in the Million Women Study. *Lancet* **2003**, *362*, 419–427. [CrossRef]
4. Adlecreutz, H.L.; Mazur, W. Phyto-estrogen and western disease. *Ann. Med.* **1997**, *29*, 95–120. [CrossRef]
5. Horiuchi, T.; Onouchi, T.; Takahashi, M.; Ito, H.; Orimo, H. Effect of soy protein on bone metabolism in postmenopausal Japanese women. *Osteoporos. Int.* **2000**, *11*, 721–724. [CrossRef] [PubMed]
6. Marini, H.; Minutoli, L.; Polito, F.; Bitto, A.; Altavilla, D.; Atteritano, M.; Gaudio, A.; Mazzaferro, S.; Frisina, A.; Frisina, N.; et al. Effects of the phytoestrogen genistein on bone metabolism in osteopenic postmenopausal women: A randomized trial. *Ann. Intern. Med.* **2007**, *146*, 839–847. [CrossRef] [PubMed]
7. Marini, H.; Minutoli, L.; Polito, F.; Bitto, A.; Altavilla, D.; Atteritano, M.; Gaudio, A.; Mazzaferro, S.; Frisina, A.; Frisina, N.; et al. OPG and sRANKL serum concentrations in osteopenic, postmenopausal women after 2-year genistein administration. *J. Bone Miner. Res.* **2008**, *23*, 715–720. [CrossRef] [PubMed]
8. Marini, H.; Bitto, A.; Altavilla, D.; Burnett, B.P.; Polito, F.; Di Stefano, V.; Minutoli, L.; Atteritano, M.; Levy, R.M.; D'Anna, R.; et al. Breast safety and efficacy of genistein aglycone for postmenopausal bone loss: A follow-up study. *J. Clin. Endocrinol. Metab.* **2008**, *93*, 4787–4796. [CrossRef] [PubMed]
9. Bitto, A.; Polito, F.; Squadrito, F.; Marini, H.; D'Anna, R.; Irrera, N.; Minutoli, L.; Granese, R.; Altavilla, D. Genistein Aglycone: A Dual Mode of Action Anti-Osteoporotic Soy Isoflavone Rebalancing Bone Turnover Towards Bone Formation. *Curr. Med. Chem.* **2010**, *27*, 3007–3018. [CrossRef]
10. Atteritano, M.; Mazzaferro, S.; Frisina, A.; Cannata, M.L.; Bitto, A.; D'Anna, R.; Squadrito, F.; Macrì, I.; Frisina, N.; Buemi, M. Genistein effects on quantitative ultrasound parameters and bone mineral density in osteopenic postmenopausal women. *Osteoporos. Int.* **2009**, *20*, 1947–1954. [CrossRef] [PubMed]
11. Atteritano, M.; Mazzaferro, S.; Bitto, A.; Cannata, M.L.; D'Anna, R.; Squadrito, F.; Macrì, I.; Frisina, A.; Frisina, N.; Bagnato, G. Genistein effects on quality of life and depression symptoms in osteopenic postmenopausal women: A 2-year randomized, double-blind, controlled study. *Osteoporos. Int.* **2014**, *25*, 1123–1129. [CrossRef] [PubMed]
12. Atteritano, M.; Pernice, F.; Mazzaferro, S.; Mantuano, S.; Frisina, A.; D'Anna, R.; Cannata, M.L.; Bitto, A.; Squadrito, F.; Frisina, N.; et al. Effects of phytoestrogen genistein on cytogenetic biomarkers in postmenopausal women: 1 year randomized, placebo-controlled study. *Eur. J. Pharmacol.* **2008**, *28*, 22–26. [CrossRef] [PubMed]
13. Harkness, L.S.; Fiedler, K.; Sehgal, A.R.; Oravec, D.; Lerner, E. Decreased bone resorption with soy isoflavone supplementation in postmenopausal women. *J. Womens Health* **2004**, *13*, 1000–1007. [CrossRef] [PubMed]
14. Kreijkamp-Kaspers, S.; Kok, L.; Grobbee, D.E.; de Haan, E.H.; Aleman, A.; Lampe, J.W.; van der Schouw, Y.T. Effect of soy protein containing isoflavones on cognitive function, bone mineral density, and plasma lipids in postmenopausal women: A randomized controlled trial. *JAMA* **2004**, *292*, 65–74. [CrossRef] [PubMed]
15. Lydeking-Olsen, E.; Beck-Jensen, J.E.; Setchell, K.D.; Holm-Jensen, T. Soymilk or progesterone for prevention of bone loss—A 2 years randomized, placebo-controlled trial. *Eur. J. Nutr.* **2004**, *43*, 246–257. [CrossRef] [PubMed]
16. Newton, K.M.; LaCroix, A.Z.; Levy, L.; Li, S.S.; Qu, P.; Potter, J.D.; Lampe, J.W. Soy protein and bone mineral density in older men and women: A randomized trial. *Maturitas* **2006**, *55*, 270–277. [CrossRef] [PubMed]
17. Sehmisch, S.; Uffenorde, J.; Maehlmeyer, S.; Tezval, M.; Jarry, H.; Stuermer, K.M.; Stuermer, E.K. Evaluation of bone quality and quantity in osteoporotic mice—The effects of genistein and equol. *Phytomedicine* **2010**, *17*, 424–430. [CrossRef] [PubMed]
18. Bitto, A.; Burnett, B.P.; Polito, F.; Levy, R.M.; Marini, H.; Di Stefano, V.; Irrera, N.; Armbruster, M.A.; Minutoli, L.; Altavilla, D.; et al. Genistein aglycone reverses glucocorticoid-induced osteoporosis and increases bone breaking strength in rats: A comparative study with alendronate. *Br. J. Pharmacol.* **2009**, *156*, 1287–1295. [CrossRef] [PubMed]

19. FRAX. Fracture Risk Assessment Tool. Available online: http://www.shef.ac.uk/FRAX (accessed on 7–11 March 2016).
20. Kanis, J.A.; Johnell, O.; Oden, A.; Johansson, H.; McCloskey, E. FRAX and the assessment of fracture probability in men and women from the UK. *Osteoporos. Int.* **2008**, *19*, 385–397. [CrossRef] [PubMed]
21. Kanis, J.A.; Burlet, N.; Cooper, C. European Society for Clinical and Economic Aspects of Osteoporosis and Osteoarthritis (ESCEO) European guidance for the diagnosis and management of osteoporosis in postmenopausal women. *Osteoporos. Int.* **2008**, *19*, 399–428. [CrossRef] [PubMed]
22. Kanis, J.A.; Johnell, O. Requirements for DXA for the management of osteoporosis in Europe. *Osteoporos. Int.* **2005**, *16*, 229–238. [CrossRef] [PubMed]
23. Palacios, S. Advances in hormone replacement therapy: Making the menopause manageable. *BMC Womens Health* **2008**, *8*, 22. [CrossRef] [PubMed]

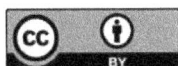

nutrients

Article

Maternal Consumption of Hesperidin and Naringin Flavanones Exerts Transient Effects to Tibia Bone Structure in Female CD-1 Offspring

Sandra M. Sacco [1,2], Caitlin Saint [2,3], Paul J. LeBlanc [2,3] and Wendy E. Ward [1,2,3,*]

[1] Department of Kinesiology, Faculty of Applied Health Sciences, Brock University, St. Catharines, ON L2S 3A1, Canada; ssacco@brocku.ca
[2] Centre for Bone and Muscle Health, Brock University, St. Catharines, ON L2S 3A1, Canada; caitlinsaint@trentu.ca (C.S.); pleblanc@brocku.ca (P.J.L.)
[3] Department of Health Sciences, Faculty of Applied Health Sciences, Brock University, St. Catharines, ON L2S 3A1, Canada
*   Correspondence: wward@brocku.ca; Tel.: +1-905-688-5550 (ext. 3024)

Received: 24 January 2017; Accepted: 3 March 2017; Published: 8 March 2017

Abstract: Hesperidin (HSP) and naringin (NAR), flavanones rich in citrus fruits, support skeletal integrity in adult and aging rodent models. This study determined whether maternal consumption of HSP and NAR favorably programs bone development, resulting in higher bone mineral density (BMD) and greater structure and biomechanical strength (i.e., peak load) in female offspring. Female CD-1 mice were fed a control diet or a HSP + NAR diet five weeks before pregnancy and throughout pregnancy and lactation. At weaning, female offspring were fed a control diet until six months of age. The structure and BMD of the proximal tibia were measured longitudinally using in vivo micro-computed tomography at 2, 4, and 6 months of age. The trabecular bone structure at two and four months and the trabecular BMD at four months were compromised at the proximal tibia in mice exposed to HSP and NAR compared to the control diet ($p < 0.001$). At six months of age, these differences in trabecular structure and BMD at the proximal tibia had disappeared. At 6 months of age, the tibia midpoint peak load, BMD, structure, and the peak load of lumbar vertebrae and femurs were similar ($p > 0.05$) between the HSP + NAR and control groups. In conclusion, maternal consumption of HSP and NAR does not enhance bone development in female CD-1 offspring.

Keywords: bone development; flavanones; hesperidin; mice; naringin; structure

---

1. Introduction

Bioactives, naturally present in foods, may provide a dietary strategy to support healthy bone development. In a developing mouse model, exposure to soy isoflavones during early postnatal life, but not maternal exposure, sets a trajectory for higher bone mineral density (BMD), improved bone structure, and greater bone strength in female offspring at adulthood [1–4]. Other bioactives such as citrus flavanones (i.e., hesperidin (HSP) and naringin (NAR)) have been shown to exert bone-sparing effects in adult and aging rodents [5–11], but whether maternal consumption of citrus flavanones during pregnancy and lactation changes the trajectory of bone development of offspring, resulting in stronger, healthier bones at adulthood has not been investigated. Given that the metabolites of citrus flavanones (i.e., hesperetin and naringenin) can be transferred to human offspring via mother's milk [12], it is of interest to examine whether maternal exposure to HSP and NAR programs the bone tissue in adult female mouse offspring.

HSP (hesperetin-7-rutinoside) and NAR (naringenin-7-neohesperidoside) are flavanone glycosides found in high amounts in citrus fruits. HSP is found in particularly rich amounts in oranges while

NAR is present at high levels in grapefruits [13–15]. When consumed by humans and rodents, HSP and NAR are hydrolyzed into the aglycones, hesperetin and naringenin, and metabolized mainly into glucuronide forms by intestinal and liver conjugation [9,13,14,16,17]. The conjugated and aglycone metabolites circulate the body and modulate bone cell activity; in rat primary osteoblasts, hesperetin and hesperitin-7-*O*-glucuronide, at levels that are physiologically achievable through dietary consumption, increased osteoblast differentiation [18,19], and increased the mRNA expression of bone morphogenic proteins (BMPs) [18,19], runt-related transcription factor 2 (Runx2) [19], and osterix [18,19] that promote osteoblast differentiation. In murine MC3T3-E1 osteoblast cells [20] and rat [10] and human [21] bone mesenchymal stem cells, NAR increased osteoblast differentiation and proliferation and increased the expression of BMP-2 [20], osteopontin [21], and osteocalcin [10]. No data exists on the ability for HSP, NAR, or their metabolites to epigenetically regulate the transcriptions of genes involved in bone development. However, that HSP and NAR stimulate signaling pathways implicated in stimulating bone formation provides biological plausibility for HSP and NAR to support bone development and skeletal integrity.

The majority of our knowledge on the positive effects of HSP and NAR on bone is derived from rodent models of bone loss (i.e., ovariectomy, orchidectomy) [5–8,10,11] and aging (i.e., senescence) [9]. While intake of HSP and NAR is reported to benefit bone health in male and female rodents, most research has been performed in females. These studies demonstrate that dietary HSP and NAR protect against the loss of bone mineral and the deterioration of bone structure and strength during ovariectomy [6–8,10,11]. However, one study [7] in younger (3 months old) intact female rats reported gains in femoral BMD, which agrees with other work demonstrating that HSP supports bone cell function via modulating signaling proteins and bone cell differentiation to increase bone formation [18]. However, no studies have assessed whether maternal consumption of HSP and NAR affects bone development in growing and adult offspring. Given that treatment with HSP, NAR, or their combination stimulates bone formation [10,18], supports bone mineral accrual [7], and protects against bone loss in ovariectomized [6–8,10,11] female rodents, we hypothesized that maternal consumption of HSP and NAR before and during pregnancy and throughout lactation would set a trajectory for better bone health in female offspring. Thus, the objective of the present study was to determine whether maternal consumption of HSP and NAR results in higher BMD, improved bone structure, and greater bone strength in female CD-1 offspring at adulthood.

2. Materials and Methods

2.1. Animals and Diets

The experimental protocol (AUP 14-04-01, 2014) was approved by the Animal Care Committee at Brock University, St. Catharines, ON, Canada. Five-week-old female (n = 17) and 8-week-old male (n = 8) CD-1 mice were purchased from Charles River Canada (St. Constant, QC, Canada) and housed with 4–5 mice per cage at 22 °C–24 °C, 50% humidity with a 12:12-h light:dark cycle. Female mice were randomized to the American Institute of Nutrition-93 (AIN-93G) control diet (CON, n = 9) for growth, pregnancy and lactation [22] or the CON diet supplemented with 0.5% HSP + 0.25% NAR (HSP + NAR, n = 8). These doses reflect a moderate (400 mL) to high (1 L) daily intake of orange or grapefruit juices in humans [14,17] and represent doses that have been shown to exert protection to bone health in adult and aging rodents [5–9]. The AIN-93G diet used in the present study was modified to contain alcohol-extracted casein (TD. 06706, Harlan Teklad, Mississauga, ON, Canada) to remove vitamins that are naturally-occurring in casein and that may influence bone development. HSP (H5254, Sigma Aldrich, Oakville, ON, Canada) and NAR (N1376, Sigma Aldrich, Oakville, ON, Canada) were added to the CON diet at the expense of cornstarch. All mice had free access to food and water throughout the study, and food intake was measured twice per week using an electronic scale.

2.2. Study Design

At 10 weeks of age, mice were mated harem-style by housing 2–3 females with one male. Mating pairs were maintained on the female's respective diets, and, once identified as pregnant, female mice were housed individually and remained on their respective diets during the remainder of pregnancy and throughout lactation. Offspring were weighed at post-natal day (PND) 9, PND 16, and PND 21 using an electronic scale. At weaning, female offspring were housed with five mice per cage and switched to the CON diet for the remainder of the study duration. Food intake was measured twice per week and body weights measured weekly to monitor growth.

2.3. In Vivo Analysis of Structure of Tibias by μCT

At 2, 4, and 6 months of age, mouse offspring were anesthetized using 2%–5% isoflurane dissolved in 100% oxygen, and the right tibias were scanned in vivo using micro-computed tomography scanning (μCT) (Skyscan 1176, Bruker microCT, Kontich, Belgium) and host software (1176 version 1.1, Skyscan 1176, Bruker microCT, Kontich, Belgium), as previously described [23]. Scanning of the right proximal tibia was performed using an isotropic voxel size of 9 μm^3, 1 mm aluminum filter, 40 kV tube voltage, 300 μA amperage, a rotation step of 0.8°, 3350 ms integration time, and over 180° with no frame averaging. Each scan lasted 16 min 23 s and resulted in 460 mGy exposure per scan to the scanned tibias (TN-502RD-H, Best Medical Canada, Ottawa, ON, Canada). This dose of radiation does not affect tibial bone structure when tibias are repeatedly exposed at 2, 4, and 6 months of age [23]. At 6 months of age, animals were euthanized within five days after receiving their last scan by exsanguination under anesthesia (5% isoflurane dissolved in 100% oxygen), followed by cervical dislocation. Tibias, femurs, and lumbar vertebrae (LV 1–6) were excised, cleaned of soft tissue, and then wrapped in saline soaked gauze and stored at −80 °C for future analyses.

2.4. Ex Vivo Analysis of Structure of Femurs and Lumbar Vertebrae by μCT

Right femurs and the second lumber vertebra (LV2) were scanned ex vivo using μCT scanning (Skyscan 1176, Bruker microCT, Kontich, Belgium). These sites were scanned ex vivo to minimize the level of radiation exposure to each mouse. The bones were wrapped in parafilm to retain moisture during scanning and placed axially in a foam holder. The foam holder containing the bones was then secured to a mouse bed for ex vivo scanning using a 9 μm^3 isotropic voxel size, 0.25 mm aluminum filter, voltage of 45 kVp, tube current of 545 μA, 850 ms exposure time, and 0.2° rotation step. Scans were performed over 180° without using frame averaging.

2.5. Reconstruction of In Vivo and Ex Vivo Images Obtained Using μCT

Graphics Processing Unit (GPU)-acceleration (GPUReconServer, Skyscan, Bruker microCT, Kontich, Belgium) and NRecon Reconstruction 64-bit software (Skyscan, Bruker microCT, Kontich, Belgium) were used to reconstruct scanned images. Except for variable misalignment compensations, all scanned samples within each skeletal site received the same corrections to smoothing, ring artifacts, beam hardening, and defect pixel masking. Reconstructed images were then reoriented (DataViewer software, version 1.5.0, Skyscan, Bruker microCT, Kontich, Belgium), and the transaxial images were saved.

2.6. Regions of Interest (ROI) and Segmentation of In Vivo and Ex Vivo Images Obtained Using μCT

ROIs were selected from transaxial images and saved as new datasets using CTAnalyzer software (Skyscan Bruker microCT, Kontich, Belgium). At the proximal tibia, the ROI consisted of the trabecular and cortical bone and began 0.967 mm (110 slices) away from the metaphyseal side of the growth plate and extended 0.510 mm (58 transaxial slices) towards the ankle [23]. At the femur neck, an ROI of the trabecular region was manually drawn to a few pixels away from the endocortical boundary and consisted of 1.680 mm (191 slices), starting at the distal edge of the femur head and extending towards the diaphysis of the femur. At the distal femur, the ROI of the trabecular region was manually drawn a few pixels away from the endocortical boundary and consisted of 0.879 mm (100 slices), starting 0.616 (70 slices) proximal to the metaphyseal edge of the growth plate and extending toward the femur neck. Another ROI was manually drawn around the midpoint region of the femur, rich in cortical bone, and consisted of 0.879 mm (100 slices) spanning above and below the femur midpoint. At the LV2, ROIs of the trabecular and cortical regions of the vertebral bodies were manually and consisted of 115 transverse slices (1.011 mm), spanning above and below the midpoint of LV2.

Task lists were generated and applied (CTAnalyzer software, Skyscan Bruker microCT, Kontich, Belgium) to the saved datasets to segment bone from the background and to analyze trabecular or cortical bone structure at each skeletal site. At the proximal tibia, an automated task list was generated [23] to segment the trabecular bone from the cortical bone. Trabecular and cortical bone were then segmented as previously described [23]. At the femur neck, femur midpoint, distal femur, and LV, task lists were generated to segment the trabecular and cortical bones from the background. Local thresholding was used to segment the trabecular bone from the background (femur neck: lower threshold = 74, upper threshold = 255, radius = 6, constant = 0; distal femur: lower threshold = 71, upper threshold = 255, radius = 6, constant = 0; LV: lower threshold = 80, upper threshold = 255, radius = 7, constant = 0) and global thresholding (femur: lower threshold = 124, upper threshold = 255; LV2: lower threshold = 122, upper threshold = 255) for segmenting the cortical bone from the background at the femur midpoint and LV2 [24].

The trabecular bone outcome measures determined at the proximal tibia, femur neck, distal femur, and LV included bone volume (BV, mm^3), total volume (TV, mm^3), bone volume fraction (BV/TV, %), trabecular thickness (Tb.Th, mm), trabecular number (Tb.N, mm-1), trabecular separation (Tb.Sp, mm), degree of anisotropy (DA, no unit), and connectivity density (Conn.D, 1/mm^3). Cortical bone outcome measures at the tibia, femur midpoint and LV included total cross-sectional area inside the periosteal envelope (Tt.Ar, mm^2), cortical bone area (Ct.Ar, mm^2), cortical area fraction (Ct.Ar/Tt.Ar, %), average cortical thickness (Ct.Th, mm), periosteal perimeter (Ps.Pm, mm), endocortical perimeter (Ec.Pm, mm), marrow area (Ma.Ar, mm^2), and eccentricity (no unit).

2.7. Bone Mineral Density (BMD) and Peak Load of Tibias, Femurs and LV1-3

To determine the trabecular BMD and cortical tissue mineral density (TMD) at the proximal tibia that were scanned in vivo at 2, 4, and 6 months of age, calibration phantoms consisting of 0.25 and 0.75 g/cm^3 calcium hydroxyapatite were scanned and reconstructed using the exact same parameters as all in vivo scans. BMD was then calibrated against the attenuation coefficient, and the trabecular BMD and cortical TMD at the proximal tibia were then measured against the attenuation coefficient [25]. Since measurement of BMD using μCT scanning is often not possible in excised samples due to the introduction of air bubbles from storage [25], BMD of the right femurs and LV1-3 was measured by dual energy X-ray absorptiometry (DXA) (Orthometrix, White Plains, NY, USA) and a specialized software program (Host Software version 3.9.4; Scanner Software version 1.2.0, Orthometrix, White Plains, NY, USA). Calibration of the DXA was performed daily using a calibration phantom. Femurs and LV1-3 were scanned using a resolution of 0.01 mm × 0.01 mm and at a speed of 2 mm/s. To determine bone strength at skeletal sites rich in cortical bone, the peak load at the midpoint of the right tibia and right femur was determined by 3-point bending using a Materials Testing System (Model 4442, Instron Corp., Norwood, MA, USA) and specialized software (Bluehill 2, Instron Corp., Norwood, MA, USA) [26]. The peak load at skeletal sites rich in trabecular bone was determined by compression testing at the femur neck and LV2 [26].

2.8. Statistical Analyses

All statistical analyses were performed using SPSS Statistics (version 22, IBM, Armonk, NY, USA). The effects of diet, age, and their interaction on food intake, body weight, and in vivo trabecular and cortical bone structure were determined using a repeated measures analysis of variance (ANOVA) (general linear model). Comparisons on all bone outcome measures between CON and HSP + NAR groups within each time point were assessed by unpaired two-tailed *t*-tests. A repeated measures ANOVA (general linear model) with a Bonferroni post-hoc test was used to determine longitudinal changes within the trabecular and cortical bone structural outcomes within each group. The primary outcome included BV/TV at the proximal tibia, with a total of seven mice per treatment group required to achieve a power of 0.8 and an alpha of 0.5. Missing values that resulted from mouse leg movement during the scan or due to computer error were replaced with the series mean. This occurred a total of four times (once in the CON group at 2 months of age, twice in the CON group at 4 months of age, and once in the HSP + NAR group at 4 months of age). Results are expressed as mean ± standard error of the mean (SEM) and the significance level was set at $p < 0.05$.

3. Results

3.1. Food Intake and Body Weight

Litter sizes (CON = 14 ± 2 pups/L, HSP + NAR= 13 ± 2 pups/L) were similar between the CON and HSP + NAR groups ($p > 0.05$). In addition, no differences ($p > 0.05$) in litter weight at PND9 (CON = 83 ± 10 g, HSP + NAR = 82 ± 6 g), PND16 (CON = 118 ± 10 g, HSP + NAR = 118 ± 5 g), or at weaning (PND21, CON = 162 ± 17 g, HSP + NAR = 160 ± 13 g) were observed between the groups. These results demonstrate that maternal consumption of HSP + NAR does not affect the growth patterns of female CD-1 offspring during suckling.

After weaning, an effect of time was observed for the mean daily food intake ($p < 0.01$) (Figure 1A) and weekly body weight ($p < 0.001$) (Figure 1B), which was expected because the mice were growing. There was no diet or time x diet effect on daily food intake or body weight throughout the study ($p > 0.05$). At the end of the study, the final body weights in 6-month-old offspring did not differ between CON and HSP + NAR groups. Thus, the food intake or growth characteristics of female offspring from weaning until six months of age were not affected by maternal and suckling exposure to HSP + NAR.

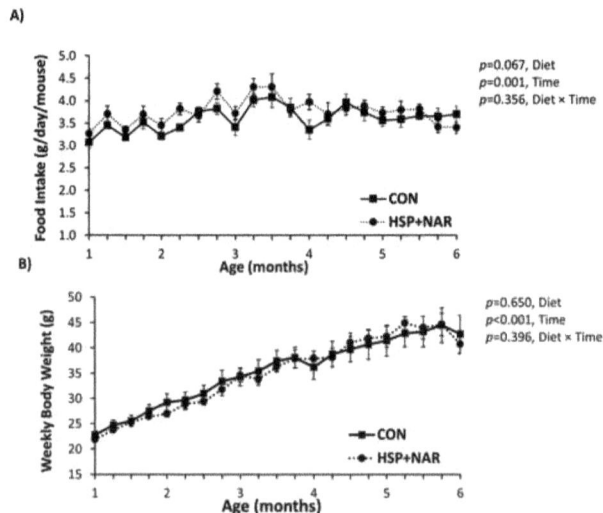

Figure 1. Mean daily food intake (**A**) and body weight (**B**) of female mice whose mothers were fed a control diet (CON) or a diet consisting of a combination of 0.5% hesperidin (HSP) and 0.25% naringin (NAR) before and during pregnancy and lactation, *n* = 8–9 per group. Mean ± standard error of the mean (SEM).

3.2. In Vivo Measurements of Trabecular and Cortical Bone Mineral Density (BMD) and Bone Structure at the Proximal Tibia

At the proximal tibia, a significant effect of diet ($p < 0.05$) was observed for several trabecular structural outcomes, whereby HSP + NAR resulted in lower BV, BV/TV, Tb.N, and Conn.D and higher Tb.Sp compared to CON at both 2 and 4 months of age (Table 1, Figure 2). A significant interaction between diet and time ($p < 0.05$) was observed for BMD and Tb.Sp, whereby HSP + NAR resulted in lower BMD at 4 months of age and higher Tb.Sp at 2 and 4 months of age compared to the CON group. No effects of diet on the trabecular bone structure at the proximal tibia was observed at 6 months of age. Thus, maternal consumption of HSP + NAR during pregnancy and lactation compromises trabecular BMD and bone structure at the proximal tibia in developing female CD-1 offspring; however, this effect does not persist into adulthood. In addition to an effect of diet, an effect of time ($p < 0.001$) was observed, whereby offspring from both the CON and HSP + NAR groups experienced a decrease in TV, BV, BV/TV, Tb.N, and Conn.D and an increase in Tb.Th and Tb.Sp from 2 to 4 months of age (Table 1, Figure 2). Similar to these changes, trabecular BMD from HSP + NAR exposure decreased from 2 to 4 months of age, while BMD decreased in the CON group after 4 months of age ($p < 0.001$). Diminutions in BV, BV/TV, Tb.N, and Conn.D within the CON group persisted to 6 months of age, resulting in trabecular bone structural outcomes that were significantly lower compared to both the 2- and 4-month time points ($p < 0.05$). In the HSP + NAR group, changes in trabecular BMD and bone structure were maintained from 4 to 6 months of age. Thus, female CD-1 offspring achieve peak trabecular BMD and bone structure before 4 months of age, a finding that agrees with previous work [23].

With regards to the cortical bone structure at the proximal tibia, Ct.Ar was significantly lower ($p < 0.05$) in the HSP + NAR group compared to the CON group at 4 months of age (Table 1, Figure 2). In addition, a time x diet effect was observed ($p < 0.05$) for Ps.Pm at the proximal tibia, whereby HSP + NAR resulted in lower Ps.Pm at 2 months of age compared to CON ($p < 0.05$). However, this effect was not apparent at 4 and 6 months of age. No effects ($p > 0.05$) from HSP + NAR exposure on cortical TMD were observed. Thus, maternal exposure during pregnancy and lactation to a combined 0.5% HSP and 0.25% NAR diet delays some characteristics of cortical bone development in female CD-1 offspring. In addition to an effect of diet on cortical bone structure, an effect of time ($p < 0.001$) was observed, whereby augments to the cortical bone TMD and structure, including Ct.Ar, Ct.Ar/Tt.Ar, and Ct.Th, were observed from 2 to 6 months of age in the CON and HSP + NAR groups (Table 1, Figure 2). In addition, diminution of Tt.Ar, Ec.Pm, and Ma.Ar were observed in both groups. These findings agree with our previous work showing that cortical bone structure reaches its peak at a later time point compared to trabecular bone in female CD-1 mice [23].

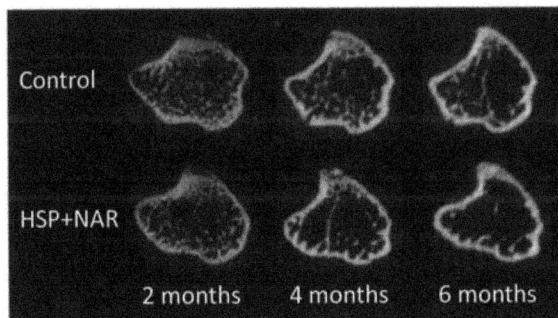

Figure 2. Representative grayscale transaxial images of right proximal tibias of female CD-1 mouse offspring at 2, 4, and 6 months of age.

Table 1. Bone mineral density (BMD) and structure at the proximal tibia at 2, 4, and 6 months of age in female CD-1 mice whose mothers were exposed to control (CON) or 0.5% hesperidin (HSP) and 0.25% naringin (NAR) diets through pregnancy and lactation.

Outcomes	CON			HSP + NAR			p Value		
	Age (Months)			Age (Months)					
	2	4	6	2	4	6	Time	Diet	Time × Diet
Trabecular Structure									
BMD (g/cm³)	0.212 ± 0.007 [a]	0.198 ± 0.003 [a]	0.154 ± 0.006 [b]	0.190 ± 0.010 [a]	0.162 ± 0.008 [t,b]	0.142 ± 0.008 [b]	<0.001	0.007	0.015
TV (mm³)	1.185 ± 0.064 [a]	0.936 ± 0.045 [b]	0.898 ± 0.046 [b]	1.022 ± 0.065 [a]	0.853 ± 0.052 [b]	0.831 ± 0.058 [b]	<0.001	0.184	0.151
BV (mm³)	0.097 ± 0.010 [a]	0.050 ± 0.006 [b]	0.025 ± 0.004 [c]	0.061 ± 0.009 [t,a]	0.029 ± 0.005 [t,b]	0.017 ± 0.004 [b]	<0.001	0.013	0.099
BV/TV (%)	8.177 ± 0.645 [a]	5.282 ± 0.464 [b]	2.764 ± 0.298 [c]	5.782 ± 0.698 [t,a]	3.260 ± 0.434 [t,b]	2.018 ± 0.526 [b]	<0.001	0.011	0.161
Tb.Th (mm)	0.059 ± 0.001 [b]	0.070 ± 0.001 [a]	0.073 ± 0.001 [a]	0.059 ± 0.001 [b]	0.068 ± 0.002 [a]	0.069 ± 0.002 [a]	<0.001	0.243	0.406
Tb.N (1/mm)	1.386 ± 0.105 [a]	0.751 ± 0.058 [b]	0.379 ± 0.42 [c]	0.976 ± 0.104 [t,a]	0.479 ± 0.063 [t,b]	0.284 ± 0.071 [b]	<0.001	0.009	0.094
Tb.Sp (mm)	0.297 ± 0.010 [c]	0.386 ± 0.003 [b]	0.429 ± 0.006 [a]	0.350 ± 0.015 [t,b]	0.430 ± 0.008 [t,a]	0.445 ± 0.006 [a]	<0.001	0.002	0.004
DA (no unit)	2.334 ± 0.095 [a]	1.970 ± 0.072 [b]	2.150 ± 0.116 [a,b]	2.562 ± 0.087	2.212 ± 0.126	2.962 ± 0.401	<0.001	0.030	0.305
Conn.D (1/mm³)	46.6 ± 4.7 [a]	20.0 ± 2.1 [b]	7.9 ± 1.8 [c]	30.1 ± 2.1 [t,a]	11.3 ± 3.1 [t,b]	8.5 ± 2.3 [b]	<0.001	0.004	0.051
Cortical Structure									
TMD (g/cm³)	0.802 ± 0.007 [c]	0.941 ± 0.112 [b]	0.996 ± 0.010 [a]	0.810 ± 0.007 [c]	0.932 ± 0.004 [b]	0.995 ± 0.007 [a]	<0.001	0.969	0.298
Ct.Ar (mm²)	1.295 ± 0.041 [b]	1.396 ± 0.025 [a,b]	1.456 ± 0.021 [a]	1.230 ± 0.035 [b]	1.299 ± 0.037 [t,a]	1.367 ± 0.049 [a]	<0.001	0.061	0.798
Tt.Ar (mm²)	3.951 ± 0.127 [a]	3.493 ± 0.104 [b]	3.517 ± 0.107 [b]	3.544 ± 0.158 [a]	3.236 ± 0.137 [b]	3.284 ± 0.159 [b]	<0.001	0.119	0.085
Ct.Ar/Tt.Ar (%)	33.1 ± 1.6 [b]	40.2 ± 1.1 [a]	41.6 ± 1.1 [a]	35.0 ± 1.0 [b]	40.4 ± 0.9 [a]	41.9 ± 1.2 [a]	<0.001	0.634	0.384
Ct.Th (mm)	0.110 ± 0.005 [c]	0.164 ± 0.005 [b]	0.187 ± 0.004 [a]	0.120 ± 0.004 [c]	0.167 ± 0.005 [b]	0.185 ± 0.003 [a]	<0.001	0.492	0.139
Ps.Pm (mm)	8.231 ± 0.123 [a]	7.851 ± 0.104 [b]	7.939 ± 0.097 [b]	7.780 ± 0.169 [t]	7.609 ± 0.159	7.731 ± 0.179	<0.001	0.135	0.046
Ec.Pm (mm)	6.535 ± 0.178 [a]	5.804 ± 0.153 [b]	5.724 ± 0.154 [b]	6.005 ± 0.193 [a]	5.457 ± 0.184 [b]	5.440 ± 0.214 [b]	<0.001	0.134	0.231
Ma.Ar (mm²)	2.656 ± 0.139 [a]	2.097 ± 0.097 [b]	2.061 ± 0.099 [b]	2.314 ± 0.131 [a]	1.937 ± 0.106 [b]	1.917 ± 0.125 [b]	<0.001	0.196	0.116
Ecc (no unit)	0.459 ± 0.032 [a,b]	0.370 ± 0.026 [b]	0.426 ± 0.021 [a]	0.459 ± 0.028	0.458 ± 0.034	0.502 ± 0.034	0.041	0.054	0.452

[t] denotes significantly different ($p < 0.05$) compared to CON within the same month. Different letters in a row denote statistical significance ($p < 0.05$) within a group over time by repeated measures analysis of variance (ANOVA). Data are expressed as mean ± standard error of the mean (SEM), $n = 8$–9/group. BV = bone volume, BV/TV = bone volume fraction, Conn.D = connectivity density, Ct.Ar = cortical bone area, Ct.Ar/Tt.Ar = cortical area fraction, Ct.Th = cortical thickness, DA = degree of anisotropy, Ecc = mean eccentricity, Ec.Pm = endocortical perimeter, Ma.Ar = marrow area, Ps.Pm = periosteal perimeter, Tb.Th = trabecular thickness, Tb.N = trabecular number, Tb.Sp = trabecular separation, TMD = tissue mineral density, Tt.Ar = total cross sectional area inside the periosteal envelope, and TV = total volume.

3.3. Ex Vivo Measurements of Trabecular and Cortical Bone Structure

At the femur neck, there were no significant differences between the CON and HSP + NAR groups for BV/TV, Tb.Th, Tb.N, and Tb.Sp (Table 2, Figure 3A). Other trabecular parameters including BV, TV, Conn.D, and DA did not differ between groups. In addition, no differences in trabecular bone properties ($p > 0.05$) were observed at the distal metaphyseal region of the femur (Table 2). At the femur midpoint, there were no differences in cortical bone properties including Ct.Ar and Ct.Th (Table 2, Figure 3A), as well as Tt.Ar, Ct.Ar/Tt.Ar, Ps.Pm, Ec.Pm, Ma.Ar, or Ecc between the CON and HSP + NAR groups.

Table 2. Ex vivo bone mineral density (BMD), structure and peak load of the femur in 6-month-old female mice whose mothers were exposed to control (CON) or 0.5% hesperidin (HSP) + 0.25% naringin (NAR) diets through pregnancy and lactation.

	CON	HSP + NAR	*p* Value
Femur BMD (g/cm^2)	0.092 ± 0.002	0.090 ± 0.003	0.427
Femur Neck Trabecular Structure			
BV/TV (%)	15.6 ± 0.7	15.0 ± 0.9	0.621
Tb.Th (mm)	0.098 ± 0.002	0.099 ± 0.002	0.835
Tb.N (1/mm)	1.591 ± 0.083	1.523 ± 0.102	0.610
Tb.Sp (mm)	0.426 ± 0.014	0.440 ± 0.013	0.462
Femur Midpoint Cortical Structure			
Ct.Ar (mm^2)	1.312 ± 0.034	1.181 ± 0.076	0.101
Ct.Th (mm)	0.264 ± 0.009	0.252 ± 0.010	0.422
Distal Femur Trabecular Structure			
BV/TV (%)	11.0 ± 0.9	10.8 ± 2.8	0.932
Tb.Th (mm)	0.081 ± 0.002	0.078 ± 0.005	0.520
Tb.N (1/mm)	1.361 ± 0.105	1.294 ± 0.292	0.813
Tb.Sp (mm)	0.463 ± 0.031	0.544 ± 0.069	0.324
Femur Neck Peak Load (N)	23.5 ± 1.2	24.3 ± 1.8	0.697
Midpoint Peak Load (N)	25.5 ± 1.1	25.4 ± 2.4	0.602

There were no significant differences in femur outcomes between CON and HSP + NAR groups. Data are expressed as mean $\pm$ standard error of the mean (SEM), n = 5–9/group. BV/TV = bone volume fraction, Ct.Ar = cortical bone area, Ct.Th = cortical thickness, Tb.Th = trabecular thickness, Tb.N = trabecular number, Tb.Sp = trabecular separation.

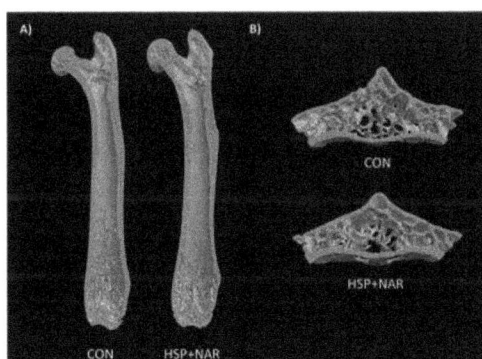

Figure 3. Representative images of the right femur (**A**) and the second lumbar vertebra (LV2) (**B**) of 6-month-old female mice whose mothers were exposed to control (CON) or 0.5% hesperidin (HSP) and 0.25% naringin (NAR) diets through pregnancy and lactation. Coronal sections consisting of the ventral half of the femur are depicted in (**A**); Transverse sections consisting of 1.011 mm of the vertebral body midsection are depicted in (**B**).

At LV2, there were no significant differences between CON and HSP + NAR with regards to BV/TV, Tb.Th, Tb.N, Tb.Sp (Table 3, Figure 3B), or other trabecular parameters. Similar to the trabecular bone, the cortical bone structural properties at LV2, including Ct.Ar and Ct.Th, were similar ($p < 0.05$) between the CON and HSP + NAR groups (Table 3). No other differences in cortical bone structure were observed between the groups. Collectively, these data indicate that maternal exposure to HSP and NAR does not result in long-term consequences to the trabecular or cortical bone structure at multiple skeletal sites in female CD-1 offspring.

Table 3. Ex vivo bone mineral density (BMD), structure and peak load of the lumbar vertebra (LV) in 6-month-old female CD-1 mice whose mothers were exposed to control (CON) or 0.5% hesperidin (HSP) + 0.25% naringin (NAR) diets through pregnancy and lactation.

	CON	HSP + NAR	*p* Value
LV1-3 BMD (g/cm^2)	0.075 ± 0.002	0.078 ± 0.004	0.490
LV2 Trabecular Structure			
BV/TV (%)	25.1 ± 1.6	22.5 ± 2.3	0.360
Tb.Th (mm)	0.081 ± 0.001	0.087 ± 0.005	0.304
Tb.N (1/mm)	3.106 ± 0.179	2.619 ± 0.228	0.110
Tb.Sp (mm)	0.296 ± 0.012	0.315 ± 0.017	0.359
LV2 Cortical Structure			
Ct.Ar (mm^2)	0.525 ± 0.013	0.523 ± 0.032	0.957
Ct.Th (mm)	0.083 ± 0.002	0.085 ± 0.005	0.706
LV2 Peak Load (N)	32.2 ± 2.7	35.8 ± 6.3	0.544

There were no significant differences in bone structure or strength between CON and HSP + NAR groups. Data are expressed as mean $\pm$ standard error of the mean (SEM), n = 5–9/group. BV/TV = bone volume fraction, Ct.Ar = cortical bone area, Ct.Th = cortical thickness, Tb.Th = trabecular thickness, Tb.N = trabecular number, Tb.Sp = trabecular separation.

3.4. Ex Vivo Measurement of Bone Mineral Density (BMD) and Peak Load

No significant differences ($p > 0.05$) in BMD at the whole femur (Table 2) or LV1-3 (Table 3) were observed between the CON and HSP + NAR groups at six months of age. The peak load at the tibia midpoint (CON = 18.1 ± 1.3 N, HSP + NAR= 18.1 ± 1.2) and at the femur midpoint, femur neck, and LV2 did not differ ($p > 0.05$) between the CON and HSP + NAR groups (Tables 2 and 3).

4. Discussion

Our data demonstrates that maternal consumption of HSP and NAR compromises trabecular structure at the proximal tibia in female CD-1 offspring at two and four months of age and trabecular BMD at four months of age; however, these differences do not persist to six months of age. At the femur and LV, the trabecular and cortical BMD and structure were not affected by dietary HSP and NAR. Moreover, the peak load was not altered by dietary HSP and NAR at the three skeletal sites measured (i.e. tibia midpoint, femur midpoint, and LV2). Thus, maternal consumption of HSP and NAR during pregnancy and lactation exerts transient effects on trabecular BMD and bone structure in female CD-1 offspring post-weaning, but these effects do not result in long-term detriments to skeletal integrity and strength at adulthood.

A novel aspect of this study included the timing of exposure to HSP and NAR. Previous studies have not investigated the effect of maternal exposure to these citrus flavanones on offspring. Thus, findings from the present study suggest that there is a critical period before and/or during pregnancy and/or lactation that transiently compromises the trabecular bone structure in female offspring. Determining which of these period(s) are critical for the effects of HSP and/or NAR on skeletal development is an area of future research interest. In addition, our findings suggest that HSP + NAR exerts differential effects on bone tissue that is dependent on the timing of exposure, as others have demonstrated that HSP, NAR, or their aglycones support bone health in mouse and rat models of adulthood, aging, or surgically- or senescent-induced bone loss [5–11]. For example, in 3-month-old female rats, a daily intake of 0.5% HSP increased femoral BMD by six months of age [7]. In ovariectomized mouse [8,11] and rat [6,7,10] models of postmenopausal bone loss, HSP, NAR or their combination protected against the deterioration of BMD, bone structure, and biomechanical strength. The protective effects of HSP and NAR on the trabecular bone have also been observed in orchidectomized mice [5] and senescent rats [9]. Collectively, these studies demonstrate that HSP, NAR, or their combination support the accrual and maintenance of BMD, bone structure, and strength in both adult and aging rodents at doses [5–9] similar to those used in the present study.

The mechanism of action is currently unknown. Studies have not investigated the effects of HSP, NAR, or their metabolites on their potential to regulate the transcription of genes involved in bone development through epigenetic mechanisms. The action of HSP and NAR on bone cell function is largely positive and attributed to their aglycone or glucuronide forms acting to increase the mRNA expression of BMP-2, BMP-4, Runx2, and osterix, which are involved in driving osteoblast differentiation and facilitating bone formation [18–20]. HSP and NAR may also decrease osteoclast activity and bone resorption [9,11]. While some literature has indicated HSP and NAR metabolites as exhibiting estrogenic properties [11,27], others have demonstrated that they do not activate estrogen receptor-alpha- (ER-alpha) or ER-beta-mediated transcription of genes [11] and that their binding affinities to estrogen receptors are low [28]. Thus, the estrogenic or anti-estrogenic potential of HSP and NAR is uncertain. Moreover, whether HSP and/or NAR metabolites can cross the placenta or be transferred to the offspring via the mother's milk in CD-1 mice is an area of future investigation. It is possible that maternal exposure to HSP and/or NAR modulates circulating levels of calciotropic hormones in the mother to result in alterations to calcium availability to the fetus in utero or to offspring during suckling; however, this remains to be determined. Further investigation is necessary to determine the mechanisms whereby HSP + NAR compromises trabecular bone structure at the proximal tibia in two- and four-month-old female offspring. Moreover, further investigation is warranted to determine whether the skeletal tissue of male offspring also responds to maternal exposure to HSP + NAR.

Among the strengths of the present study is the comprehensive assessment that was performed on BMD, structure, and strength at multiple skeletal sites. That HSP + NAR exposure did not induce effects at 6 months of age on bone mineral, structure, and biomechanical strength at the tibias, femurs, and LV demonstrates consistency among all skeletal sites examined and provides strong evidence that HSP + NAR does not have long-lasting effects on skeletal integrity in female CD-1 offspring when mothers are exposed before and during pregnancy and throughout lactation. Another strength is that that changes in tibial BMD and bone structure were evaluated within the same mice throughout the course of the study. This longitudinal evaluation of BMD and bone structure within the same mice resulted in a statistically powerful design and reduced the number of animals required to conduct the present study. A limitation of the present study is the uncertainty of whether the compromised bone structure with HSP + NAR treatment at two and four months of age is due to the combined action of HSP and NAR or if one of these flavanones is responsible for these observed effects. As we are the first to examine the efficacy HSP and NAR in a programming model of bone development, we chose to provide HSP and NAR in combination at levels that have established effects in aging rodent models [8,9,11] as a proof of efficacy. Moreover, identifying whether the critical period is preconception, and/or during pregnancy, and/or lactation remains unknown.

5. Conclusions

In conclusion, maternal consumption of HSP + NAR exerts transient effects on trabecular bone development at the proximal tibia in female CD-1 offspring. That BMD, structure, and strength at the tibia, femur, and LV were similar between the CON and HSP + NAR groups at six months of age suggests that maternal consumption of HSP + NAR does not favorably program bone health in female CD-1 offspring.

Acknowledgments: W.E.W. holds a Canada Research Chair in Bone and Muscle Development. We thank the Canadian Institutes of Health Research for funding this research (grant number 130544) and the Canada Foundation for Innovation (grant number 222084) for the purchase of the micro-computed tomography system.

Author Contributions: S.M.S. and W.E.W. conceptualized the study and designed the experiments. S.M.S. and C.S. conducted the in vivo portion of the study, including the in vivo micro-computed tomography scanning of mice. P.J.L. provided insight into the study. S.M.S. performed the bone analyses. S.M.S. wrote the initial drafts of the manuscript with W.E.W., and all authors contributed to and approved the final version.

Conflicts of Interest: The authors declare no conflict of interest.

References

1. Kaludjerovic, J.; Ward, W.E. Bone-specific gene expression patterns and whole bone tissue of female mice are programmed by early life exposure to soy isoflavones and folic acid. *J. Nutr. Biochem.* **2015**, *26*, 1068–1076. [CrossRef] [PubMed]
2. Kaludjerovic, J.; Ward, W.E. Neonatal administration of isoflavones attenuates deterioration of bone tissue in female but not male mice. *J. Nutr.* **2010**, *140*, 766–772. [CrossRef] [PubMed]
3. Dinsdale, E.C.; Kaludjerovic, J.; Ward, W.E. Isoflavone exposure throughout suckling results in improved adult bone health in mice. *J. Dev. Orig. Health Dis.* **2012**, *3*, 271–275. [CrossRef] [PubMed]
4. Kaludjerovic, J.; Ward, W.E. Neonatal exposure to daidzein, genistein, or the combination modulates bone development in female CD-1 mice. *J. Nutr.* **2009**, *139*, 467–473. [CrossRef] [PubMed]
5. Chiba, H.; Kim, H.; Matsumoto, A.; Akiyama, S.; Ishimi, Y.; Suzuki, K.; Uehara, M. Hesperidin prevents androgen deficiency-induced bone loss in male mice. *Phytother. Res.* **2014**, *28*, 289–295. [CrossRef] [PubMed]
6. Habauzit, V.; Nielsen, I.L.; Gil-Izquierdo, A.; Trzeciakiewicz, A.; Morand, C.; Chee, W.; Barron, D.; Lebecque, P.; Davicco, M.J.; Williamson, G.; et al. Increased bioavailability of hesperetin-7-glucoside compared with hesperidin results in more efficient prevention of bone loss in adult ovariectomised rats. *Br. J. Nutr.* **2009**, *102*, 976–984. [CrossRef] [PubMed]
7. Horcajada, M.N.; Habauzit, V.; Trzeciakiewicz, A.; Morand, C.; Gil-Izquierdo, A.; Mardon, J.; Lebecque, P.; Davicco, M.J.; Chee, W.S.; Coxam, V.; et al. Hesperidin inhibits ovariectomized-induced osteopenia and shows differential effects on bone mass and strength in young and adult intact rats. *J. Appl. Physiol. (1985)* **2008**, *104*, 648–654. [CrossRef] [PubMed]
8. Chiba, H.; Uehara, M.; Wu, J.; Wang, X.; Masuyama, R.; Suzuki, K.; Kanazawa, K.; Ishimi, Y. Hesperidin, a citrus flavonoid, inhibits bone loss and decreases serum and hepatic lipids in ovariectomized mice. *J. Nutr.* **2003**, *133*, 1892–1897. [PubMed]
9. Habauzit, V.; Sacco, S.M.; Gil-Izquierdo, A.; Trzeciakiewicz, A.; Morand, C.; Barron, D.; Pinaud, S.; Offord, E.; Horcajada, M.N. Differential effects of two citrus flavanones on bone quality in senescent male rats in relation to their bioavailability and metabolism. *Bone* **2011**, *49*, 1108–1116. [CrossRef] [PubMed]
10. Li, N.; Jiang, Y.; Wooley, P.H.; Xu, Z.; Yang, S.Y. Naringin promotes osteoblast differentiation and effectively reverses ovariectomy-associated osteoporosis. *J. Orthop. Sci.* **2013**, *18*, 478–485. [PubMed]
11. Pang, W.Y.; Wang, X.L.; Mok, S.K.; Lai, W.P.; Chow, H.K.; Leung, P.C.; Yao, X.S.; Wong, M.S. Naringin improves bone properties in ovariectomized mice and exerts oestrogen-like activities in rat osteoblast-like (UMR-106) cells. *Br. J. Pharmacol.* **2010**, *159*, 1693–1703. [CrossRef] [PubMed]
12. Song, B.J.; Jouni, Z.E.; Ferruzzi, M.G. Assessment of phytochemical content in human milk during different stages of lactation. *Nutrition* **2013**, *29*, 195–202. [CrossRef] [PubMed]
13. Zeng, X.; Bai, Y.; Peng, W.; Su, W. Identification of naringin metabolites in human urine and feces. *Eur. J. Drug Metab. Pharmacokinet.* **2016**. [CrossRef] [PubMed]
14. Manach, C.; Morand, C.; Gil-Izquierdo, A.; Bouteloup-Demange, C.; Remesy, C. Bioavailability in humans of the flavanones hesperidin and narirutin after the ingestion of two doses of orange juice. *Eur. J. Clin. Nutr.* **2003**, *57*, 235–242. [CrossRef] [PubMed]
15. Rouseff, R.L.; Martin, S.F.; Youtsey, C.O. Quantitative survey of narirutin, naringin, hesperidin, and neohesperidin in citrus. *J. Agric. Food Chem.* **1987**, *35*, 1027–1030. [CrossRef]

16. Booth, A.N.; Jones, F.T.; Deeds, F. Metabolic and glucosuria studies on naringin and phloridzin. *J. Biol. Chem.* **1958**, *233*, 280–282. [PubMed]

17. Erlund, I.; Meririnne, E.; Alfthan, G.; Aro, A. Plasma kinetics and urinary excretion of the flavanones naringenin and hesperetin in humans after ingestion of orange juice and grapefruit juice. *J. Nutr.* **2001**, *131*, 235–241. [PubMed]

18. Trzeciakiewicz, A.; Habauzit, V.; Mercier, S.; Lebecque, P.; Davicco, M.J.; Coxam, V.; Demigne, C.; Horcajada, M.N. Hesperetin stimulates differentiation of primary rat osteoblasts involving the bmp signalling pathway. *J. Nutr. Biochem.* **2010**, *21*, 424–431. [CrossRef] [PubMed]

19. Trzeciakiewicz, A.; Habauzit, V.; Mercier, S.; Barron, D.; Urpi-Sarda, M.; Manach, C.; Offord, E.; Horcajada, M.N. Molecular mechanism of hesperetin-7-o-glucuronide, the main circulating metabolite of hesperidin, involved in osteoblast differentiation. *J. Agric. Food Chem.* **2010**, *58*, 668–675. [CrossRef] [PubMed]

20. Wu, J.B.; Fong, Y.C.; Tsai, H.Y.; Chen, Y.F.; Tsuzuki, M.; Tang, C.H. Naringin-induced bone morphogenetic protein-2 expression via PI3K, Akt, c-Fos/c-Jun and AP-1 pathway in osteoblasts. *Eur. J. Pharmacol.* **2008**, *588*, 333–341. [CrossRef] [PubMed]

21. Zhang, P.; Dai, K.R.; Yan, S.G.; Yan, W.Q.; Zhang, C.; Chen, D.Q.; Xu, B.; Xu, Z.W. Effects of naringin on the proliferation and osteogenic differentiation of human bone mesenchymal stem cell. *Eur. J. Pharmacol.* **2009**, *607*, 1–5. [CrossRef] [PubMed]

22. Reeves, P.G.; Nielsen, F.H.; Fahey, G.C., Jr. AIN-93 purified diets for laboratory rodents: Final report of the American institute of nutrition ad hoc writing committee on the reformulation of the AIN-76A rodent diet. *J. Nutr.* **1993**, *123*, 1939–1951. [PubMed]

23. Sacco, S.M.; Saint, C.; Longo, A.B.; Wakefield, C.B.; Salmon, P.L.; LeBlanc, P.J.; Ward, W.E. Repeated irradiation from micro-computed tomography scanning at 2, 4 and 6 months of age does not induce damage to tibial bone microstructure in male and female CD-1 mice. *BoneKEy Rep.* **2017**. [CrossRef]

24. Otsu, N. A threshold selection method from gray-level histograms. *IEEE Trans. Syst. Man. Cyber.* **1979**, *9*, 62–66. [CrossRef]

25. Bruker. *Method Note: Bone Mineral Density (BMD) and Tissue Mineral Density (TMD) Calibration and Measurement by Micro-CT Using Bruker-MicroCT CT-Analyser*; Bruker microCT: Kontich, Belgium, 2014.

26. Fonseca, D.; Ward, W.E. Daidzein together with high calcium preserve bone mass and biomechanical strength at multiple sites in ovariectomized mice. *Bone* **2004**, *35*, 489–497. [CrossRef] [PubMed]

27. Breinholt, V.; Larsen, J.C. Detection of weak estrogenic flavonoids using a recombinant yeast strain and a modified MCF7 cell proliferation assay. *Chem. Res. Toxicol.* **1998**, *11*, 622–629. [CrossRef] [PubMed]

28. Kuiper, G.G.; Lemmen, J.G.; Carlsson, B.; Corton, J.C.; Safe, S.H.; van der Saag, P.T.; van der Burg, B.; Gustafsson, J.A. Interaction of estrogenic chemicals and phytoestrogens with estrogen receptor beta. *Endocrinology* **1998**, *139*, 4252–4263. [PubMed]

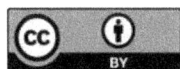

nutrients

MDPI

Review

Dried Plums, Prunes and Bone Health: A Comprehensive Review

Taylor C. Wallace [1,2]

[1] Department of Nutrition and Food Studies, George Mason University, Fairfax, VA 22030, USA; taylor.wallace@me.com; Tel.: +1-270-839-1776
[2] Think Healthy Group, Inc., Washington, DC 20001, USA

Received: 15 March 2017; Accepted: 17 April 2017; Published: 19 April 2017

Abstract: The 2015–2020 Dietary Guidelines for Americans advocate for increasing fruit intake and replacing energy-dense foods with those that are nutrient-dense. Nutrition across the lifespan is pivotal for the healthy development and maintenance of bone. The National Osteoporosis Foundation estimates that over half of Americans age 50+ have either osteoporosis or low bone mass. Dried plums, also commonly referred to as prunes, have a unique nutrient and dietary bioactive profile and are suggested to exert beneficial effects on bone. To further elucidate and summarize the potential mechanisms and effects of dried plums on bone health, a comprehensive review of the scientific literature was conducted. The PubMed database was searched through 24 January 2017 for all cell, animal, population and clinical studies that examined the effects of dried plums and/or extracts of the former on markers of bone health. Twenty-four studies were included in the review and summarized in table form. The beneficial effects of dried plums on bone health may be in part due to the variety of phenolics present in the fruit. Animal and cell studies suggest that dried plums and/or their extracts enhance bone formation and inhibit bone resorption through their actions on cell signaling pathways that influence osteoblast and osteoclast differentiation. These studies are consistent with clinical studies that show that dried plums may exert beneficial effects on bone mineral density (BMD). Long-term prospective cohort studies using fractures and BMD as primary endpoints are needed to confirm the effects of smaller clinical, animal and mechanistic studies. Clinical and prospective cohort studies in men are also needed, since they represent roughly 29% of fractures, and likewise, diverse race and ethnic groups. No adverse effects were noted among any of the studies included in this comprehensive review. While the data are not completely consistent, this review suggests that postmenopausal women may safely consume dried plums as part of their fruit intake recommendations given their potential to have protective effects on bone loss.

Keywords: dried plum; prune; bone

---

1. Introduction

The 2015–2020 Dietary Guidelines for Americans (DGA) advocate for healthy eating patterns that include a variety of fruits. This includes all fresh, frozen, canned and dried fruits and fruit juices [1]. The recommended intake of fruit in the Healthy US-Style Eating Pattern at the 2000-kcal level is two cup-equivalents of fruit per day. Increasing the amount and variety of fruits Americans consume is a strategy that helps individuals meet a wide range of nutrient requirements. However, per the 2015–2020 DGA, average intake of fruit is well below recommendations for almost all age-sex groups, except in children ages 1–8 years [1]. Average intake of fruit is lowest among girls ages 14–18 years and in women age 51+ years [1], two critical time points in bone development and maintenance.

Osteoporosis is a rising public health concern, given the aging population and suboptimal dietary intakes of dairy, fruits, vegetables and whole grains, which provide a variety of essential nutrients that influence bone accretion and maintenance across the lifespan. The National Osteoporosis Foundation estimates that 10.3% of Americans over the age of 50 years have osteoporosis (*t*-score $\leq$ 2.5), and 43.9% have low bone mass (also commonly referred to as osteopenia; *t*-score $\leq$ 1.0), a risk factor for osteoporosis [2]. The risk of fractures increases with age among individuals age 50+, and differs by sex, race and ethnicity [2,3]. Although many factors contribute to this debilitating event, the most significant causes are reduction in bone mass, structural deterioration and increased frequency of falls. It 2005, it was estimated that the over two million incident osteoporotic fractures occurring annually in the U.S. had an economic burden of $16.9 billion, which is anticipated grow to three million fractures at a cost of $25.3 billion by 2025 [4]. Men account for 29% of these fractures and 25% of the cost burden [4]. Optimization of lifestyle factors known to influence bone mass and strength is an important strategy aimed at reducing the risk of fractures later in life.

Plums are a type of drupe fruit that belong to the subgenus *Prunus* (family Rosaceae). They differ from other subgenera of drupe fruits (cherries, peaches, etc.) since the shoots have a terminal bud and unclustered single side buds, flowers combine in groups of one to five on short stems, the fruit has a crease running down one side and a smooth seed. There are over 40 species of plums currently documented, although two species, the European plum (*Prunus domestica*) and Japanese plum (*Prunus salicina* and hybrids) are of commercial significance globally [5]. The origin of European plum is thought to have been near the Caspian Sea, while Japanese plums originated in China, but derived their name from the country where they were cultivated. European plums were introduced in the U.S. by pilgrims in the 17th century, while Japanese plums were introduced to the U.S. in the late 19th century. China, Serbia and Romania are the world's leading producers of plums. Worldwide, greater than 11.2 million metric tons of plums were harvested in 2014 per the Food and Agriculture Organization (FAO) of the United Nations [6]. While all prunes originate from fresh plums, not all plum varieties are considered prunes. Commercialized prunes, also commonly known as dried plums, are the dehydrated version of the cultivar *Prunus domestica* L. cv d'Agen. This specific variety has a naturally-occurring sugar content that enables it to be dried while still containing the pit, without being fermented. The State of California produces ~99% of the plums in the U.S. and ~40% of the world's dried plums [7].

Dried plums are widely known for their laxative effect, which is commonly attributed to their dietary fiber content [8], but is also likely influenced by the significant amounts of phenolics (e.g., chlorogenic acid) and sorbitol present in the fruit. Dried plums are not only a source of dietary fiber, but also a good source of potassium and vitamin K (Table 1). One serving or ~4 dried plums is 92 kilocalories and provides 2.4 g of dietary fiber, 280 mg of potassium and 22.8 µg of vitamin K. Dried plums also contain several dietary bioactives, including phenolic compounds, such as 3-caffeoylquinic acid, 4-caffeoylquinic acid, 5-caffeoylquinic acid, 3-p-coumarolylquinic acid, caffeic acid, p-coumaric acid and quercetin-3-*O*-rutinoside [9], whose benefits may extend beyond the basic nutrition requirements of humans. There is an emerging body of evidence from laboratory, animal and human studies that suggests that dried plums may exert an effect on bone health. Hooshmand and others found that two servings (100 g) of dried plums per day slowed the rate of bone turnover and helped to improve bone mineral density (BMD) in a clinical study of 160 randomized postmenopausal women (100 completed the study) not receiving hormone replacement therapy [10]. A more recent clinical study by the same group confirmed the bone protective effects in postmenopausal women receiving one serving of dried plums per day [11]. However, a comprehensive review of dried plums and bone health is not currently present in the peer-reviewed scientific literature.

Table 1. Nutritional profile of dried plums per 100 g.

Nutrient	Unit	DV	Plums, Dried (Prunes) (09291) [a]
Macronutrients			
Water	g	ND	30.92
Energy	Kcal	2000	240
Protein	g	50	2.18
Fat	g	78	0.38
Carbohydrate	g	275	63.88
Fiber	g	28	7.1
Minerals			
Calcium	mg	1300	43
Iron	mg	18	0.93
Magnesium	mg	400	41
Phosphorus	mg	1000	69
Potassium	mg	4700	732
Sodium	mg	2300	2.0
Zinc	mg	15	0.44
Copper	mg	2	0.281
Manganese	mg	2	0.299
Selenium	µg	70	0.3
Vitamins			
Vitamin C	mg	60	0.6
Thiamin	mg	1.5	0.51
Riboflavin	mg	1.7	0.186
Niacin	mg	20	1.882
Pantothenic acid	mg	10	0.422
Vitamin B6	mg	2	0.205
Folate	µg	400	4.0
Choline	mg	550	10.1
Vitamin B12	µg	6	0.0
Vitamin A	IU	5000	781
Vitamin D	µg	20	0.0
Vitamin E	mg	30	0.43
Vitamin K	µg	80	59.5

[a] Nutrient Database Number (NDB No.) in the USDA Food Composition Databases. DV = daily value; ND = not defined by FDA.

2. Methods

2.1. Literature Search

A comprehensive literature search was conducted as of 24 January 2017 using the PubMed database. The search methodology is outlined in Table 2. A systematic literature search was not conducted for lack of clinical and observational evidence and since the focus was to evaluate potential mechanisms from various types of data.

Included in the review were cell, animal, population and clinical studies in the English language that assessed the effects of dried plums or extracts of the former on markers of bone health. All articles were screened by title/abstract and, in some cases, full-text. A complete manual search of reference lists of original studies was also conducted. Excluded studies (*n* = 26) were those of any kind that did not assess dried plum (prune) or plum intake on one or more markers or clinical endpoints of bone health.

Table 2. Search strategy.

Search No.	Search	Results	Search Type
1	bone and bones (MeSH Terms)	536,127	Advanced
2	bone AND (fracture* OR density OR resorption OR development)	340,163	Advanced
3	osteoporosis	73,977	Advanced
4	osteoblasts	36,771	Advanced
5	osteoclasts	19,477	Advanced
6	#1 OR #2 OR #3 OR #4 OR #5	762,438	Advanced
7	Prune(TIAB) OR plum(TIAB) OR dried plum(tiab)	2460	Advanced
8	#6 AND #7	50	

MeSH = medical subject heading; TIAB = title/abstract.

2.2. Data Extraction

Quantitative and qualitative data information from each study, including author and year of study, geographic study location, study design, product information, intervention, population, markers measured, duration and results, were extracted (Tables 3–5).

Table 3. Clinical trials.

Reference	Location	Design	Plum Product	Intervention	Population	Markers Measured	Duration	Results
Arjmandi et al. 2002 [12]	USA	RCT	Dried plum (P. domestica)	100 g/day DP or 75 g/day dried apple	Postmenopausal women (n = 58)	IFG-1, IGFBP-3, AP, BSAP, TRAP, phosphorus, magnesium, calcium, urine-DPD, urine-HP	3 months	DP led to borderline significant increases in AP and IGF-1. Borderline significant increase in BSAP No significant differences on other markers measured.
Hooshmand et al. 2011 [10]; Hooshmand et al. 2014 [13]	USA	RCT	Dried plum (P. domestica)	100 g/day DP or 75 g/day dried apple	Postmenopausal women with osteopenia (n = 160 enrolled; 100 completed)	BMD (spine, ulna, total hip and whole body), RANKL, OPG, sclerostin, osteocalcin, TRAP-5b, BALP, DPD, phosphorus, calcium	1 year	Significant increase in BMD at the spine and ulna in both groups, however increases were significantly greater in the DP group compared to dried apple control. Borderline significant increase in RANKL and OPG on DP group. Significant decrease in sclerostin, BSAP and TRAP-5b. No significant differences on other markers measured.
Simonthsnavice et al. 2014 [14]	USA	Intervention	Dried plum (P. domestica)	90 g/day DP with combination resistance training vs. resistance training alone.	Female breast cancer survivors (n = 23)	BMD (lumbar spine, femur and forearm), TRAP-5b, BSAP, CRP	6 months	No significant differences between groups or any group-by-time interaction.
Hooshmand et al. 2016 [11]	USA	RCT	Dried plum (P. domestica)	0, 50 g/day or 100 g/day DP.	Postmenopausal women (n = 48)	BMD (total body, total hip, L1-L4 and ulna), BAP, TRAP-5b, BAP/TRAP-5b ratio, hs-CRP, IGF-1, sclerostin, RANKL, OPG, RANKL/OPG ratio, 25(OH)D, calcium, phosphorus	6 months	Compared to controls: Both doses of DP prevented loss of total body BMD but not hip, spine or ulna BMD as compared to the control group. TRAP-5b decreased at 3 months and this was sustained at 6 months in both 50 and 100 g DP groups. BAP/TRAP-5b ratio was significantly greater at 6 months in both DP groups. No significant differences on other markers measured.

25(OH)D = 25-hydroxyvitamin D; AP = alkaline phosphatase; BAP = bone alkaline phosphatase; BMD = bone mineral density; BSAP = bone-specific alkaline phosphatase; DP = dried plums; DPD = deoxypyridinoline; HS = hydroxylysylpyridinoline; hs-CRP = high sensitivity C-reactive protein; IGF-1 = insulin-like growth factor-1; IGFBP-3 = insulin-like growth factor-binding protein-3; OPG = osteoprotegerin; RANKL = receptor activator of nuclear factor kappa-B ligand; TRAP = tartrate-resistant acid phosphatase; TRAP-5b = tartrate-resistant acid phosphatase-5b.

Table 4. Animal studies.

Reference	Location	Animal Model	Plum Product	Methods	Markers Measured	Duration	Results
Arjmandi et al. 2010 [15]	USA	Sprague-Dawley rats	Dried plum (*P. domestica*), DP puree, DP juice, DP pulp/skin, DPP	After surgery to establish bone loss, rats placed on various diets supplemented with 13 different combinations of fructooligosaccharides and DP vs. a control diet.	BMD and BMC (whole body, right femur, 4th lumbar vertebrae), calcium loss (4th lumbar), TbS, serum OC, serum IGF-1, calcium, phosphorus, and magnesium.	60 days	Compared to the other treatments, diets supplemented with 5% FOS and 7.5% DP was most effective in reversing both right femur and fourth lumbar BMD and fourth lumbar calcium loss while significantly decreasing TbS. No significant effects of treatment on serum or urine measures of bone turnover.
Bu et al. 2007 [16]	USA	Male Sprague-Dawley rats	Dried plum (*P. domestica*) vs. parathyroid hormone	Diet supplementation of 6-month old male rats with 25% DP vs. a control diet.	BMA, BMC, BMD (whole body, femur, vertebrae), trabecular architecture, cortical bone, serum ALP, serum protein, BV/TV, TbN, TbSp, femur and vertebral (connectivity density, SMI, linear attenuation), total force, stiffness, physiological force.	90 days	DPs induced a significant increase in vertebra and femoral BMD compared to controls. DPs induced a significant increase in femur BMC compared to controls. The DP group had significantly: • Higher femur and vertebra BV/TV, TbN. • Higher femur connectivity density, femur and vertebral linear attenuation. • Higher cortical thickness and cortical area. • Lower TbSp and femur SMI. • Higher total force, stiffness, and physiological force. • Lower average von Mises stresses.
Deyhim et al. 2005 [17]	USA	Sprague-Dawley rats	Dried plum (*P. domestica*)	Dietary supplementation of adult osteopenic rats with 5%, 15% or 25% DP vs. a control diet.	Serum ALP, TRAP activities, calcium, magnesium, IGF-1, BMD (femur, tibia, vertebra), trabecular microarchitecture, urinary DPD, L4 BMD, BV/TV, connectivity density, TbSp, and TbTh.	60 days	Compared to OVX controls: • All DP groups had significantly higher femur BMD, tibia BMD, as well as lower TbSp. • 25% DP groups had significantly higher L4 BMD, BV/TV, and connectivity density. • 15% and 25% DP groups had significantly higher TbN and lower TbTh.

Table 4. *Cont.*

Reference	Location	Animal Model	Plum Product	Methods	Markers Measured	Duration	Results
Franklin et al. 2006 [18]	USA	Male Sprague–Dawley rats	Dried plum (*P. domestica*)	Dietary supplementation of male rats with 5%, 15% or 25% DP vs. a control diet.	Whole body BMC, BMA, BMD), BMC (femur, L4 vertebra), trabecular bone microarchitecture markers (BV/TV, TbN, TbSp), serum ALP, osteocalcin, IGF-I, RANKL, OPG, cortical strength, cortical area, medullary area, cortical porosity, distal femur and L4 vertebral (SMI, connectivity density, LinAtt), IGF, DPD, OPG, RANKL.	90 days	15% and 25% DP groups significantly prevented a reduction in whole body BMD, as well as femur and L4 vertebra BMC. 15% and 25% DP groups protected against the decrease in mechanical strength required to break the femur bone. Compared to controls: • 5% and 25% DP groups had significantly higher distal femur BV/TV. • 25% DP group had significantly higher L4 vertebra BV/TV, TbN and significantly lower L4 vertebra TbSp. • All DP groups had significantly higher distal femur TbN and lower distal femur TbSp, DPD, RANKL. • 15% and 25% DP groups had significantly higher cortical strength and lower vertebral SMI and OPG. • 25% DP group had significantly lower femur SMI and higher femur and vertebral connectivity density, vertebral LinnAtt, and IGF. • 5% and 25% DP groups had significantly higher LinAtt. No significant differences on other markers measured.
Halloran et al. 2010 [19]	USA	Harlan Sprague Dawley mice	Dried plum (*P. domestica*)	Dietary supplementation of adult and old male mice with 15%, 25% DP vs. a control diet.	BV/TV, TbN, TbSp, P1NP, SMI, connective density, degree of anisotropy, ObS, OcS, BFR, cortical thickness, bone area, cortical area, Medullary area, BMD and PYD.	6 months	Within both adult and old mice, increasing DP supplementation was associated with greater BV. Mice fed 25% DP had significantly greater BV compared to controls. Mice fed 25% DP had significantly greater BV compared to those fed 15%. The differences in magnitude of the percent changes between control mice and those fed 25% DP were significantly greater in adult vs. old mice. Compared to controls: • Adult mice fed 25%DP had higher BV/TV, TbN, connective density, and lower SMI. • Old mice fed 25% DP had higher degree of anisotropy and cortical thickness, and lower medullary area and PYD. • Old mice fed 15% DP had higher cortical area. No significant differences on other markers measured.

Table 4. *Cont.*

Reference	Location	Animal Model	Plum Product	Methods	Markers Measured	Duration	Results
Johnson et al. 2011 [20]	USA	Sprague-Dawley rats	Dried plum (*P. domestica*)	Female ovarian hormone deficient rats a fed control, soy, soy + FOS, soy + 7.5% DP, and soy + 7.5% DP + FOS diet vs. a control diet.	BMD, BMC (Whole body, right femur, 4th lumbar vertebrae), serum ALP, urinary creatinine, urinary DPD, femur strength, TbN, BV/TV, TbTh, and TbSp.	60 days	Whole body and 4th lumbar BMD were significantly higher in diets with DP + FOS compared to the control and soy diets. No significant differences on other markers measured.
Leotoing et al. 2016 [21]	France	Wistar rats	High and low chlorogenic acid dried plum (*P. domestica*) and DP juice concentrate (15%)	Female rats High and low chlorogenic acid dried plum (*P. domestica*) and DP juice concentrate (15%) diets vs. a control diet.	Urinary DPD, OC, CPII, CTX-II, BMD (Total femoral, metaphyseal), BMC, urine calcium, primary pre-osteoblasts (proliferation, ALP), bone remodeling index, and cartilage remodeling index.	90 days (in vivo), 7 days (ex vivo)	10 and 50 µmol/L concentrations of neochlorogenic, chlorogenic, or caffeic acid significantly decreased pre-osteoblast ALP activity and increased pre-osteoblast proliferation. The low chlorogenic acid DP juice and DP juice concentrate groups showed significantly higher trabecular distal BMD, significantly increased cortical BMD, and increased total BMC compared to control. High chlorogenic acid DP juice group had significantly higher trabecular distal BMD compared to controls. High chlorogenic acid DP juice, low chlorogenic acid DP juice + fiber and low chlorogenic acid DP juice concentrate significantly prevented increase in OC. Low chlorogenic acid DP juice + fiber and low chlorogenic acid DP juice concentrate significantly prevented increase in DPD. Both high and low chlorogenic acid DP juice and DP juice concentrate lead to higher urinary calcium excretion compared to controls. Only high chlorogenic acid DP juice significantly counteracted the decrease in CPII. Only the high chlorogenic acid DP juice group had significantly higher CRI.
Monsefi et al. 2013 [22]	Iran	Pregnant mice	Dried plum (*P. domestica*) extract (8 mL/kg) and DP hydroalcoholic extracts (1.6 g/kg)	Pregnant mice were fed DP extracts vs. a control diet and outcomes measured on their fetuses.	Serum calcium, magnesium, ALP, bone calcium, and phosphorus.	30 days	Non-pregnant mice fed DP extract had significantly higher bone calcium compared to non-pregnant controls. Non-pregnant mice fed DP hydroalcoholic extracts had significantly higher bone phosphorus compared to non-pregnant controls. Non-pregnant mice fed both DP extract and DP hydroalcoholic extract had significantly higher bone calcium compared to non-pregnant controls.

Table 4. *Cont.*

Reference	Location	Animal Model	Plum Product	Methods	Markers Measured	Duration	Results
Pawlowski et al. 2014 [23]	USA	Sprague-Dawley rats	Dried plum powder extract (0.20% and 0.45% w/w total dietary polyphenols)	Randomized, crossover intervention trial to evaluate 12 different polyphenolics containing diets on bone turnover.	Urine calcium (total and ^{45}Ca), NTx and ALP.	10 days	Bone calcium retention was significantly improved due to dietary intervention with 0.45% DP extract compared to baseline. 0.45% DP extract improved bone calcium retention compared with the 0.20% DP extract. No significant effect on other outcomes.
Rendina et al. 2012 [24]	USA	Adult female C57BL/6J mice	Dried plum (*Prunus domestica*)	Adult female mice placed on 5%, 15% or 25% DP intervention vs. a control diet.	BMA, BMC and BMD of the 4th to 5th lumbar vertebrae (L4-L5), TbN, BV/TV, TbTh, TbSp, connectivity density, SMI, PINP, IGF-I, NFATc, Runx2, biomechanical properties of trabecular bone, OC, IL-6, and TNF-α.	4 weeks	Mean BMC and BMA were significantly higher in the 25% DP group compared to the control. 15% DP group had a significantly higher plasma IGF-1 compared to the control. 15% and 25% DP groups significantly increased BV/TV compared to the control. 15% and 25% DP groups significantly decreased TbSp beyond that of the control group. 15% and 25% DP groups experienced a significant increase in vertebra TbTh compared to the control. 15% and 25% DP groups had significantly lower Von Mises stress distribution compared to the control. 15% and 25% DP groups had significantly higher vertebral connective density and tibia apparent mean/density, and lower vertebral SMI and OC expression and TNF-α. 25% DP group had significantly higher apparent mean/density and tibia connective density, and significantly lower tibia SMI. 25% DP group significantly increased TbN compared to the control. All doses of DP groups had significantly lower plasma PINP, NFATc and Runx2 compared to the control.

Table 4. *Cont.*

Reference	Location	Animal Model	Plum Product	Methods	Markers Measured	Duration	Results
Rendina et al. 2013 [25]	USA	Adult osteopenic ovariectomized C57BL/6 mice	Dried plum (*Prunus domestica*), 25%	This study was designed to compare the efficacy of DP, apple, apricot, grape, and mango vs. a control in the restoration of bone in an osteopenic mouse model.	Whole body and L4-5 (BMA, BMC, BMD), TbN, BV/TV, TbTh, TbSp, SMI, biomechanical testing of vertebra and tibia, connective density, NFATc1, ALP, Col1a1, OC, Bak1, Casp3, and Casp9.	8 weeks	Compared to the control the DP group had significantly higher whole body and spine BMA, BMD and BMC. DP group had significantly higher vertebral BV/TV, TbN, TbTh, connective density, SMI, and trabecular density compared to the control group. DP group had significantly higher proximal tibia BV/TV compared to the control group. DP group had significantly higher vertebral total force, stiffness, size independent stiffness compared to the control group. DP group had significantly lower NFATc1 compared to the control group. DP group had significantly higher Bak1 and lower Casp3 and compared to the control group. No significant differences on other markers.
Schreurs et al. 2016 [26]	USA	Male C57BL/6J mice	Dried plum (*Prunus domestica*), 25%	This study randomized mice to 25% DP intervention vs. a control to protect from bone loss and then later exposed them to ionizing radiation.	Nfe2l2, RANKL, MCP-1, OPG, TNF-α, TbN, BV/TV, TbTh, TbSp,	7–21 days	Compared to the irradiated controls, levels of Nfe2l2, RANKL, MCP-1, OPG, and TNF-α in the DP group were not statistically different. After exposure to radiation, DP mice did not have any significant decrease in TbN, BV/TV, TbTh or TbSp indicating a radio-protective effects against cancellous bone loss compared to irradiated controls. DP fed mice had significantly higher BV/TV, TbTh and TbN after being exposed to simulated space radiation compared to control diet.

Table 4. *Cont.*

Reference	Location	Animal Model	Plum Product	Methods	Markers Measured	Duration	Results
							BV/TV and TbTh significantly increased and SMI significantly decreased after 2 and 4 weeks of DP. TbN significantly increased after 4 weeks of DP. After 2 and 4 weeks of DP: • OcS, ObS, MAR, MS/BS, BFR/BS decreased significantly. • Osteoclasts significantly decreased. DP fed mice had significantly lower: • Ctsk gene expression. • Immune-related cytokines (IL-1a, IL-1b, IL-10, IL-12, IL-13, IL-17, TNF-α, and MCP-1). • CTX
Shahnazari et al. 2016 [27]	USA	C57Bl/6 mice	Dried plum (*Prunus domestica*)	Skeletally mature (6-month-old) and growing (1- and 2-month-old) male mice were placed on a 5%, 15% or 25% DP intervention vs. a control diet.	BV/TV, TbTh, TbN, SMI, OcS, ObS, MAR, MS/BS, BFR/BS, Ctsk, OPG, RANKL, CTX, and P1NP.	1–4 weeks	BV/TV increased significantly in mice fed 5%, 15% or 25% DP. TbTh increased significantly among mice fed 25% DP. TbN increased significantly in mice fed 5%, 15% or 25% DP. SMI decreased significantly for mice fed 15% and 25% DP. Among 2-month-old mice, ObS increased significantly among mice fed 5%, 15% or 25% DP. Among 3-month-old mice, ObS increased significantly among mice fed 5% DP. No significant differences on other markers.

Table 4. *Cont.*

Reference	Location	Animal Model	Plum Product	Methods	Markers Measured	Duration	Results
Smith et al. 2014b [28]	USA	Female Sprague-Dawley rats	Dried plum (*Prunus domestica*)	Osteopenic rats were placed on 5%, 15% or 25% DP intervention vs. a control diet.	BMD (whole body, femur and vertebra), BV/TV, TbN, TbSp, connective density, TbTh (proximal tibia, vertebra), Cortical thickness, cortical area, medullary area, cortical porosity, DPD, P1NP, cancellous BFR and MS/BS, MAR, MS/bone area, BFR/BV, Periosteal (BFR, MS, MAR), endocortical (BFR, MS, MAR), Bmp2, Bmp4, ColIIa, IGF-1, Nfatc1, and RANKL.	6 weeks	Compared to controls: • Vertebral BMD increased significantly in 15% and 25% DP groups • Femur BMD increased significantly in 5%, 15%, and 25% DP groups • Whole body BMD increased significantly in 5%, 15%, and 25% DP groups Within the vertebra and when compared to controls: • BV/TV, TbN, TbSp, connective density increased significantly in 5%, 15% and 25% DP groups. • TbTh increased significantly in 15% and 25% DP groups. Within the proximal tibia and when compared to controls: TbSp decreased significantly in 15% and 25% DP groups. When compared to controls: cortical thickness increased significantly in 5%, 15%, and 25% DP groups. 25% of DP significantly suppressed increase in urinary DPD excretion. 5%, 15%, and 25% DP groups significantly suppressed serum P1NP.Compared to controls: • 15% and 25% DP groups significantly suppressed increase in cancellous BFR and MS/BS. • 15% and 25% DP groups significantly suppressed increase in cancellous BFR and MS/BS. • 15% DP groups significantly suppressed increase in MAR • MS/bone area, BFR/BV, Periosteal BFR levels were significantly decreased in 5%, 15%, and 25% DP groups. • All groups of DP increased significantly Bmp4 expression. • 25% group significantly increased IGF-1 expression. • Relative abundance of NFATc1 mRNA was significantly lower in all DP groups. No significant differences on other markers.

Table 4. *Cont.*

Reference	Location	Animal Model	Plum Product	Methods	Markers Measured	Duration	Results
							At 4 weeks: • Whole body BMD, vertebra (BMD, BMC) were significantly higher in the DP group. • Lumbar BV/TV, connective density, femur cortical thickness, were significantly higher in the DP group. SMI was significantly lower in the DP group. At 12 weeks: • Whole body BMA, BMC and BMD, as well as vertebra BMD and BMC were significantly higher in the DP group. • BV/TV (lumbar and distal femur), trabecular number (lumbar and distal femur), connectivity density (lumbar and distal femur), and femur cortical thickness, were significantly higher in the DP group.
Smith et al. 2014a [29]	USA	Male C57BL/6 mice	Dried plum (*Prunus domestica*)	Osteopenic rats were placed on 25% DP intervention vs. a control diet.	Whole-body and vertebral (BMD, BMC, BMA) lumbar vertebra, distal femur, femur mid-diaphysis (BV/TV, TbN, TbTh, TbS, connective density, SMI), PINP, PYD, glutathione peroxidase activity, OcS, ObS, MS, BFR, MAR, Pparc, Osx, Bmp2, Bmp4, ALP, Col1a1, OC, RANKL, OPG, NFATc1, and Ctsk.	4 or 12 weeks	• Trabecular separation (lumbar and distal femur), SMI (lumbar and distal femur) were significantly lower in the DP group. At 4 and 12 weeks, serum PINP of DP group were significantly reduced compared to controls. At 12 weeks, serum PYD was significantly lower in the DP group. The DP group had significantly higher glutathione peroxidase activity than the control at 12 weeks. At 4 weeks, the DP group had significantly lower OcS, ObS, MS, and BMR. At 4 weeks, the DP group had significantly higher Pparc; lower Osx, Bmp4, ALP, Col1a1, Bglap2, RANKL, and NFATc1.

Table 4. *Cont.*

Reference	Location	Animal Model	Plum Product	Methods	Duration	Markers Measured	Results
Arjmandi et al. 2001 [30]	USA	Female Sprague-Dawley rats	(*Prunus domestica*)	Female rats were either ovariectomized or sham operated. The ovariectomized groups were then fed either a 5% or 25% DP supplemented diet vs. a control diet.	45 days	Trabecular (total area, bone area, % bone area). Cortical (total area, bone area, marrow space, endosteal perimeter, and periosteal perimeter.	Compared to the controls the 25% DP group had significantly higher trabecular BA. Unreported results (data not shown): • DP diets dose-dependently enhanced IGF-1.

ALP = alkaline phosphatase; BAK1 = BRI1-associated kinase 1; BFR = bone formation rate; BMA = bone mineral area; BMC = bone mineral content; BMD = bone mineral density; BMP2 = bone morphogenetic protein-2; BMP4 = bone morphogenetic protein-4; BS = bone surface; BS = bone surface; BV = bone volume; Casp3 = caspase-3; Casp9 = caspase-9; Col1a1 = collagen type 1a1; Col11a = collagen type 1; CPII = C-propeptide of type II collagen; Ctsk = cathepsin K; CTX = C-terminal telopeptide of type II collagen; DP = dried plum; DPD = deoxypyridinoline; DPP = dried plum polyphenols; FOS = fructooligosaccharides; IGF = insulin-like growth factor; IGF-1 = insulin-like growth factor-1; IL-6 = Interleukin-6; LinAtt = Linear X-ray attenuation coefficient; MAR = Mineral absorption rate; MCP-1 = Monocyte chemoattractant 1; MS = Mineralizing surface; NFATc = Nuclear factor of activated T cells; NFATc1 = Nuclear factor of activated T cells-1; Nfe212 = Nuclear factor erythroid derived 212; NTx = N-telopeptides of type-1 collagen; ObS = Osteoblast surface; OC = osteocalcin; OcS = Osteoclast surface; OPG = osteoprotegerin; Osx = osterix; PINP = procollagen type I N-terminal propeptide; Pparc = proliferator-activated receptor gamma; PYD = pyridinoline; RANKL = receptor activator of nuclear factor kappa-B ligand; Runx2 = Runt-related protein 2; SMI = structural model index;TbN = trabecular bone number; TbSp = trabecular bone separation; TbTh = trabecular thickness; TNF-a = tumor necrosis factor-alpha; TRAP = tartrate-resistant acid phosphatase; TV = trabecular volume.

Table 5. Cell studies.

Reference	Location	Cell Type	Plum Product	Dose	Methods	Markers Measured	Results
Bu et al. 2008 [31]	USA	RAW 264.7 murine macrophage cells	DPE (*P. domestica*)	0, 10, 20, or 30 µg/mL dried plum polyphenols	Cells were cultured and treated with various doses of dried plum extract.	Osteoclast differentiation and activity.	DPE suppressed osteoclast differentiation and activity under normal, oxidative stress, and inflammatory conditions.
Bu et al. 2009 [32]	USA	MC3T3-E1 cells	DPP (*P. domestica*)	0, 2.5, 5, 10 and 20 µg/mL	Cells were plated and pretreated with dried plum extracts and later stimulated with TNF-α.	Osteoblast function, mineralized nodule formation, and ALP.	DPP significantly increased intracellular ALP activity under normal conditions and significantly restored the TNF-α-induced suppression of intracellular ALP activity. DPP increased mineralized nodule formation under normal and inflammatory conditions. DPP increased osteoblast activity and function.
Hooshmand et al. 2015 [33]	USA	RAW 264.7 cells	DPP (*Prunus domestica* L)	0, 0.1, 1, 10, 100, 1000 µg/mL DPP	Cells were treated to different doses of DPP.	NO, COX-2, and MA	In comparison to LPS-treated control cells: • 1000 µg/mL DPP significantly reduced NO production. • 100 and 1000 µg/mL DPP significantly decreased reduced protein level of COX-2. • 1000 µg/mL DPP significantly prevented oxidation-induced increase in MA level.

ALP = alkaline phosphatase; COX-2 = cyclooxygenase-1; DPE = dried plum extract; DPP = dried plum polyphenols; MA = malondialdehyde; NO = nitric oxide; TNF-a = tumor necrosis factor-alpha.

3. Results

The literature search of the PubMed database yielded 50 articles [10–61]. After title/abstract review, 22 articles were screened in full-text and included in this comprehensive review [10–29,31,32]. Two additional studies [30,33] were included after examination of the reference lists of the 22 studies identified in the literature search. Data and results from each of the 24 included studies are listed in Tables 3–5.

Four clinical trials were identified in this comprehensive review [10–14]. Most the studies retrieved for full-text review were animal studies involving either rats or mice (16 total) [15–30], although three (cell) studies were also identified [31–33]. No observational studies were identified in the PubMed literature search or after examination of the reference lists of included studies.

4. Discussion

Dried plums are being increasingly recognized for their role in bone health. This comprehensive review supports that consumption of dried plums is safe and may be a bone healthy option for postmenopausal women wishing to satisfy daily requirement for fruit as outlined by the 2015–2020 DGA. It is important to note that dried plums contain a higher amount of vitamin K as compared to other commonly-consumed fruits, which may influence bone health by helping to improve calcium balance.

The quality of clinical studies included in this comprehensive review was acceptable, noting that none utilized a sample size based on a priori power calculation, nor were the treatment allocations able to be concealed from the participants and/or investigators. All four clinical studies identified were derived from the same laboratory group [10–14], meriting the need for replication by additional investigators. Clinical studies included in this review had several limitations, such as a short duration of 3–12 months, which is a narrow window to see significant changes in BMD. All four clinical studies were un-blinded, and only the Hooshmand et al. 2016 [11] had an inactive placebo group. The Hooshmand et al. 2011 [10] and Hooshmand et al. 2014 [13] manuscripts used dried apples as the control group and represent the same study population with additional biomarkers being measured for the latter publication post hoc (BMD data are presented twice). Participants in this study also received 500 mg of calcium and 400 IU of vitamin D during the intervention [10,13], even though administration of these supplements was equal across both arms. Simonavice et al., 2014 [14], assessed the effects of dried plums and resistance training vs. resistance training alone on blood markers of bone and inflammation in female breast cancer survivors. While this study found null effects, these results are likely not generalizable to healthy postmenopausal women experiencing normal hormone-related bone loss. Resistance training has been shown to have a larger effect on preventing bone loss as compared to most dietary interventions and could have masked the much smaller the effects, if present, exerted by dried plums. The Hooshmand et al., 2016 [11], found that dried plum consumption at 50–100 g/day for a period of six months prevented loss of total body BMD, but not spine, hip or ulna BMD, likely due to its shorter duration.

Consistent improvements in BMD at several sites were noted in animal studies designed to model conditions at or before peak bone mass, pregnancy, post-menopause, osteopenia and/or osteoporosis. Rat models of ovarian hormone deficiency have been used for over 25 years to simulate postmenopausal bone loss in humans. Ovarian hormone deficient rats and postmenopausal women have many similar characteristics when it comes to bone loss. These characteristics include increased rates of bone turnover with resorption exceeding formation, an initial rapid phase of bone loss followed by a slower phase due to the ovariectomy, greater loss of trabecular vs. cortical bone, decreased intestinal absorption of calcium and a similar response to drug (e.g., bisphosphonate therapy) and lifestyle interventions (e.g., physical activity) [41]. Indeed, animal studies show that dried plums and/or their polyphenol-rich extracts can beneficially affect both BMD and bone biomarkers. The animal and cell studies presented in this comprehensive review are consistent with and supportive of the theory that a diet high in phenolics and/or flavonoids may enhance bone formation and inhibit bone resorption through their actions on cell signaling pathways that influence osteoblast and osteoclast differentiation [62]. Total body BMD and BMD at specific sites, as well as several blood biomarkers, including AP, BAP, BSAP, OPG, RANKL and TRAP-5b, have been shown to be consistently and beneficially impacted across both clinical and animal studies. Animal studies also collectively support that dried plums may beneficially influence bone area and micro-architecture.

Several bone turnover markers seemed to be improved among clinical studies; however, there was a lack of consistency among many of the markers across and between both clinical and animal studies. For instance, Arjmandi et al., 2002 [12], found significant increases in bone alkaline phosphatase (BAP), but the latter larger study Hooshmand et al., 2011 [10], reported a decrease in BAP. Noting the abundance of bone turnover markers measured in both research and the clinical setting, the International Osteoporosis Foundation (IOF) and International Federation of Clinical Chemistry and Laboratory Medicine (IFCC) Bone Markers Working group recently reviewed the scientific literature to determine the clinical potential of bone turnover markers, which includes the prediction of fracture risk and monitoring treatments for osteoporosis [63]. The IOF/IFCC working group identified one bone resorption marker (s-CTX, serum C-terminal telopeptide of type I collagen) and one bone formation marker (s-PINP, serum procollagen type 1 N propeptide) to be used as reference markers and measured by standardized assays in observational and intervention studies [63]. While only one animal study assessed the effects of dried plums on CTX [27] and two on PINP [27,28], collectively, the animal studies included in this review showed beneficial effects of dried plums and/or their polyphenol-rich extracts on most, but not all, markers of bone turnover. Nevertheless, bone turnover markers are likely too premature in their standardization and clinical utility to accurately predict small changes in bone, as expected in dietary interventions. Differences in study design, dose and duration may also contribute to the inconsistencies in the bone turnover markers measured across and between rodent and cell studies.

Future Research

Identification of the active components, particularly individual phenolics, and their potential modes of action are necessary to fully understand the overall effect of dried plums on bone health across the lifespan. While existing data indicate that consumption of dried plums may be beneficial in postmenopausal women with ongoing bone loss, future clinical and prospective cohort studies in premenopausal women, men and adolescents prior to peak bone mass accrual are necessary to confirm their effects across the population and to make generalizable dietary guidance statements.

Recent epidemiological studies show that phenolic compounds may have a stronger association with bone than general fruit and vegetable consumption [62]. Even though BMD is a validated biomarker of bone health, fractures represent the most significant clinical endpoint of bone health across the lifespan. Prospective cohort studies designed to assess potential associations of dried plum intake on both fracture risk and changes in BMD across the population and various subpopulations are greatly needed to confirm the findings of studies included in this comprehensive review.

5. Conclusions

Dried plums are an easy means to help individuals meet their daily recommendations for fruit intake. The beneficial effects of dried plums on bone health may be in part due to the unique variety of phenolics and nutrients present in the fruit. Animal and cell studies suggest that dried plums and/or their extracts enhance bone formation and inhibit bone resorption through their actions on cell signaling pathways that influence osteoblast and osteoclast differentiation; however, results on specific markers are not consistent across and between studies. Animal studies are somewhat consistent with small clinical interventions that show dried plums may exert beneficial effects on total body and site-specific BMD. Long-term prospective cohort studies using fractures and BMD as primary endpoints are needed to confirm the effects of smaller clinical, animal and mechanistic studies. No adverse effects were noted among any of the studies included in this comprehensive review. While the data are not completely consistent, this review suggests that postmenopausal women may safely consume dried plums as part of their fruit intake recommendations given their potential to have protective effects on bone loss.

Acknowledgments: Funding for the development of the manuscript was provided through an unrestricted educational grant from the California Dried Plum Board.

Author Contributions: T.C.W. analyzed data and wrote the manuscript.

Conflicts of Interest: The California Dried Plum Board had no role in the design of the study; in the collection, analyses or interpretation of data; in the writing of the manuscript; nor in the decision to publish the results. T.C.W. recused himself of all editorial involvement in the manuscript's review process.

References

1. US Department of Health and Human Services and US Department of Agriculture. 2015–2020 Dietary Guidelines for Americans. Available online: http://health.gov/dayietaryguidelines/2015/guidelines (accessed on 15 March 2017).
2. Wright, N.C.; Looker, A.C.; Saag, K.G.; Curtis, J.R.; Delzell, E.S.; Randall, S.; Dawson-Hughes, B. The recent prevalence of osteoporosis and low bone mass in the United States based on bone mineral density at the femoral neck or lumbar spine. *J. Bone Min. Res.* **2014**, *29*, 2520–2526. [CrossRef] [PubMed]
3. Looker, A.C.; Borrud, L.G.; Dawson-Hughes, B.; Shepherd, J.A.; Wright, N. Osteoporosis or low bone mass at the femur neck or lumbar spine in older adults: United States, 2005–2008. *NCHS Data Brief* **2012**, *93*, 1–8.
4. Burge, R.; Dawson-Hughes, B.; Solomon, D.H.; Wong, J.B.; King, A.; Tosteson, A. Incidence and economic burden of osteoporosis-related fractures in the United States, 2005–2025. *J. Bone Min. Res.* **2007**, *22*, 465–475. [CrossRef] [PubMed]
5. Topp, L.F.; Russell, D.M.; Neumuller, M.; Dalbo, M.A.; Liu, W. Plum. In *Fruit Breeding*; Springer: New York, NY, USA, 1991.
6. Food and Agriculture Organization of the United Nations. FAOSTAT 2013. Available online: http://faostat.fao.org (accessed on 27 October 2016).
7. US Department of Agriculture, Foreign Agriculture Service. Data & Analysis. Available online: https://www.fas.usda.gov/data (accessed on 29 March 2016).
8. Tinker, L.F.; Schneeman, B.O.; Davis, P.A.; Gallaher, D.D.; Waggoner, C.R. Consumption of prunes as a source of dietary fiber in men with milk hypercholesterolemia. *Am. J. Clin. Nutr.* **1991**, *53*, 1259–1265. [PubMed]
9. Rothwell, J.A.; Perez-Jimenez, J.; Vos, F.; Crespy, V.; du Chaffaut, L.; Mennen, L.; Knox, C.; Eisner, R.; Cruz, J.; Wishart, D.; et al. Phenol-Explorer 3.0: A Major Update of the Phenol-Explorer Database to Incorporate Data on the Effects of Food Processing on Polyphenol Content. Database. Available online: http://phenol-explorer.eu/contents/food/51 (accessed on 15 March 2017).
10. Hooshmand, S.; Chai, S.C.; Saadat, R.L.; Payton, M.E.; Brummel-Smith, K.; Arjmandi, B.H. Comparative effects of dried plum and dried apple on bone in postmenopausal women. *Br. J. Nutr.* **2011**, *106*, 923–930. [CrossRef] [PubMed]
11. Hooshmand, S.; Kern, M.; Metti, D.; Shamloufard, P.; Chai, S.C.; Johnson, S.A.; Payton, M.E.; Arjmandi, B.H. The effect of two doses of dried plum on bone density and bone biomarkers in osteopenic postmenopausal women: A randomized, controlled trial. *Osteoporos. Int.* **2016**, *27*, 2271–2279. [CrossRef] [PubMed]
12. Arjmandi, B.H.; Khalil, D.A.; Lucas, E.A.; Georgis, A.; Stoecker, B.J.; Hardin, C.; Payton, M.E.; Wild, R.A. Dried plums improve indices of bone formation in postmenopausal women. *J. Womens Health Gend Based Med.* **2002**, *11*, 61–68. [CrossRef] [PubMed]
13. Hooshmand, S.; Brisco, J.R.Y.; Arjmandi, B.H. The effect of dried plum on serum levels of receptor activator of NF-kappaB ligand, osteoprotegerin and sclerostin in osteopenic postmenopausal women: A randomised controlled trial. *Br. J. Nutr.* **2014**, *112*, 55–60. [CrossRef] [PubMed]
14. Simonavice, E.; Liu, P.-Y.; Ilich, J.Z.; Kim, J.-S.; Arjmandi, B.; Panton, L.B. The effects of a 6-month resistance training and dried plum consumption intervention on strength, body composition, blood markers of bone turnover, and inflammation in breast cancer survivors. *Appl. Physiol. Nutr. Metab.* **2014**, *39*, 730–739. [CrossRef] [PubMed]

15. Arjmandi, B.H.; Johnson, C.D.; Campbell, S.C.; Hooshmand, S.; Chai, S.C.; Akhter, M.P. Combining fructooligosaccharide and dried plum has the greatest effect on restoring bone mineral density among select functional foods and bioactive compounds. *J. Med. Food* **2010**, *13*, 312–319. [CrossRef] [PubMed]
16. Bu, S.Y.; Lucas, E.A.; Franklin, M.; Marlow, D.; Brackett, D.J.; Boldrin, E.A.; Devareddy, L.; Arjmandi, B.H.; Smith, B.J. Comparison of dried plum supplementation and intermittent PTH in restoring bone in osteopenic orchidectomized rats. *Osteoporos. Int.* **2007**, *18*, 931–942. [CrossRef] [PubMed]
17. Deyhim, F.; Stoecker, B.J.; Brusewitz, G.H.; Devareddy, L.; Arjmandi, B.H. Dried plum reverses bone loss in an osteopenic rat model of osteoporosis. *Menopause* **2005**, *12*, 755–762. [CrossRef] [PubMed]
18. Franklin, M.; Bu, S.Y.; Lerner, M.R.; Lancaster, E.A.; Bellmer, D.; Marlow, D.; Lightfoot, S.A.; Arjmandi, B.H.; Brackett, D.J.; Lucas, E.A. Dried plum prevents bone loss in a male osteoporosis model via IGF-I and the RANK pathway. *Bone* **2006**, *39*, 1331–1342. [CrossRef] [PubMed]
19. Halloran, B.P.; Wronski, T.J.; VonHerzen, D.C.; Chu, V.; Xia, X.; Pingel, J.E.; Williams, A.A.; Smith, B.J. Dietary dried plum increases bone mass in adult and aged male mice. *J. Nutr.* **2010**, *140*, 1781–1787. [CrossRef] [PubMed]
20. Johnson, C.D.; Lucas, E.A.; Hooshmand, S.; Campbell, S.; Akhter, M.P.; Arjmandi, B.H. Addition of fructooligosaccharides and dried plum to soy-based diets reverses bone loss in the ovariectomized rat. *Evid. Based Complement. Alternat. Med.* **2011**. [CrossRef] [PubMed]
21. Leotoing, L.; Wauquier, F.; Davicco, M.-J.; Lebecque, P.; Gaudout, D.; Rey, S.; Vitrac, X.; Massenat, L.; Rashidi, S.; Wittrant, Y. The phenolic acids of Agen prunes (dried plums) or Agen prune juice concentrates do not account for the protective action on bone in a rat model of postmenopausal osteoporosis. *Nutr. Res.* **2016**, *36*, 161–173. [CrossRef] [PubMed]
22. Monsefi, M.; Parvin, F.; Farzaneh, M. Effects of plum extract on skeletal system of fetal and newborn mice. *Med. Princ. Pract.* **2013**, *22*, 351–356. [CrossRef] [PubMed]
23. Pawlowski, J.W.; Martin, B.R.; McCabe, G.P.; Ferruzzi, M.G.; Weaver, C.M. Plum and soy aglycon extracts superior at increasing bone calcium retention in ovariectomized Sprague Dawley rats. *J. Agric. Food Chem.* **2014**, *62*, 6108–6117. [CrossRef] [PubMed]
24. Rendina, E.; Lim, Y.F.; Marlow, D.; Wang, Y.; Clarke, S.L.; Kuvibidila, S.; Lucas, E.A.; Smith, B.J. Dietary supplementation with dried plum prevents ovariectomy-induced bone loss while modulating the immune response in C57BL/6J mice. *J. Nutr. Biochem.* **2012**, *23*, 60–68. [CrossRef] [PubMed]
25. Rendina, E.; Hembree, K.D.; Davis, M.R.; Marlow, D.; Clarke, S.L.; Halloran, B.P.; Lucas, E.A.; Smith, B.J. Dried plum's unique capacity to reverse bone loss and alter bone metabolism in postmenopausal osteoporosis model. *PLoS ONE* **2013**, *8*, e60569. [CrossRef] [PubMed]
26. Schreurs, A.-S.; Shirazi-Fard, Y.; Shahnazari, M.; Alwood, J.S.; Truong, T.A.; Tahimic, C.G.T.; Limoli, C.L.; Turner, N.D.; Halloran, B.; Globus, R.K. Dried plum diet protects from bone loss caused by ionizing radiation. *Sci. Rep.* **2016**, *6*, 21343. [CrossRef] [PubMed]
27. Shahnazari, M.; Turner, R.T.; Iwaniec, U.T.; Wronski, T.J.; Li, M.; Ferruzzi, M.G.; Nissenson, R.A.; Halloran, B.P. Dietary dried plum increases bone mass, suppresses proinflammatory cytokines and promotes attainment of peak bone mass in male mice. *J. Nutr. Biochem.* **2016**, *34*, 73–82. [CrossRef] [PubMed]
28. Smith, B.J.; Bu, S.Y.; Wang, Y.; Rendina, E.; Lim, Y.F.; Marlow, D.; Clarke, S.L.; Cullen, D.M.; Lucas, E.A. A comparative study of the bone metabolic response to dried plum supplementation and PTH treatment in adult, osteopenic ovariectomized rat. *Bone* **2014**, *58*, 151–159. [CrossRef] [PubMed]
29. Smith, B.J.; Graef, J.L.; Wronski, T.J.; Rendina, E.; Williams, A.A.; Clark, K.A.; Clarke, S.L.; Lucas, E.A.; Halloran, B.P. Effects of dried plum supplementation on bone metabolism in adult C57BL/6 male mice. *Calcif. Tissue Int.* **2014**, *94*, 442–453. [CrossRef] [PubMed]
30. Arjmandi, B.H.; Lucas, E.A.; Juma, S.; Soliman, A.; Stoecker, B.J.; Khalil, D.A.; Smith, B.J.; Wang, C. Dried plums prevent ovariectomy-induced bone loss in rats. *J. Am. Nutraceut. Assoc.* **2001**, *4*, 50–56.
31. Bu, S.Y.; Lerner, M.; Stoecker, B.J.; Boldrin, E.; Brackett, D.J.; Lucas, E.A.; Smith, B.J. Dried plum polyphenols inhibit osteoclastogenesis by downregulating NFATc1 and inflammatory mediators. *Calcif. Tissue Int.* **2008**, *8*, 475–488. [CrossRef] [PubMed]
32. Bu, S.Y.; Hunt, T.S.; Smith, B.J. Dried plum polyphenols attenuate the detrimental effects of TNF-alpha on osteoblast function coincident with up-regulation of Runx2, Osterix and IGF-I. *J. Nutr. Biochem.* **2009**, *20*, 35–44. [CrossRef] [PubMed]

33. Hooshmand, H.; Kumar, A.; Zhang, J.Y.; Johnson, S.A.; Chai, S.C.; Arjmandi, B.H. Evidence for anti-inflammatory and antioxidative properties of dried plum polyphenols in macrophage RAW 264.7 cells. *Food Funct.* **2015**, *6*, 1719–1725. [CrossRef] [PubMed]

34. Barone, C.M.; Marion, R.; Shanske, A.; Argamaso, R.V.; Shprintzen, R.J. Craniofacial, limb, and abdominal anomalies in a distinct syndrome: Relation to the spectrum of Pfeiffer syndrome type 3. *Am. J. Med. Genet.* **1993**, *45*, 745–750. [CrossRef] [PubMed]

35. Bracero, L.A.; Clark, D.; Pieffer, M.; Fakhry, J. Sonographic findings in a case of cloverleaf skull deformity and prune belly. *Am. J. Perinatol.* **1988**, *5*, 239–241. [CrossRef] [PubMed]

36. Frydman, M.; Cohen, H.A.; Ashkenazi, A.; Varsano, I. Familial segregation of cervical ribs, Sprengel anomaly, preaxial polydactyly, anal atresia, and urethral obstruction: A new syndrome? *Am. J. Med. Genet.* **1993**, *45*, 717–720. [CrossRef] [PubMed]

37. Fuentes, J.M.; Bouscarel, C.; Choucair, Y.; Roquefeuil, B.; Vlahovitch, B.; Blanchet, P. Monitoring of intracranial pression in acute neurotrauma by extra-dural screw (author's transl). *Anesth. Analg.* **1979**, *36*, 429–433.

38. Gambacorta, D.; Biancotti, R.; Consorti, P.; Zei, E. Clinical aspects of the prognosis of skull and brain injuries. A study of 108 cases. *Minerva Anestesiol.* **1980**, *46*, 703–708. [PubMed]

39. Gearhart, J.P.; Albertsen, P.C.; Marshall, F.F.; Jeffs, R.D. Pediatric applications of augmentation cystoplasty: The Johns Hopkins experience. *J. Urol.* **1986**, *136*, 430–432. [PubMed]

40. Gofton, W.T.; Macdermid, J.C.; Patterson, S.D.; Faber, K.J.; King, G.J.W. Functional outcome of AO type C distal humeral fractures. *J. Hand Surg. Am.* **2003**, *28*, 294–308. [CrossRef] [PubMed]

41. Hooshmand, S.; Arjmandi, B.H. Viewpoint: Dried plum, an emerging functional food that may effectively improve bone health. *Ageing Res. Rev.* **2009**, *8*, 122–127. [CrossRef] [PubMed]

42. Hublin, J.J. Paleoanthropology: Homo erectus and the limits of a paleontological species. *Curr. Biol.* **2014**, *24*, R82–R84. [CrossRef] [PubMed]

43. Kostka, V.M.; Krautwald-Junghanns, M.E.; Balks, E. Polyostotic hyperostosis in a plum-headed parakeet (*Psittacula cyanocephala* L., 1766). *Tierarztl. Prax* **1996**, *24*, 36–40. [PubMed]

44. Loh, K.C.; Salisbury, S.R.; Accott, P.; Gillis, R.; Crocker, J.F. Central precocious puberty and chronic renal failure: A reversible condition post renal transplantation. *J. Pediatr. Endocrinol. Metab.* **1997**, *10*, 539–545. [CrossRef] [PubMed]

45. Oostenbroek, H.J.; Brand, R.; van Roermund, P.M. Lower limb deformity due to failed trauma treatment corrected with the Ilizarov technique: Factors affecting the complication rate in 52 patients. *Acta Orthop.* **2009**, *80*, 435–439. [CrossRef] [PubMed]

46. Pagon, R.A.; Smith, D.W.; Shepard, T.H. Urethral obstruction malformation complex: A cause of abdominal muscle deficiency and the "prune belly". *J. Pediatr.* **1979**, *94*, 900–906. [CrossRef]

47. Robicsek, F.; Watts, L.T. Pectus carinatum. *Thorac. Surg. Clin.* **2010**, *20*, 563–574. [CrossRef] [PubMed]

48. Romero Otero, J.; Gomez Fraile, A.; Feltes Ochoa, J.; Blanco Carballo, O.; Aransay Bramtot, A.; Lopez Vazquez, F.; Alonso, L. Megalourethra in association with VACTER syndrome. *Actas Urol. Esp.* **2006**, *30*, 412–414. [CrossRef]

49. Sacco, S.M.; Horcajada, M.-N.; Offord, E. Phytonutrients for bone health during ageing. *Br. J. Clin. Pharmacol.* **2013**, *75*, 697–707. [CrossRef] [PubMed]

50. Shah, D.; Sharma, S.; Faridi, M.M.A.; Mishra, K. VACTERL association with Prune-Belly syndrome. *Indian Pediatr.* **2004**, *41*, 845–847. [PubMed]

51. Shamberger, R.C.; Welch, K.J. Surgical repair of pectus excavatum. *J. Pediatr. Surg.* **1988**, *23*, 615–622. [CrossRef]

52. Shen, C.-L.; von Bergen, V.; Chyu, M.-C.; Jenkins, M.R.; Mo, H.; Chen, C.-H.; Kwun, I.-S. Fruits and dietary phytochemicals in bone protection. *Nutr. Res.* **2012**, *32*, 897–910. [CrossRef] [PubMed]

53. Shen, W.; Wang, G.; Cui, J.; He, J. Skull plasty to correct congenital craniosynostosis. *Zhonghua Zheng Xing Wai Ke Za Zhi* **2007**, *23*, 284–287. [PubMed]

54. Shen, W.; Wang, G.; Cui, J.; He, J.; Chen, J. Cranial vault reconstruction of plagiocephaly. *Zhonghua Zheng Xing Wai Ke Za Zhi* **2007**, *23*, 459–462. [PubMed]

55. Shen, W.; Wang, G.; Wu, Y.; Cui, J.; He, J. Total calvarial reconstruction for sagittal synostosis. *Zhonghua Zheng Xing Wai Ke Za Zhi* **2006**, *22*, 172–174. [PubMed]

56. Smolkin, T.; Soudack, M.; Goldstein, I.; Sujov, P.; Makhoul, I.R. Prune belly syndrome: Expanding the phenotype. *Clin. Dysmorphol.* **2008**, *17*, 133–135. [CrossRef] [PubMed]

57. Stacewicz-Sapuntzakis, M. Dried plums and their products: Composition and health effects–An updated review. *Crit. Rev. Food Sci. Nutr.* **2013**, *53*, 1277–1302. [CrossRef] [PubMed]

58. Wang, L.; Gao, W.; Xiong, K.; Hu, K.; Liu, X.; He, H. VEGF and BFGF expression and histological characteristics of the bone-tendon junction during acute injury healing. *J. Sports Sci. Med.* **2014**, *13*, 15–21. [PubMed]

59. Wheeler, P.G.; Weaver, D.D. Adults with VATER association: Long-term prognosis. *Am. J. Med. Genet. Part A* **2005**, *138A*, 212–217. [CrossRef] [PubMed]

60. Zeng, H.; Liu, Y. Electro-acupuncture combined with plum-blossom needle tapping for treatment of supraorbital neuritis-a clinical observation of 59 cases. *J. Tradit. Chin. Med.* **2003**, *23*, 193–194. [PubMed]

61. Zhao, R.; Liu, Z.; Wang, J.; Xie, G. Combination of acupuncture with cupping increases life quality of patients of osteoporosis. *Zhongguo Zhen Jiu* **2008**, *28*, 873–875. [PubMed]

62. Weaver, C.M.; Alekel, D.L.; Ward, W.E.; Ronis, M.J. Flavonoid intake and bone health. *J. Nutr. Gerontol. Geriatr.* **2012**, *31*, 239–253. [CrossRef] [PubMed]

63. Vasikaran, S.; Eastell, R.; Bruyere, O.; Foldes, A.J.; Garnero, P.; Griesmacher, A.; McClung, M.; Morris, H.A.; Silverman, S.S.; Trenti, T.; et al. Markers of bone turnover for the prediction of fracture risk and monitoring of osteoporosis treatment: a need for international reference standards. *Osteoporos. Int.* **2011**, *22*, 391–420. [CrossRef] [PubMed]

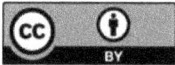

nutrients

MDPI

Article

Palmitoleic Acid Inhibits RANKL-Induced Osteoclastogenesis and Bone Resorption by Suppressing NF-κB and MAPK Signalling Pathways

Bernadette van Heerden [1,†], Abe Kasonga [1,†], Marlena C. Kruger [2,3] and Magdalena Coetzee [1,3,*]

[1] Department of Physiology, University of Pretoria, Pretoria 0001, South Africa;
    bernadettevanheerden@ymail.com (B.v.H.); abe.kasonga@up.ac.za (A.K.)
[2] School of Food and Nutrition, Massey Institute of Food Science and Technology, Massey University,
    Palmerston North 4442, New Zealand; m.c.kruger@massey.ac.nz
[3] Institute for Food, Nutrition and Well-being, University of Pretoria, Pretoria 0001, South Africa
* Correspondence: magdalena.coetzee@up.ac.za; Tel.: +27-12-319-2445; Fax: +27-12-321-1679
† These authors contributed equally to this work.

Received: 7 February 2017; Accepted: 19 April 2017; Published: 28 April 2017

Abstract: Osteoclasts are large, multinucleated cells that are responsible for the breakdown or resorption of bone during bone remodelling. Studies have shown that certain fatty acids (FAs) can increase bone formation, reduce bone loss, and influence total bone mass. Palmitoleic acid (PLA) is a 16-carbon, monounsaturated FA that has shown anti-inflammatory properties similar to other FAs. The effects of PLA in bone remain unexplored. Here we investigated the effects of PLA on receptor activator of nuclear factor kappa B (NF-κB) ligand (RANKL)-induced osteoclast formation and bone resorption in RAW264.7 murine macrophages. PLA decreased the number of large, multinucleated tartrate resistant acid phosphatase (TRAP) positive osteoclasts and furthermore, suppressed the osteolytic capability of these osteoclasts. This was accompanied by a decrease in expression of resorption markers (*Trap*, matrix metalloproteinase 9 (*Mmp9*), cathepsin K (*Ctsk*)). PLA further decreased the expression of genes involved in the formation and function of osteoclasts. Additionally, PLA inhibited NF-κB activity and the activation of mitogen activated protein kinases (MAPK), c-Jun N-terminal kinase (JNK) and extracellular signal–regulated kinase (ERK). Moreover, PLA induced apoptosis in mature osteoclasts. This study reveals that PLA inhibits RANKL-induced osteoclast formation in RAW264.7 murine macrophages through suppression of NF-κB and MAPK signalling pathways. This may indicate that PLA has potential as a therapeutic for bone diseases characterized by excessive osteoclast formation.

Keywords: palmitoleic acid; osteoclasts; bone resorption; fatty acid

1. Introduction

Bone resorption and formation are tightly coupled in healthy individuals in a process known as bone remodelling [1]. However, when there is an imbalance between formation and resorption, many bone pathologies may arise such as osteoporosis, osteopetrosis, and rheumatoid arthritis [2]. There are three main bone cell types involved in bone remodelling namely; osteocytes; osteoblasts, and osteoclasts. Osteocytes remain embedded within the mineralized matrix of bone and are thought to translate mechanical loading into biochemical signals that affect bone remodelling [3]. Osteoblasts are responsible for the synthesis and mineralization of bone as well as modulating the differentiation of osteoclasts [4]. Osteoclasts are large, multinucleated cells that are responsible for the resorption of bone. They are formed by the fusion of mononuclear hematopoietic cells of the monocyte-macrophage lineage in the presence of differentiation factors, macrophage colony-stimulating factor (M-CSF) and receptor activator of nuclear factor kappa B (NF-κB) ligand (RANKL), both produced by osteoblasts [5,6].

Osteoclasts resorb bone by developing a microenvironment in which the mineral part of the bone is dissolved and the organic part is degraded [7]. The osteoclast forms a sealing zone and creates a tight seal with the matrix of the bone. This sealing zone encircles the ruffled border responsible for increasing the surface area for resorption [7]. Binding of RANKL to the receptor activator of nuclear factor kappa B (RANK) on osteoclast precursors will trigger the NF-κB pathway and the mitogen activated kinase (MAPK) pathways, c-Jun N-terminal kinase (JNK), extracellular signal–regulated kinase (ERK), and p-38. Activation of these pathways will promote the expression of nuclear factor activator T-cells, cytoplasmic 1 (NFATc1) through Fos proto-oncogene (cFos). NFATc1 is known as the master regulator of osteoclast formation and function. NFATc1 will increase expression of dendritic cell-specific transmembrane protein (DC-STAMP), which plays an important role in osteoclast formation through cell-to-cell fusion; the release of collagenolytic enzymes (matrix metalloproteinase 9 (MMP-9), cathepsin K (CTSK), and tartrate resistant acid phosphatase (TRAP)); and the acidification of the resorption lacuna through carbonic anhydrase 2 (CAR2). Long-chain polyunsaturated fatty acids (LCPUFAs) such as alpha-linolenic acid (ALA), docosahexaenoic acid (DHA), and eicosapentaenoic acid (EPA) have been studied for their protective effects on bone health [8]. Studies have shown that these fatty acids (FAs) can increase bone formation, reduce bone loss, and influence total bone mass [9]. EPA and DHA have further been shown to decrease osteoclast formation and activity [8,10–12], possibly explaining their bone protective effects. Similar anti-osteoclastogenic effects have been reported in vitro with the use of oleic acid (OA), an anti-inflammatory monounsaturated fatty acid (MUFA) [13].

Palmitoleic acid (PLA) is an omega-7, 16-carbon, MUFA obtained from dietary sources, such as macadamia oil, and can be synthesized endogenously by adipocytes [14,15]. PLA is formed by the dehydrogenation of palmitic acid—a saturated 16-carbon fatty acid. PLA has been shown to have anti-inflammatory properties similar to other fatty acids such as DHA, EPA, and OA [14]. Several studies on PLA have revealed a wide array of effects on health [15–18]. Results from these studies have shown that PLA downregulates and inhibits lipogenesis, therefore controlling fat production in bovine adipocytes; increases low-density lipoprotein-cholesterol and lowers high-density lipoprotein-cholesterol, but also reduces total cholesterol levels in hypercholesterolemic men; increases basal glucose uptake in skeletal muscles of rats by increasing the number of glucose transporter (GLUT) 1 and GLUT4 transporters in the plasma membrane, hence controlling insulin resistance; and reduces the accumulation of hepatic lipids in mice with Type 2 diabetes [15–18]. Further studies have found that PLA increases insulin sensitivity and is a strong predictor of insulin sensitivity in humans [19]. However, the effects of PLA on insulin sensitivity have proven controversial, as other studies have revealed contradictory results [20,21]. These conflicting studies underlie the need for further research into the effects of PLA on health. Despite its anti-inflammatory properties and other health benefits, the effects of PLA on bone are largely unexplained. In this study, we investigated the effects of PLA on RANKL-induced osteoclast formation in RAW264.7 murine macrophages. To the best of our knowledge, no previous studies have been conducted on the effects of PLA in osteoclasts.

2. Materials and Methods

2.1. Reagents and Materials

Dulbecco's Modified Eagle's medium (DMEM) was purchased from GIBCO (Invitrogen Corp, Carlsbad, CA, USA) and heat inactivated fetal bovine serum (FBS) was bought from Amersham (Little Chalfont, UK). Palmitoleic acid (PLA) was acquired from Cayman Chemical Company (Ann Arbor, MI, USA). RANKL was obtained from Research and Diagnostic Systems (R&D Systems, Minneapolis, MN, USA) while TRI Reagent, Trypan blue, and all other chemicals of research grade were obtained from Sigma-Aldrich Inc. (St. Louis, MO, USA). The Alamar blue reagent, 4–12% NuPAGE Novex Bis-Tris polyacrylamide gels, cell extraction buffer, iBlot Gel Transfer Device and the iBlot Western Detection Chromogenic Kit were all supplied by Life Technologies (Carlsbad, CA, USA). M-MuLV reverse transcriptase was purchased from New England Biolabs (Ipswich, MA,

USA). Roche FastStart Essential DNA Green Master was acquired from Roche (Basel, Switzerland). The bicinchoninic acid (BCA) protein assay kit was purchased from Thermo Scientific (Rockford, IL, USA) and the rabbit polyclonal antibodies against glyceraldehyde 3-phosphate dehydrogenase (GAPDH), JNK, pJNK, ERK, and pERK were supplied by Abcam (Cambridge, MA, USA).

2.2. Fatty Acid Preparation

PLA was prepared at a stock concentration of 100 mM in ethanol, aliquoted, and stored at $-80\,°C$ in the dark until required. The stock solution was then freshly diluted to the required working concentrations of 20, 40, 60, 80, and 100 µM in complete culture medium [8]. The highest concentration of ethanol did not exceed 0.1% during the experiments, and this was used for the vehicle control.

2.3. Cell Culture

RAW264.7 murine macrophages (#TIB-71) were purchased from American Type Culture Collection (ATCC, Rockville, MD, USA) and were cultured in a flask with DMEM supplemented with 10% FBS and 1% antibiotic solution containing fungizone (0.25 µg/mL), streptomycin (100 µg/mL), and penicillin (100 µg/mL). The cells were incubated at 37 °C and humidified at 5% CO_2.

2.4. Alamar Blue Assay for Cell Viability

RAW264.7 murine macrophages were plated in a sterile 96-well plate at a density of 5×10^3 cells per well. After 24 h for attachment, the cells were exposed to PLA (20–100 µM) or vehicle (0.1% ethanol) for a further 48 h. At the end of the culture period, cells were assessed for cell viability using an Alamar Blue assay as per the manufacturer's instructions (Life Technologies). Absorbance values were measured using an Epoch Micro-plate spectrophotometer (BioTek, Winooski, VT, USA) at a wavelength of 570 nm and using 600 nm as the reference [22]. Results are expressed as percentage of control.

2.5. Osteoclast Formation and TRAP Activity Assay

RAW264.7 murine macrophages were seeded into a sterile 96-well plate at a density of 5×10^3 cells per well in complete culture medium with increasing concentrations of PLA (20–100 µM) or vehicle (0.1% ethanol) in combination with 15 ng/mL of RANKL for 5 days. The cell culture media and compounds were replaced on day 3. At the end of the culture period, TRAP activity was measured in conditioned media while the cells were stained for the presence of TRAP. Assessment of TRAP activity was done as previously described [8] and was quantified by optical absorbance at 405 nm using an Epoch Micro-plate Spectrophotometer (BioTek). The results are expressed as percentage of the control. TRAP staining of the cells was performed as previously described [8]. TRAP-positive (pink) multinucleated cells that contained more than three nuclei were regarded as osteoclasts and were counted [22]. Photographs were taken of these cells with a Discovery V20 StereoMicroscope using an AxioCam MRc5 camera (Carl Zeiss, Oberkochen, Germany).

2.6. Actin Ring Formation

RAW264.7 murine macrophages were seeded into a sterile 96-well plate at a density of 5×10^3 cells per well in complete culture medium with increasing concentrations of PLA (20–100 µM) or vehicle (0.1% ethanol) in combination with 15 ng/mL of RANKL for 5 days. The cell culture media and compounds were replaced on day 3. At the end of the culture period, the cells were fixed with 3.7% formaldehyde solution in PBS for 10 min and then permeabilized with 0.1% Triton X-100 for 10 min. The cells were then stained with Alexa fluor 568 phalloidin (Life Technologies) for 40 min, followed by 35 µg mL^{-1} Hoechst 33342 solution for 10 min to stain the nuclei. Photomicrographs were then taken using a Zeiss inverted Axiovert CFL40 microscope equipped with a Zeiss Axiovert MRm monochrome camera (Carl Zeiss, Oberkochen, Germany). The following filters were used: Hoechst (Excitation: 352 nm, Emission: 455 nm); Phalloidin (Excitation: 502 nm. Emission: 525 nm).

2.7. Bone Resorption Assay

RAW264.7 murine macrophages were seeded into a sterile 24-well osteoassay plate (Corning Inc., Corning, NY, USA) at a density of 1×10^4 cells per well, in the presence of RANKL (30 ng/mL) and varying concentrations of PLA (40–100 µM) or vehicle (0.1% ethanol) for 5 days [23]. At the end of the culture period, a modified von Kossa stain was performed and photomicrographs of the resorbed areas were taken as previously described [23]. Resorption was quantified using ImageJ software [24].

2.8. Polymerase Chain Reaction (PCR)

RAW264.7 murine macrophages were seeded into a sterile 24-well plate at a density of 1.5×10^4 cells per well and were exposed to PLA (100 µM) or vehicle (0.1% ethanol) in combination with RANKL (15 ng/mL) for 5 days. TRI reagent was used to extract the total cellular RNA and 1 µg of this RNA was reverse transcribed into cDNA using M-MuLV reverse transcriptase. Roche FastStart Essential DNA Green Master was used for the quantitative real time PCR (qT-PCR). Gene expression was analysed using the $2^{-\Delta\Delta CT}$ method after results were normalized to *Gapdh* [23]. The primers used in this study were synthesized by Inqaba Biotec (Pretoria, South Africa) and are shown in Table 1.

Table 1. Primers that were used in this study.

Gene	Forward Primer Sequence (5′–3′)	Reverse Primer Sequence (5′–3′)
Gapdh	GATGACATCAAGAAGGTGGTGAAGC	ATACCAGGAAATGAGCTTGACAAAG
Mmp9	GTCATCCAGTTTGGTGTCGCG	AGGGGAAGACGCACAGCTC
Ctsk	CTGGAGGGCCAACTCAAGA	CCTCTGCATTTAGCTGCCTT
Trap	CAGCTGTCCTGGCTCAA	GTAGGCAGTGACCCCGT
cFos	CCCATCGCAGACCAGAGC	ATCTTGCAGGCAGGTCGGT
Dcstamp	ATGACTTGCAACCTAAGGGCAAAG	GTCTGGTTCCAAGAAACAAGGTCAT
Nfatc1	GTGGAGAAGCAGAGCAC	ACGCTGGTACTGGCTTC
Car2	GAGTTTGATGACTCTCAGGACAA	CATATTTGGTGTTCCAGTGAACCA

Gapdh: glyceraldehyde 3-phosphate dehydrogenase; *Mmp9*: matrix metalloproteinase 9; *Ctsk*: cathepsin K; *Trap*: tartrate resistant acid phosphatase; *cFos*: Fos proto-oncogene; *Dcstamp*: dendritic cell-specific transmembrane protein; *Nfatc1*: cytoplasmic 1; *Car2*: carbonic anhydrase 2.

2.9. Western Blotting

RAW264.7 murine macrophages were seeded in a sterile six-well plate at a density of 1×10^6 cells per well and incubated at 37 °C for 24 h. Thereafter, the cells were pre-exposed to PLA (100 µM) or the vehicle (0.1% ethanol) for 4 h. Thereafter, cells were exposed to RANKL (15 ng/mL) in combination with PLA (100 µM) or vehicle (0.1% ethanol) for 30 min. The cells were then lysed in ice-cold radioimmunoprecipitation assay (RIPA) buffer that was already supplemented with protease and phosphatase inhibitors. A bicinchoninic acid (BCA) protein assay kit was used to quantify the purified proteins and equal amounts of protein were resolved on a 12% polyacrylamide gel. Proteins were then electrotransferred onto nitrocellulose membranes with Tris glycine transfer buffer containing 192 mM glycine, 25 mM Tris, and 20% methanol and then probed with specific rabbit antibodies at 4 °C overnight. This was followed by incubation with Immun-Star goat anti-rabbit-horseradish peroxidase conjugate secondary antibody (Bio-Rad, Hercules, CA, USA) and a ChemiDoc MP (Bio-Rad) was then used to obtain digital images of the blots.

2.10. NF-κB/SEAP Assay

RAW264.7 macrophages were stably transfected with pNiFty2-SEAP (Invivogen, San Diego, CA, USA), an NF-κB-inducible reporter plasmid containing $5\times$ NF-κB repeated transcription factor binding sites as well as a reporter gene—secreted embryonic alkaline phosphatase (SEAP), with GeneCellin transfection reagent [25]. Transfected RAW264.7 murine macrophages were seeded into a sterile 96-well plate at a density of 5×10^3 cells per well in serum-free selection medium supplemented with Zeocin. The cells were exposed to PLA (20–100 µM) or vehicle (0.1% ethanol) in combination with RANKL (30 ng/mL) and incubated for 48 h at 37 °C and 5% CO_2. After the culture period, the supernatant was transferred to a separate 96-well plate and heated to 65 °C for 10 min to inhibit endogenous alkaline phosphatase. SEAP assay was conducted as per the manufacturer's instructions.

2.11. Mature Osteoclasts

RAW264.7 murine macrophages were seeded into two sterile 96-well plates at a density of 5×10^3 cells per well for 5 days in the presence of RANKL (15 ng/mL) to allow differentiation. The medium was changed on day 3. On day 5, varying concentrations of PLA (20–100 μM) were added to both plates and incubated for 24 h and 48 h, respectively.

2.11.1. LDH Assay

Necrosis causes permeabilisation of cell plasma membranes, which allows for cellular components such as lactate dehydrogenase (LDH) to leak out of these damaged cells [26]. After the culture period, LDH release was determined as previously mentioned [27]. Readings were taken on a spectrophotometer at an optical absorbance of 490–520 nm.

2.11.2. Hoechst Staining

After the culture period, the cells were washed with PBS and stained with Hoechst in the dark for 5 min. Photomicrographs were taken using a Zeiss inverted Axiovert CFL40 microscope equipped with a Zeiss Axiovert MRm monochrome camera using the following filters: Hoechst (Excitation: 352 nm, Emission: 455 nm) (Carl Zeiss, Oberkochen, Germany).

2.11.3. Statistical Analysis

Three independent experiments were performed in 6-fold, unless otherwise stated, and exposed cells were compared to the vehicle control. Results are displayed as the mean ± the standard deviations. Statistical analysis was done by one-way analysis of variance (ANOVA) followed by a Bonferroni post hoc test using GraphPad Prism software. All p-values ≤ 0.05 were considered significant.

3. Results

3.1. The Effect of PLA on Cell Viability

RAW264.7 murine macrophages were exposed to a concentration gradient of 20–100 μM of PLA for 48 h. These concentrations were not found to be cytotoxic to the cells and were used for further testing (Figure 1).

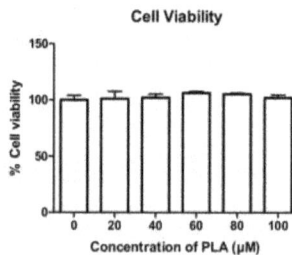

Figure 1. Effect of palmitoleic acid (PLA) on cell viability. Cells were exposed to varying concentrations of PLA (20–100 μM) for 48 h and an Alamar Blue assay was performed to test cell viability. Results are shown as percentage of control and expressed as mean ± standard deviation.

3.2. PLA Inhibits Osteoclast Formation

RAW264.7 murine macrophages were differentiated with RANKL for 5 days in the presence of varying concentrations of PLA. TRAP activity levels (Figure 2A) and number of osteoclasts counted (Figure 2B) were significantly reduced at all concentrations tested. TRAP stain images (Figure 2C) show large, well developed osteoclasts in the RANKL only cells, whereas the size and number of mature osteoclasts reduce with an increase in PLA concentration. The highest reduction was shown at 100 μM, therefore for the PLA concentration of 100 μM only a few multinucleated cells were present. This concentration was used for further experiments.

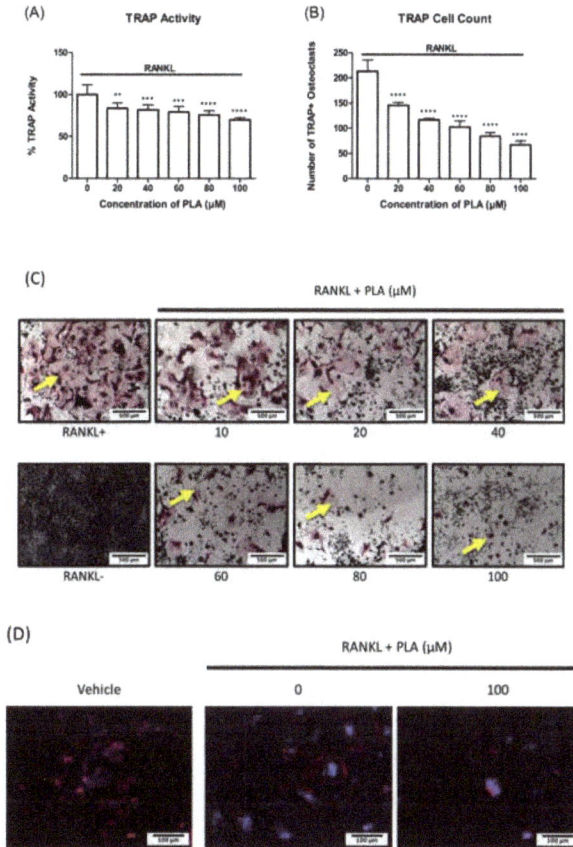

Figure 2. Effect of PLA on tartrate resistant acid phosphatase (TRAP) activity and osteoclastogenesis. RAW264.7 murine macrophages were differentiated into osteoclasts in the presence of receptor activator of NF-κB ligand (RANKL) (15 ng/mL) and PLA (20–100 μM) for five days. (**A**) TRAP activity was determined as described in the methods. Results are shown as percentage of control and expressed as mean ± standard deviation; (**B**) Number of TRAP positive osteoclasts counted at different concentrations; (**C**) Effect of varying concentrations of PLA on osteoclast formation. TRAP positive (pink) osteoclasts are shown by yellow arrows. (Scale bar = 500 μm); (**D**) RAW264.7 murine macrophages were seeded onto glass coverslips with or without of PLA (100 μM) in combination with RANKL (15 ng/mL). Cells were stained for actin (red) and nuclei (blue) using Alexa fluor 568 phalloidin and Hoechst, respectively. (Scale bar = 100 μm). ** $p < 0.01$; *** $p < 0.001$; **** $p < 0.0001$ compared to control.

3.3. The Effect of PLA on RAW264.7 Murine Macrophage Morphology

Actin rings were detected by fluorescent microscopy in order to visualize the structure of the actin rings in mature osteoclasts after treatment with PLA. Large multinucleated cells with clear actin rings are seen in wells exposed to RANKL only. PLA reduced the size and number of the osteoclasts with actin rings (Figure 2D). Furthermore, the actin rings that formed are smaller and incomplete after exposure to PLA.

3.4. PLA Suppresses Bone Resorption

RAW264.7 murine macrophages were seeded onto a 24-well osteoassay plate coated with a layer of bone mimetic substrate. The cells were exposed to RANKL alone or in combination with PLA for 5 days. A decrease in bone resorption was observed with an increase in PLA concentration (Figure 3A). ImageJ software was used to quantify the percentage of bone resorption (Figure 4B). Decreases in bone resorption were shown to be statistically significant.

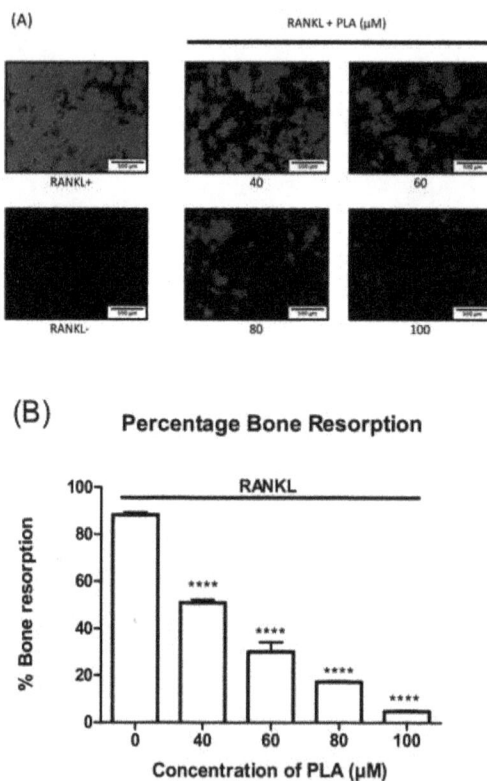

Figure 3. Effect of PLA on bone resorption. RAW264.7 macrophages were seeded onto bone mimetic plates in the presence of RANKL (15 ng/mL) and PLA (40–100 μM) for five days (**A**) Effect of PLA on bone resorption in RAW264.7 murine macrophages. The white areas are where the osteoclasts have resorbed the bone mimetic plate. (Scale bar = 500 μm); (**B**) Resorbed areas were quantified using ImageJ software and expressed as mean ± standard deviation. Results are shown as percentage of control. (**** $p < 0.0001$) compared to control.

3.5. PLA Suppresses the Expression of Osteoclast-Specific Gene Expression

The binding of RANKL to the RANK receptor induces the expression of downstream signalling molecules that play a major role in the formation of osteoclasts as well as the bone resorbing function of mature osteoclasts. PLA (100 µM) treatment significantly reduced the expression of all osteoclast-specific genes tested in this study (Figure 4).

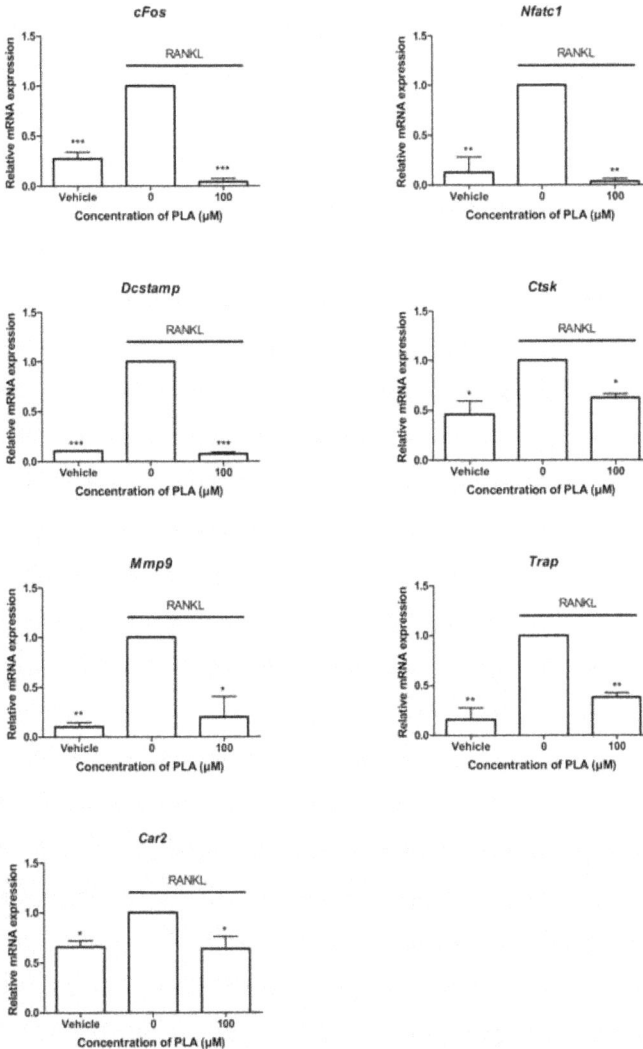

Figure 4. Effect of PLA on osteoclast specific gene expression. RAW264.7 murine macrophages were seeded at 1.5×10^4 cells per well in the presence or absence of PLA (100 µM) in combination with RANKL (15 ng/mL) for five days. RNA was isolated and reverse transcribed into cDNA and relative expression of osteoclast specific genes was determined by quantitative-PCR. Results are expressed relative to the RANKL treated control. (* $p < 0.05$; ** $p < 0.01$; *** $p < 0.001$).

3.6. PLA Inhibits RANKL-Induced Activation of NF-κB and MAPK Pathways

Activation of both the NF-κB and MAPK pathways is integral in the formation and function of osteoclasts. To elucidate the effects of PLA on RANKL-induced NF-κB activation, RAW264.7 macrophages were stably transfected with NF-κB-SEAP reporter plasmid. Cells were treated with PLA (20–100 μM) in combination with RANKL (35 ng/mL) for 24 h. PLA at 80 and 100 μM significantly reduced RANKL-induced NF-κB activation after 24 h (Figure 5A).

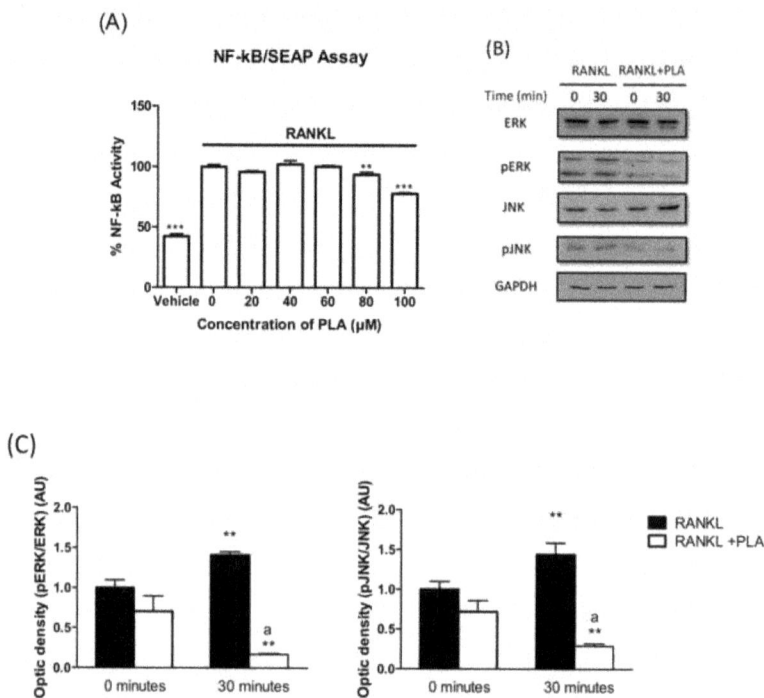

Figure 5. (**A**) RAW264.7 murine macrophages were transfected with nuclear factor kappa B (NF-κB)-SEAP reporter plasmid and exposed to RANKL (35 ng/mL) with or with PLA (20–100 μM) in serum-free selection media for 24 h. Secreted embryonic alkaline phosphatase (SEAP) reporter assay was performed as per the manufacturer's instructions. Results are expressed as percent of positive control. (** $p < 0.01$; *** $p < 0.001$); (**B**). RAW264.7 cells were seeded at 1×10^6 cells per well. Cells were exposed to RANKL (15 ng/mL) and PLA (100 μM) for 30 min. Thereafter cell lysates were prepared and western blot was performed to determine the activation of mitogen activated protein kinase (MAPK) proteins (ERK and JNK). Glyceraldehyde 3-phosphate dehydrogenase (GAPDH) was used as a loading control; (**C**) Densitometry analysis of bands was conducted using ImageJ software. Results are expressed as mean ± standard deviation; $n = 3$ per group (** $p < 0.01$ vs. 0 min RANKL) ([a] $p < 0.001$ vs. 30 min RANKL).

Western blotting was conducted to test the effects of PLA on the activation of the MAPKs: JNK and ERK. After pre-exposing cells to PLA (100 μM) or vehicle for 4 h, cells were treated with RANKL (15 ng/mL) for 30 min. Vehicle control cells showed an increase in the phosphorylated form of the MAPK proteins, indicating activation of these proteins (Figure 5B). PLA suppressed the phosphorylation of both ERK and JNK, indicating inhibition of these pathways (Figure 5C).

3.7. Induction of Apoptosis by PLA in Mature Osteoclasts

To elucidate the action of PLA on mature osteoclasts, RAW264.7 murine macrophages were differentiated in sterile 96-well plates. LDH release for necrosis and Hoechst staining for apoptosis was performed after 24 h and 48 h exposure to PLA. There was no significant increase in LDH release after 24 h or 48 h (Figure 6A). An increase in nuclear condensation and fragmentation was detected in the PLA exposed cells compared to the control (Figure 6B,C).

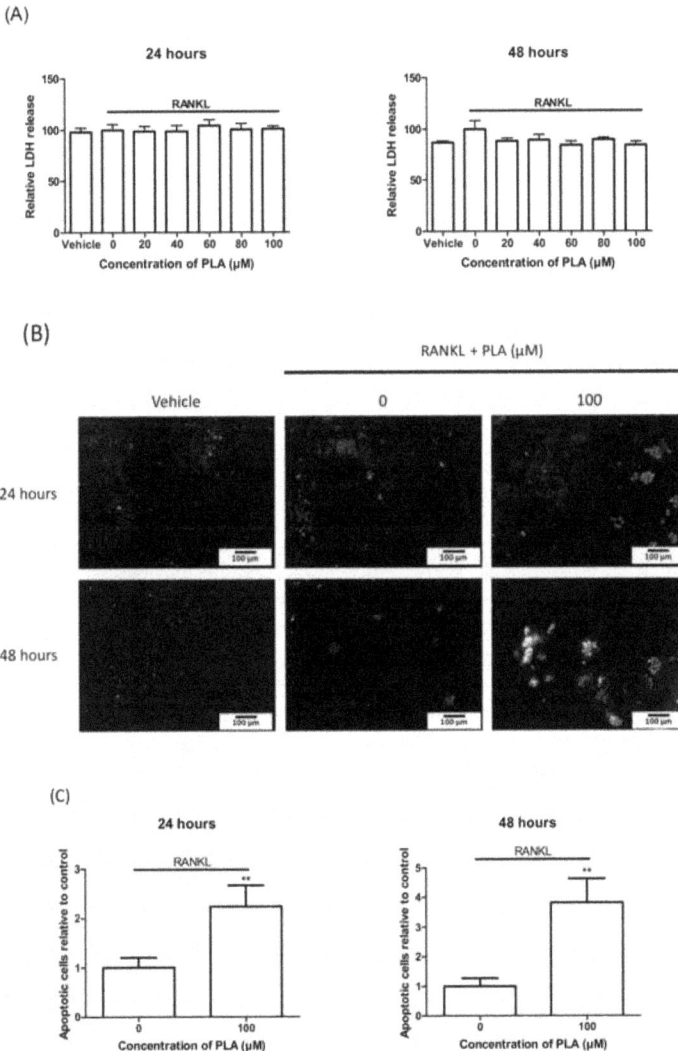

Figure 6. RAW 264.7 murine macrophages were matured in 96-well plates for 5 days followed by exposure to PLA (100 μM) for 24 h or 48 h. (**A**) Lactate dehydrogenase (LDH) results obtained 24 h and 48 h after treatment with PLA. Results are shown as percentage of positive control; (**B**) Hoechst staining performed on mature osteoclasts to visualize nuclear condensation and fragmentation. Scale bar = 100 μm; (**C**) Number of cells with nuclear fragmentation were counted. Results are expressed relative to the control. (** $p < 0.01$).

4. Discussion

Fatty acids (FAs) are key dietary nutrients crucial for health and well-being. FAs are commonly found in nuts, oils, seafood, and various other widely consumed food sources. Several studies have focused on the importance of unsaturated FAs in bone metabolism [8,10,11,28–31]. Chronic inflammatory diseases are known to increase the risk of bone fractures, as pro-inflammatory cytokines amplify the formation of osteoclasts [32]. Therefore, targeting osteoclast formation with anti-inflammatory compounds has been used as a strategy to combat bone diseases characterized by excessive osteoclast activity. For this reason, the effects of ω-3 long-chain polyunsaturated FAs (LCPUFAs) in particular have been studied in osteoclasts, as they are known to exert anti-inflammatory effects. Palmitoleic acid (PLA), an omega-7, 16-carbon monounsaturated FA (MUFA) is also known to possess anti-inflammatory effects [18]; however, the role of PLA on bone health remains unexplored. This study sought to investigate the effects of PLA on differentiating and mature osteoclasts in RAW264.7 murine macrophages to determine if PLA exerts any anti-osteoclastogenic potential.

In this study, the RAW264.7 murine macrophage model was used for osteoclastogenesis. RAW264.7 macrophages fuse and differentiate into mature resorbing osteoclasts in the presence of RANKL and are therefore suitable for studying in vitro effects on RANKL-induced osteoclast formation and activity [33]. Our findings show that PLA inhibited RANKL-induced osteoclastogenesis in RAW264.7 murine macrophages. Inhibition of osteoclast formation was accompanied by changes in morphology. During osteoclast differentiation, cytoskeletal rearrangement leads to the formation of actin rings. These actin rings play a crucial role in maintaining the cell structure, which is important for resorption to occur [34]. In this study, we found that actin ring formation was decreased by PLA. This was accompanied by a significant reduction in the osteolytic ability of osteoclasts derived from RAW264.7 macrophages. The decrease in actin ring formation and resorption was most likely due to inhibition of osteoclast formation by PLA. However, PLA was shown to downregulate genes that play a role in the fusion of osteoclast precursors (*Dcstamp*, dendritic cell-specific transmembrane protein) and in the resorptive process (*Ctsk*, *Mmp9*, *Trap*, *Car2*). This was most likely due to the reduction in *cFos* and *Nfatc1*, which are crucial for the expression of osteoclast specific characteristics [35]. NFATc1 is known as the master regulator of osteoclast formation and function and its activation is a key point in the RANKL signalling cascade.

RANKL-induced activation of *cFos* and *Nfatc1* is downstream of the activation of the NF-κB and MAPK pathways [36]. NF-κB deficient mice have been shown to have no osteoclasts and develop severe osteopetrosis [37]. The MAPKs, p-38 [38], JNK1 [39], and ERK have all been shown to be activated when RANK is stimulated and are critical to osteoclast formation [36]. Therefore, targeting NF-κB and MAPK may lead to decreases in osteoclastogenesis and bone loss. Rahman et al. have shown that the ω-3 LCPUFAs, docosahexaenoic acid (DHA), and eicosapentaenoic acid (EPA) can inhibit osteoclast formation through inhibition of NF-κB nuclear translocation and p-38 expression in RAW264.7 murine macrophages [12]. More recent studies on DHA have shown inhibition of JNK, ERK, and p-38 activation as well as NF-κB activity in mouse bone marrow macrophages [11]. Similar to results on ω-3 LCPUFAs, we found that PLA inhibited NF-κB activity as well as the activation of the MAPKs, JNK and ERK. Supplementation with high doses of EPA and DHA has been shown to decrease bone loss associated with breast cancer [40]. Furthermore, diets rich in ω-3 LCPUFA have been associated with increased bone mineral density and peak bone mass [30]. Our results suggest that PLA may possess bone protective effects similar to ω-3 LCPUFAs.

Additionally, we found that, not only did PLA affect osteoclast formation, it further induced apoptosis in mature osteoclasts. Nuclear condensation and fragmentation are key markers of apoptosis [41]. We report that PLA induced both nuclear condensation and fragmentation in matured osteoclasts indicating apoptosis. Quantification of cells with nuclear fragmentation revealed that exposure to PLA significantly increased the number of apoptotic cells. This result is again similar to results reported on bone marrow macrophages exposed to DHA [11]. When cells are necrotic, their plasma membranes become permeabilized and allow cellular components to leak out [27].

Lactate dehydrogenase (LDH), a soluble cytoplasmic enzyme, is one such component known to leak out of these damaged cells [26]. We found that PLA did not significantly increase LDH release, indicating that the cells were not necrotic. These results indicate that PLA induced programmed cell death in mature osteoclasts.

5. Conclusions

This study reveals the potential anti-osteoclastogenic properties of PLA for the first time. Our findings show that treatment with PLA inhibits RANKL-induced formation of osteoclasts and interfered with the expression of osteoclast-specific genes in vitro. PLA inhibited the activation of the NF-κB and MAPK pathways, offering a possible mechanism of action for its anti-osteoclastogenic effects. PLA further stimulated apoptosis in mature osteoclasts. Therefore, this study provides evidence that PLA may be developed as a nutraceutical for the treatment of diseases characterized by excessive osteoclast formation.

Acknowledgments: Research reported in this publication was supported by the South African Medical Research Council (SAMRC)—Grantholder M. Coetzee.

Author Contributions: Magdalena Coetzee and Abe Kasonga conceived the idea for the study. Bernadette van Heerden carried out the research and analysed the data. Abe Kasonga contributed in experimental design and data interpretation. Abe Kasonga and Bernadette van Heerden wrote the manuscript. Marlena C. Kruger and Magdalena Coetzee provided critical review and manuscript editing. All authors read and approved the final manuscript.

Conflicts of Interest: The authors declare no conflict of interest.

References

1. Raggatt, L.J.; Partridge, N.C. Cellular and molecular mechanisms of bone remodeling. *J. Biol. Chem.* **2010**, *285*, 25103–25108. [CrossRef] [PubMed]
2. Blair, H.C.; Athanasou, N.A. Recent advances in osteoclast biology and pathological bone resorption. *Histol. Histopathol.* **2004**, *19*, 189–199. [PubMed]
3. Bonewald, L.F.; Johnson, M.L. Osteocytes, mechanosensing and wnt signaling. *Bone* **2008**, *42*, 606–615. [CrossRef] [PubMed]
4. Baum, R.; Gravallese, E.M. Impact of inflammation on the osteoblast in rheumatic diseases. *Curr. Osteoporos. Rep.* **2014**, *12*, 9–16. [CrossRef] [PubMed]
5. Boyce, B. Advances in the regulation of osteoclasts and osteoclast functions. *J. Dent. Res.* **2013**, *92*, 860–867. [CrossRef] [PubMed]
6. Teitelbaum, S.L. Bone resorption by osteoclasts. *Science* **2000**, *289*, 1504–1508. [CrossRef] [PubMed]
7. Bar-Shavit, Z. The osteoclast: A multinucleated, hematopoietic-Origin, bone-Resorbing osteoimmune cell. *J. Cell. Biochem.* **2007**, *102*, 1130–1139. [CrossRef] [PubMed]
8. Kasonga, A.E.; Deepak, V.; Kruger, M.C.; Coetzee, M. Arachidonic acid and docosahexaenoic acid suppress osteoclast formation and activity in human cd14+monocytes, in vitro. *PLoS ONE* **2015**. [CrossRef] [PubMed]
9. Kajarabille, N.; Díaz-Castro, J.; Hijano, S.; López-Frías, M.; López-Aliaga, I.; Ochoa, J.J. A new insight to bone turnover: Role of-3 polyunsaturated fatty acids. *Sci. World J.* **2013**. [CrossRef] [PubMed]
10. Boeyens, J.C.; Deepak, V.; Chua, W.H.; Kruger, M.C.; Joubert, A.M.; Coetzee, M. Effects of omega3- and omega6- Polyunsaturated fatty acids on rankl-induced osteoclast differentiation of RAW264.7 cells: A comparative in vitro study. *Nutrients* **2014**, *6*, 2584–2601. [CrossRef] [PubMed]
11. Kim, H.-J.; Ohk, B.; Yoon, H.J.; Kang, W.Y.; Seong, S.J.; Kim, S.-Y.; Yoon, Y.-R. Docosahexaenoic acid signaling attenuates the proliferation and differentiation of bone marrow-Derived osteoclast precursors and promotes apoptosis in mature osteoclasts. *Cell Signal.* **2017**, *29*, 226–232. [CrossRef] [PubMed]
12. Rahman, M.; Bhattacharya, A.; Fernandes, G. Docosahexaenoic acid is more potent inhibitor of osteoclast differentiation in RAW 264.7 cells than eicosapentaenoic acid. *J. Cell. Physiol.* **2008**, *214*, 201–209. [CrossRef] [PubMed]

13. Drosatos-Tampakaki, Z.; Drosatos, K.; Siegelin, Y.; Gong, S.; Khan, S.; Van Dyke, T.; Goldberg, I.J.; Schulze, P.C.; Schulze-Spate, U. Palmitic acid and DGAT1 deficiency enhance osteoclastogenesis, while oleic acid-induced triglyceride formation prevents it. *J. Bone Miner. Res.* **2014**, *29*, 1183–1195. [CrossRef] [PubMed]

14. Guo, X.; Li, H.; Xu, H.; Halim, V.; Zhang, W.; Wang, H.; Ong, K.T.; Woo, S.-L.; Walzem, R.L.; Mashek, D.G. Palmitoleate induces hepatic steatosis but suppresses liver inflammatory response in mice. *PLoS ONE* **2012**, *7*, e39286. [CrossRef] [PubMed]

15. Nestel, P.; Clifton, P.; Noakes, M. Effects of increasing dietary palmitoleic acid compared with palmitic and oleic acids on plasma lipids of hypercholesterolemic men. *J. Lipid Res.* **1994**, *35*, 656–662. [PubMed]

16. Burns, T.; Duckett, S.; Pratt, S.; Jenkins, T. Supplemental palmitoleic (C16:1 *cis*-9) acid reduces lipogenesis and desaturation in bovine adipocyte cultures. *J. Anim. Sci.* **2012**, *90*, 3433–3441. [CrossRef] [PubMed]

17. Dimopoulos, N.; Watson, M.; Sakamoto, K.; Hundal, H.S. Differential effects of palmitate and palmitoleate on insulin action and glucose utilization in rat l6 skeletal muscle cells. *Biochem. J.* **2006**, *399*, 473–481. [CrossRef] [PubMed]

18. Yang, Z.-H.; Miyahara, H.; Hatanaka, A. Chronic administration of palmitoleic acid reduces insulin resistance and hepatic lipid accumulation in kk-A y mice with genetic type 2 diabetes. *Lipids Health Dis.* **2011**, *10*, 1. [CrossRef] [PubMed]

19. Stefan, N.; Kantartzis, K.; Celebi, N.; Staiger, H.; Machann, J.; Schick, F.; Cegan, A.; Elcnerova, M.; Schleicher, E.; Fritsche, A. Circulating palmitoleate strongly and independently predicts insulin sensitivity in humans. *Diabetes Care* **2010**, *33*, 405–407. [CrossRef] [PubMed]

20. Fabbrini, E.; Magkos, F.; Su, X.O.; Abumrad, N.A.; Nejedly, N.; Coughlin, C.C.; Okunade, A.L.; Patterson, B.W.; Klein, S. Insulin sensitivity is not associated with palmitoleate availability in obese humans. *J. Lipid Res.* **2011**, *52*, 808–812. [CrossRef] [PubMed]

21. Mozaffarian, D.; Cao, H.M.; King, I.B.; Lemaitre, R.N.; Song, X.L.; Siscovick, D.S.; Hotamisligil, G.S. Circulating palmitoleic acid and risk of metabolic abnormalities and new-Onset diabetes. *Am. J. Clin. Nutr.* **2010**, *92*, 1350–1358. [CrossRef] [PubMed]

22. Deepak, V.; Kasonga, A.; Kruger, M.C.; Coetzee, M. Inhibitory effects of eugenol on rankl-induced osteoclast formation via attenuation of NF-κB and mapk pathways. *Connect Tissue Res.* **2015**, *56*, 195–203. [CrossRef] [PubMed]

23. Visagie, A.; Kasonga, A.; Deepak, V.; Moosa, S.; Marais, S.; Kruger, M.C.; Coetzee, M. Commercial honeybush (*cyclopia* spp.) tea extract inhibits osteoclast formation and bone resorption in RAW264. 7 murine macrophages—an in vitro study. *Int. J. Environ. Res. Public Health* **2015**, *12*, 13779–13793. [CrossRef] [PubMed]

24. Rasband, W. *Imagej Software*; National Institutes of Health: Bethesda, MD, USA, 1997; Volume 2012.

25. Deepak, V.; Kasonga, A.; Kruger, M.C.; Coetzee, M. Carvacrol inhibits osteoclastogenesis and negatively regulates the survival of mature osteoclasts. *Biol. Pharm. Bull.* **2016**. [CrossRef] [PubMed]

26. Burd, J.; Usategui-Gomez, M. A colorimetric assay for serum lactate dehydrogenase. *Clin. Chim. Acta* **1973**, *46*, 223–227. [CrossRef]

27. Chan, F.K.-M.; Moriwaki, K.; De Rosa, M.J. Detection of necrosis by release of lactate dehydrogenase activity. *Methods Mol. Biol.* **2013**, *979*, 65–70. [PubMed]

28. Shomali, T.; Rezaian, M.; Rassouli, A.; Asadi, F. Effect of eicosapentaenoic acid on bone changes due to ethylprednisolone in rats. *Basic. Clin. Pharm. Toxicol.* **2009**, *105*, 46–50. [CrossRef] [PubMed]

29. Yang, P.; Chan, D.; Felix, E.; Cartwright, C.; Menter, D.G.; Madden, T.; Klein, R.D.; Fischer, S.M.; Newman, R.A. Formation and antiproliferative effect of prostaglandin E3 from eicosapentanoic acid in human lung cancer cells. *J. Lipid Res.* **2004**, *45*, 1030–1039. [CrossRef] [PubMed]

30. Högstrom, M.; Nördstrom, P.; Nördstrom, A. N-3 fatty acids are positively associated with peak bone mineral density and bone accrual in healthy men: The NO$_2$ study. *Am. J. Clin. Nutr.* **2007**, *85*, 803–807.

31. Shimizu, T.; Yokotani, K. Effects of centrally administered prostaglandin E3 and thromboxane A3 on plasma noradrenaline and adrenaline in rats: Comparison with prostaglandin E2 and thromboxane A2. *Eur. J. Pharm.* **2009**, *611*, 30–34. [CrossRef] [PubMed]

32. Redlich, K.; Smolen, J.S. Inflammatory bone loss: Pathogenesis and therapeutic intervention. *Nat. Rev. Drug Discov.* **2012**, *11*, 234–250. [CrossRef] [PubMed]

33. Collin-Osdoby, P.; Osdoby, P. Rankl-Mediated osteoclast formation from murine RAW 264.7 cells. *Bone Res. Protoc. Second Ed.* **2012**, *816*, 187–202.

34. Boyle, W.J.; Simonet, W.S.; Lacey, D.L. Osteoclast differentiation and activation. *Nature* **2003**, *423*, 337–342. [CrossRef] [PubMed]
35. Kim, K.; Lee, S.H.; Kim, J.H.; Choi, Y.; Kim, N. NFATc1 induces osteoclast fusion via up-Regulation of Atp6v0d2 and the dendritic cell-Specific transmembrane protein (DC-STAMP). *Mol. Endocrinol.* **2008**, *22*, 176–185. [CrossRef] [PubMed]
36. Wada, T.; Nakashima, T.; Hiroshi, N.; Penninger, J.M. Rankl-Rank signaling in osteoclastogenesis and bone disease. *Trends Mol. Med.* **2006**, *12*, 17–25. [CrossRef] [PubMed]
37. Xing, L.P.; Chen, D.; Boyce, B.F. Mice deficient in NF-κB p50 and p52 or rank have defective growth plate formation and post-Natal dwarfism. *Bone Res.* **2013**, *1*, 336–345. [CrossRef] [PubMed]
38. Matsumoto, M.; Sudo, T.; Saito, T.; Osada, A.; Tsujimoto, M. Involvement of p38 mitogen-Activated protein kinase signaling pathway in osteoclastogenesis mediated by receptor activator of NF-κB ligand (RANKL). *J. Biol. Chem.* **2000**, *275*, 31155–31161. [CrossRef] [PubMed]
39. David, J.P.; Sabapathy, K.; Hoffmann, O.; Idarraga, M.H.; Wagner, E.F. Jnk1 modulates osteoclastogenesis through both c-Jun phosphorylation-Dependent and independent mechanisms. *J. Cell Sci.* **2002**, *115*, 4317–4325. [CrossRef] [PubMed]
40. Hutchins-Wiese, H.L.; Picho, K.; Watkins, B.A.; Li, Y.; Tannenbaum, S.; Claffey, K.; Kenny, A.M. High-Dose eicosapentaenoic acid and docosahexaenoic acid supplementation reduces bone resorption in postmenopausal breast cancer survivors on aromatase inhibitors: A pilot study. *Nut. Cancer Int. J.* **2014**, *66*, 68–76. [CrossRef] [PubMed]
41. Saraste, A.; Pulkki, K. Morphologic and biochemical hallmarks of apoptosis. *Cardiovasc. Res.* **2000**, *45*, 528–537. [CrossRef]

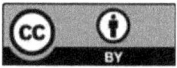

nutrients

MDPI

Article

Distribution of Constituents and Metabolites of Maritime Pine Bark Extract (Pycnogenol®) into Serum, Blood Cells, and Synovial Fluid of Patients with Severe Osteoarthritis: A Randomized Controlled Trial

Melanie Mülek [1], Lothar Seefried [2], Franca Genest [2] and Petra Högger [1,*]

[1]   Institut für Pharmazie und Lebensmittelchemie, Universität Würzburg, 97074 Würzburg, Germany;
      melanie.muelek@pharmazie.uni-wuerzburg.de
[2]   Department of Orthopedics, Orthopedic Center for Musculoskeletal Research, 97074 Würzburg, Germany;
      l-seefried.klh@uni-wuerzburg.de (L.S.); f-genest.klh@uni-wuerzburg.de (F.G.)
*   Correspondence: petra.hoegger@uni-wuerzburg.de; Tel.: +49-931-318-5468; Fax: +49-931-318-5494

Received: 17 March 2017; Accepted: 26 April 2017; Published: 28 April 2017

Abstract: The present randomized controlled study aimed to investigate the in vivo distribution of constituents or metabolites of the standardized maritime pine bark extract Pycnogenol®. Thirty-three patients with severe osteoarthritis scheduled for a knee arthroplasty were randomized to receive either 200 mg per day Pycnogenol® (P+) or no treatment (Co) over three weeks before surgery. Serum, blood cells, and synovial fluid samples were analyzed using liquid chromatography coupled to tandem mass spectrometry with electrospray ionization (LC-ESI/MS/MS). Considerable interindividual differences were observed indicating pronounced variability of the polyphenol pharmacokinetics. Notably, the highest polyphenol concentrations were not detected in serum. Catechin and taxifolin primarily resided within the blood cells while the microbial catechin metabolite δ-(3,4-dihydroxy-phenyl)-γ-valerolactone, ferulic, and caffeic acid were mainly present in synovial fluid samples. Taxifolin was detected in serum and synovial fluid exclusively in the P+ group. Likewise, no ferulic acid was found in serum samples of the Co group. Calculating ratios of analyte distribution in individual patients revealed a simultaneous presence of some polyphenols in serum, blood cells, and/or synovial fluid only in the P+ group. This is the first evidence that polyphenols distribute into the synovial fluid of patients with osteoarthritis which supports rationalizing the results of clinical efficacy studies.

Keywords: pine bark extract; LC-ESI/MS/MS; randomized controlled study; osteoarthritis; human; polyphenols

1. Introduction

Dietary polyphenols have been associated with numerous beneficial effects on human health. Studies investigating the absorption of polyphenols from the gastrointestinal tract revealed that blood concentrations of individual polyphenols are often very low [1]. Moreover, polyphenolic compounds are often subjected to an extensive metabolism [2]. Some metabolites generated by gut microbial metabolism obviously contribute to health effects [3].

One of those bioactive metabolites is δ-(3,4-dihydroxy-phenyl)-γ-valerolactone (M1) which is formed by the human intestinal flora from the procyanidins' catechin units [2]. It has been detected in urine and plasma samples after intake of Pycnogenol® [4,5]. The dietary supplement Pycnogenol® is a standardized extract of the French maritime pine, which conforms to the monograph *"Maritime pine extract"* in the United States Pharmacopeia (USP). It contains 65%–75% oligomeric procyanidins and polyphenolic monomers, phenolic, or cinnamic acids and their glycosides [6].

In numerous clinical studies Pycnogenol® demonstrated effects in different chronic diseases of, for example, inflammatory or cardiovascular origin [6,7].

Another chronic disease with high pharmacoeconomic burden and significant impact on the patients' quality of life is osteoarthritis (OA). OA is a chronic degenerative joint disease which is characterized by progressive cartilage destruction and it is the leading cause of pain and disability [8]. Treatment of OA includes pharmacological and non-pharmacological interventions and aims at pain relief and improvement of function. Severe OA might also require surgical interventions such as knee or hip arthroplasty [9]. Dietary factors or supplements have been discussed as options in the management or prevention of OA [10].

In clinical studies OA symptoms such as pain and joint stiffness have been shown to improve upon intake of Pycnogenol® [11,12]. While this clinical observation is consistent with a previously shown inhibition of nuclear factor κB (NF-κB) activation and inhibition of various matrix metalloproteinases by constituents or metabolites of this pine bark extract [13,14], it is not clear yet whether bioactive polyphenols would actually be present at the site of disease (e.g., in the joints affected by OA). After an oral intake of multiple doses of Pycnogenol® concentrations in the nanomolar range of catechin, taxifolin, caffeic acid, ferulic acid, and of a bioactive metabolite M1 have been detected in human plasma [5]. Moreover, an uptake of M1 into erythrocytes, monocytes, and endothelial cells has been observed in vitro [15,16]. The purpose of the current study was to investigate the in vivo distribution of constituents or metabolites of Pycnogenol® in serum, blood cells, and synovial fluid of patients with severe OA scheduled for a knee replacement surgery.

2. Materials and Methods

2.1. Clinical Study Design

The present study was a randomized controlled clinical trial involving patients with severe osteoarthritis (OA) according to the Western Ontario and McMaster Universities Arthritis Index (WOMAC) score, who were scheduled for an elective knee replacement surgery (Kellgren-Lawrence grade III–IV). Patients were not eligible if they regularly took non-steroidal anti-inflammatory drugs (NSAIDs) or glucocorticoids perorally within the past four weeks, if they currently received a therapy with anti-coagulants, or if they tested positive for the human immunodeficiency virus (HIV), hepatitis B or C, or if they had a previous or current infection of the affected knee joint. As rescue medication acetaminophen (paracetamol), tramadol, or a combination of tilidine and naloxone was allowed. The study was conducted in accordance with the Declaration of Helsinki, and the protocol was approved by the local Ethics Committee of the Medical Faculty of the University Würzburg (Project identification code 248/11).

A total of 33 OA patients were recruited for the study and gave informed written consent before they participated in the study. The chosen number of patients was based on a previous pharmacokinetic study with healthy volunteers receiving the pine bark extract [5]. Patients were randomized into two groups using a computer-generated randomization list which was not accessible to the physicians and nurses who were involved in the patient care and management. Study participants (n = 16) were assigned to the treatment group receiving 200 mg of the French maritime pine bark extract Pycnogenol® (Horphag Research Ltd., Geneva, Switzerland) per day (twice daily two capsules with each 50 mg) over three weeks prior to the planned surgery. The control group was comprised of 17 patients who did not receive Pycnogenol®. All patients were asked to comply with a polyphenol-free nutrition, especially two days before each blood sampling. For this purpose, they were provided with nutritional check-lists specifying food/beverages they should avoid and for recording what they ingested within the last two days before blood sampling. Adherence to the study medication was estimated based on the number of returned Pycnogenol® capsules upon hospitalization for the knee replacement surgery.

Blood samples from each study participant were collected (BD Vacutainer® SST II Advance; Becton Dickinson GmbH, Heidelberg, Germany) before oral intake of Pycnogenol® (V1, basal value);

during the intake, approximately 1–2 days before the surgery (V2); and during or shortly before knee surgery (V3), about 12 h after the last dose of Pycnogenol®. Immediately after blood sampling the serum and cellular fraction were separated under sterile conditions. On the day of the surgery residual knee cartilage and synovial fluid were also collected. All samples were shock-frozen immediately and stored at −80 °C. The outcome measure was the concentration of pine bark extract-derived polyphenols in serum, blood cells, and synovial fluid as determined by liquid chromatography coupled to tandem mass spectrometry with electrospray ionization (LC-ESI/MS/MS).

All medical procedures including enrollment of participants, surgery, patient care, and sample collection took place at the orthopedic center (Orthopädie und Orthopädische Klinik König-Ludwig-Haus, Universität Würzburg) between September 2012 and September 2014. The generation of the random allocation sequence, assignment of participants to the intervention or control group, and analysis of all patient samples took place at the Institut für Pharmazie und Lebensmittelchemie. Since the study primarily focused on pharmacokinetic/bioanalytical aspects, specifically on the analysis of polyphenols in various human specimen, an early registration was overlooked and the study was registered retroactively.

2.2. Chemicals, Reagents, and Special Materials

Analytical standards of (+)-catechin, taxifolin, ferulic acid, caffeic acid, and the internal standard (IS) 3,4-dihydroxyhydrocinnamic acid (hydrocaffeic acid) were all obtained from Sigma-Aldrich (Taufkirchen, Germany). The metabolite M1 (δ-(3.4-dihydroxy-phenyl)-γ-valerolactone) was synthesized by M. Rappold as part of his diploma thesis. Methanol (MeOH, LC-MS analyzed) from J.T.Baker Mallinckrodt and water (HiPerSolv CHROMANORM® for LC-MS) were obtained from VWR (Darmstadt, Germany). Ammonium formate (AF) and formic acid (FA) were purchased from Sigma-Aldrich. An enzymatic mixture of β-glucuronidase/sulfatase (β-Gln/Sulfa) from *Helix pomatia* (Type HP-2; Sigma-Aldrich) was used for enzymatic hydrolysis. Ethyl acetate, *tert*-butyl methyl ether (MTBE), and phosphate buffered saline (PBS, pH 7.4) were obtained from Sigma-Aldrich.

2.3. Standard Solutions

Stock solutions (1 mg/mL) of each standard substance ((+)-catechin, taxifolin, ferulic acid, caffeic acid, and M1) and of the internal standard (IS; hydrocaffeic acid) were prepared in 100% methanol and stored at −80 °C. They were diluted with methanol to yield working standards which were aliquoted and stored at −20 °C.

2.4. Human Specimen for Calibration Curves

Packed cells and serum were obtained from a blood bank (Bayerisches Rotes Kreuz (BRK), München, Germany) and handled as previously described [17,18]. Synovial fluid was collected from patients with intra-articular fluid accumulation who needed punctuation of the effusion for medical reasons. Synovial fluid samples were pooled to obtain a single batch for preparation of calibration standards for quantification of the clinical study samples.

2.5. Liquid Chromatography (LC)

Details of the LC method have been reported before [18,19]. Briefly, for the LC analysis an Agilent 1260 system was used. The chromatographic separation was carried out using a Pursuit PFP-C18 column (4.6 × 150 mm, particle size 3 μm) at 20 °C (all from Agilent Technologies, Santa Clara, CA, USA). The mobile phase consisted of 5 mM ammonium formate with 0.065% (*v/v*) formic acid (pH = 3.2; A) and methanol with 0.1% formic acid (B). The flow rate was set to 0.6 mL/min and the sample injection volume was 5 μL. The gradient elution was conducted starting at 60% B (0 min) to 95% B (2.50 min) and maintained to 95% B to 5.50 min followed by re-equilibration at 60% B. The total run time was 10.00 min with a post time of 3 min.

2.6. Mass Spectrometry (MS/MS)

Details of the MS/MS method using a G 6460 TripleQuad LC/MS with turbo electrospray ionization (ESI; Agilent Technologies, Santa Clara, CA, USA) have been previously reported [17,18]. The optimized MS/MS transitions and mass spectrometric parameters of the compounds to be quantified in human blood cell and serum samples were recently reported [18,19]; optimized parameters of additionally determined M1 metabolites in blood cells are listed in Table S1 in the electronic supplementary material. Optimized MS/MS transitions and mass spectrometric parameters of the compounds to be quantified in human synovial fluid samples are listed in Table S2.

2.7. Preparation of Human Serum Samples

Serum samples (1.5 mL) were prepared by liquid-liquid extraction with prior enzymatic incubation containing β-Gln/Sulfa to hydrolyze conjugated analytes [5], as previously described [18,19]. Additionally, 1.5 mL of serum was analyzed without prior enzymatic hydrolysis to calculate the degree of conjugation with sulfate and glucuronic acid.

2.8. Preparation of Human Blood Cell Samples

Human blood cell samples were prepared as previously detailed [18]. Therefore, 2.0 mL blood cells of each study volunteer were processed with prior enzymatic hydrolysis to determine the total concentration of the analytes.

2.9. Preparation of Human Synovial Fluid Samples

Synovial fluid samples were prepared with a newly developed and optimized liquid-liquid extraction method. Therefore, 40 µL 4% o-phosphoric acid was added to 1.0 mL human synovial fluid (pH 5.0). Afterwards, the samples were incubated with an enzyme mixture containing β-Gln/Sulfa (1500 U β-Gln and 2 U Sulfatase per mL synovial fluid) for 45 min at 37 °C on a horizontal shaker (100 rpm) to hydrolyze conjugated analytes [5]. Then, 60 µL 4% o-phosphoric acid (pH 3.2), 25 µL IS (24.85 ng/mL), and 3.0 mL extraction solvent containing ethyl acetate and *tert*-butyl methyl ether (1:1; *v/v*) were added, vortexed for 1 min (Multi-Vortex, VWR, Darmstadt, Germany), and centrifuged for 5 min at $3300 \times g$ (4 °C). Thereafter, 2.0 mL of the upper organic layer was evaporated to dryness under nitrogen. The residue was reconstituted in 75 µL of 100% MeOH and centrifuged at $18,000 \times g$ for 15 min at 4 °C before LC-MS/MS analysis.

A full validation was performed for the quantification of the analytes in human synovial fluid with the optimized liquid-liquid extraction method and prior enzymatic hydrolysis. The validation included the selectivity, linearity, lower limit of quantification (LLOQ), accuracy and precision (intra- and interday), recovery, process efficiency, matrix effects (quantitative), carry over, cross talk, and post-preparative stability. Also, the freeze- and thaw-, short-term-, and long-term stability of the analytes in human serum were investigated.

2.10. Quantification of the Samples of the Study Participants

For each patient, specimen human pooled matrix-matched calibration standards with an internal standard (structural) were used for quantification of the study samples. In case of a basal presence of an analyte in the blank matrix, the calibration curve was shifted along the y axis by the response of the zero-sample (containing the IS) [20].

2.11. Statistical Analysis

Data were analyzed using descriptive statistics. Typically, mean and standard deviation (SD) were calculated. For comparison of the study participants' basic demographic characteristics a Student's *t*-test was used to compare the patients of the treatment and control group.

3. Results

3.1. Patients and Protocol Adherence

A total of 33 patients were enrolled into the study and randomized to receive either Pycnogenol® (n = 16) or no treatment (n = 17). One patient of the control group decided against the scheduled knee replacement surgery and was excluded. During the surgical procedure, there was a failure to collect blood, synovial fluid, and cartilage samples for one patient in both the control group and the Pycnogenol® group. These patients were excluded from the analysis (Figure 1). Thus, 30 patients (66.7% female) underwent analysis after receiving Pycnogenol® ("P+"; 9 females, 6 males) or no treatment as the control group ("Co"; 11 females, 4 males). There was no statistically significant difference between the groups in any of the basic demographic characteristics (Student's *t*-test, $p > 0.05$), the mean age (± standard deviation SD) was 64.3 ± 8.2 years, height 1.69 ± 0.10 m, body weight 87.33 ± 15.66 kg (BMI 30.74 ± 5.29 kg/m^2).

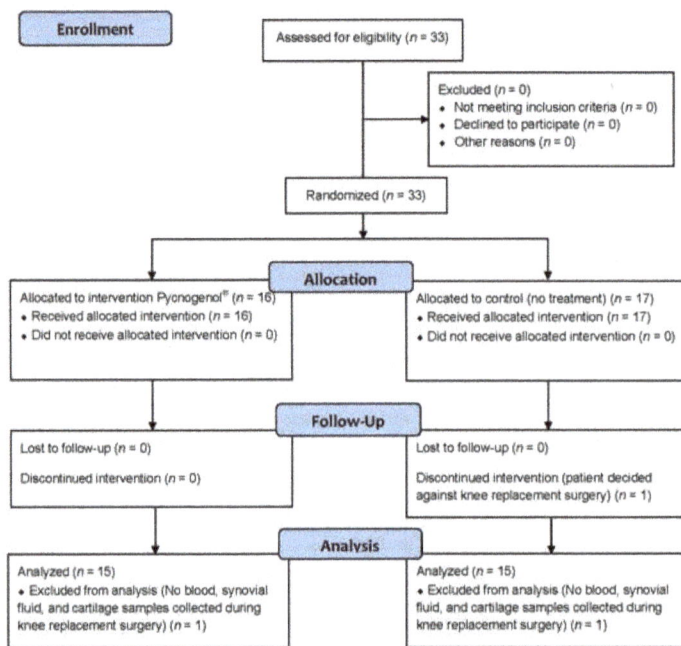

Figure 1. CONSORT (Consolidated Standards of Reporting Trials; www.consort-statement.org) 2010 Flow diagram of the study.

All study participants were requested to avoid polyphenol-rich food/beverages (e.g., coffee, green tea, wine, chocolate, some fruits and vegetables) within the last two days before the blood samplings. Analysis of the nutrition protocols revealed that the nutritional advice was not followed well and dietary violations were admitted before collecting 42% of the blood samples. Thus, concentrations of common polyphenols such as catechin or caffeic acid from other sources than Pycnogenol® were to be expected in the blood samples.

In contrast, the adherence to the study medication was excellent based on the pill count-back on returned medication containers. In the Pycnogenol® group the average adherence was 99.4% (range 96%–100%) for all but one study participant who apparently took only 76% of the capsules.

No treatment-associated adverse effects were reported except for one patient of the Pycnogenol® group who experienced flatulence.

3.2. Method for Analysis of Polyphenols in Human Synovial Fluid Samples

To the best of our knowledge, this is the first study describing the detection and quantification of polyphenols in human synovial fluid. Since concentrations in synovial fluid samples were possibly lower than in blood and based on the fact that a previous pharmacokinetic study revealed plasma concentrations of polyphenolic compounds in the nanomolar range after intake of Pycnogenol® [5], a highly sensitive method was required. In the course of method development, the main focus was the optimal detection and quantification of the metabolite M1.

Analogous to previously developed methods for analysis of Pycnogenol® polyphenols in serum and blood cells [18,19], various sample preparation techniques were compared and a liquid-liquid extraction method was chosen. For the analytes of highest interests, the lower limits of quantification (LLOQs) in synovial fluid were 0.080 ng/mL for taxifolin and 0.117 ng/mL for M1 (Table 1 and Table S9). The method was slightly less sensitive for ferulic acid (LLOQ of 1.53 ng/mL), catechin (2.14 ng/mL), and caffeic acid (3.07 ng/mL).

Table 1. Lower limits of quantification (LLOQs) of polyphenolic analytes of highest interest. Data for serum and blood cells was derived from previous work [18,19].

Analyte	LLOQ Synovial Fluid (ng/mL)	LLOQ Serum (ng/mL)	LLOQ Blood Cells (ng/mL)
Catechin	2.14	5.86	28.90
M1	0.12	0.16	0.12
Taxifolin	0.08	0.06	0.12
Caffeic Acid	3.07	8.22	48.40
Ferulic Acid	1.53	2.74	0.97

In the supplementary materials, details about the recovery, matrix effects, and process efficiency (Tables S10 and S11), as well as the internal standard normalized matrix factor (Table S12) in pooled and individual lots of synovial fluid are documented. The method was validated based on current EMA (European Medicines Agency) and FDA (US Food and Drug Administration) guidelines and complied with the requirements for selectivity, linearity (Table S3), precision and accuracy (Tables S6 and S7), robustness (Table S6), carry-over, cross-talk, and post-preparative stability (Tables S9 and S10).

Representative chromatograms of all three specimens of an individual study participant after multiple dosing of 200 mg/day Pycnogenol® over the course of three weeks (P+, V3) revealed total concentrations of 23.17 ng/mL catechin, 3.70 ng/mL ferulic acid, 0.19 ng/mL taxifolin, 0.16 ng/mL M1 in serum, 74.31 ng/mL catechin, 1.93 ng/mL ferulic acid, and 0.57 ng/mL taxifolin in blood cells, and 3.19 ng/mL ferulic acid, 0.18 ng/mL taxifolin, and 0.17 ng/mL M1 in synovial fluid (Figure 2).

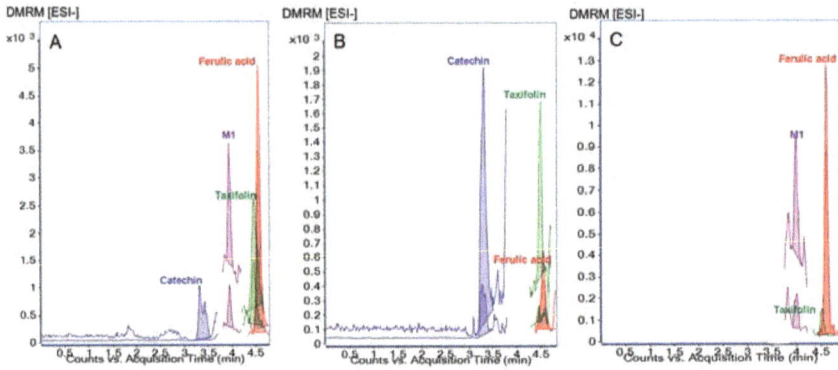

Figure 2. Example chromatograms for quantification in the three different sample matrices of one individual study participant after multiple dosing of 200 mg/day Pycnogenol® over the course of three weeks (P+, V3). (**A**) Serum; (**B**) Blood cells; (**C**) Synovial fluid.

3.3. Pycnogenol® Constituents and Metabolites in Serum Samples

In the basal serum samples (V1) the mean total concentrations (free and conjugated) of all study participants were 27.07 ± 16.39 ng/mL catechin (mean and standard deviation), 1.80 ± 2.63 ng/mL for M1, 0.07 ng/mL ($n = 1$) for taxifolin, 6.40 ± 2.58 ng/mL for ferulic acid, and 18.58 ± 6.32 ng/mL for caffeic acid. For example, catechin was detectable in 29 out of 30 V1 samples, and in 24 samples the concentrations were above 10 ng/mL. Thereby, catechin was primarily present as glucuronide-/sulfate-conjugate. When only the free concentrations were regarded, catechin was detectable in 20 out of 30 V1 samples, and in 11 samples the concentrations were above 10 ng/mL. There were no apparent differences in the basal concentrations between the participants assigned to the P+ or Co group. Even when disregarding those patients who admitted a violation of the dietary restrictions there were still considerable basal concentrations present in serum.

The analysis of serum samples obtained after three weeks (V3) of Pycnogenol® intake revealed the highest concentrations for catechin, followed by caffeic acid, ferulic acid, M1, and taxifolin (Table 2, panel A). Although there was a tendency of higher concentrations of catechin in the P+ compared to the control group, the serum concentrations of M1 and caffeic acid in the control group exceeded those in the P+ group (Table 2, panel A). When patients who admitted intake of, for example, coffee, green tea, or chocolate were excluded from the analysis the trend of higher catechin levels as well as clearly higher concentrations of M1 in the P+ group became obvious and caffeic acid was not even detectable in the control group (Table 2, panel B).

Table 2. Results of the sample analysis in serum, blood cells, and synovial fluid of patients taking Pycnogenol® 200 mg/day (P+) and control patients (Co) receiving no supplement. The population numbers (n) indicate the number of patients with detectable concentrations of the respective polyphenol. **A**: Total mean concentrations and standard deviations (SD) determined after three weeks (V3) without exclusion of patients who admitted violations of the dietary restrictions; **B**: Total mean concentrations and SD determined after three weeks (V3). Patients who admitted violations of the dietary restrictions in their nutritional protocols were excluded. n.d.: not detected; Conc.: concentration.

A		Catechin Conc. (ng/mL) ± SD		M1 Conc. (ng/mL) ± SD		Taxifolin Conc. (ng/mL) ± SD		Ferulic Acid Conc. (ng/mL) ± SD		Caffeic Acid Conc. (ng/mL) ± SD	
Serum	P+	52.53 ± 18.40	$n = 15$	0.54 ± 0.84	$n = 9$	0.20 ± 0.12	$n = 5$	3.02 ± 0.39	$n = 7$	9.28 ± 0.51	$n = 3$
	Co	45.85 ± 39.59	$n = 15$	1.07 ± 1.09	$n = 5$	n.d.	-	n.d.		14.84 ± 1.92	$n = 3$
Blood Cells	P+	71.18 ± 27.34	$n = 14$	0.19 ± 0.07	$n = 12$	0.52 ± 0.23	$n = 15$	1.86 ± 0.36	$n = 10$	n.d.	-
	Co	70.48 ± 36.22	$n = 13$	0.21 ± 0.05	$n = 5$	0.48 ± 0.32	$n = 15$	1.80 ± 0.85	$n = 7$	n.d.	-
Synovial Fluid	P+	2.99 ± 0.43	$n = 4$	0.62 ± 0.77	$n = 5$	0.21 ± 0.03	$n = 2$	4.29 ± 1.83	$n = 8$	10.32 ± 3.96	$n = 7$
	Co	3.94 ± 1.83	$n = 2$	0.78 ± 0.74	$n = 4$	n.d.	-	3.04 ± 0.79	$n = 6$	12.83 ± 8.95	$n = 10$

B		Catechin Conc. (ng/mL) ± SD		M1 Conc. (ng/mL) ± SD		Taxifolin Conc. (ng/mL) ± SD		Ferulic Acid Conc. (ng/mL) ± SD		Caffeic Acid Conc. (ng/mL) ± SD	
Serum	P+	48.41 ± 18.61	$n = 11$	0.70 ± 1.02	$n = 6$	0.20 ± 0.12	$n = 5$	3.09 ± 0.46	$n = 5$	9.78	$n = 1$
	Co	32.24 ± 17.38	$n = 8$	0.25 ± 0.05	$n = 2$	n.d.	-	n.d.		n.d.	-
Blood Cells	P+	73.75 ± 29.25	$n = 11$	0.20 ± 0.07	$n = 9$	0.56 ± 0.19	$n = 11$	1.85 ± 0.38	$n = 9$	n.d.	-
	Co	63.31 ± 31.28	$n = 7$	0.18 ± 0.05	$n = 2$	0.39 ± 0.16	$n = 8$	1.69 ± 0.10	$n = 3$	n.d.	-
Synovial Fluid	P+	3.00 ± 0.58	$n = 2$	0.92 ± 0.93	$n = 3$	0.21 ± 0.03	$n = 2$	4.31 ± 2.10	$n = 6$	10.63 ± 3.86	$n = 4$
	Co	2.65	$n = 1$	0.17 ± 0.03	$n = 2$	n.d.	-	3.16 ± 0.22	$n = 3$	10.99 ± 5.79	$n = 4$

The degree of analyte conjugation with sulfate and glucuronic acid in serum was determined for all samples (V1 and V3) and ranged from 54.29% ± 26.77% for catechin ($n = 51$) to 98.34% ± 4.40% for M1 ($n = 30$; Table 3).

Table 3. Mean and standard deviation (SD) of the conjugation degree in serum samples (both P+ and Co group; V1, V2, and V3 blood samples; in total $n = 90$ samples). Results were compared with former investigations [5].

Analytes	Conjugation Degree (%)					
	Current Study			Former Investigation		
	Mean	± SD	Sample Size	Mean	± SD	Sample Size
Catechin	54.29	26.77	$n = 51$	56.50	27.90	$n = 5$
M1	98.34	4.40	$n = 30$	100 *		
Taxifolin	96.75	7.23	$n = 11$	100 *		
Ferulic Acid	90.32	16.58	$n = 24$	100 *		
Caffeic Acid	80.95	17.95	$n = 10$	69.40	11.80	$n = 3$

* A conjugation degree of 100% was assumed because no free concentrations were detectable.

3.4. Pycnogenol® Constituents and Metabolites in Blood Cell Samples

As seen with the serum samples before, basal total concentrations of the analytes with the exception of caffeic acid were detectable at V1, with no differences between the participants assigned to the P+ or Co group. Mean concentrations of 61.38 ± 40.25 ng/mL catechin (mean ± SD), 1.68 ± 0.55 ng/mL ferulic acid, 0.40 ± 0.18 ng/mL taxifolin, and 0.19 ± 0.08 ng/mL M1 were determined.

The analysis of blood cell samples obtained after three weeks (V3) of intake of Pycnogenol® revealed the highest concentrations for catechin, followed by ferulic acid, M1, and taxifolin (Table 2, panel A). No caffeic acid was detectable in any of the samples. There were no clear differences in the concentrations determined in the P+ or Co group. When patients who admitted non-adherence to the dietary restrictions were excluded from the analysis there was a slight trend towards higher catechin, taxifolin, and ferulic acid levels in the P+ group compared to the control group (Table 2, panel B).

In the V3 samples of the P+ group, the open-chained ester form of M1 (M1-COOH; $n = 5$; Figure S1A) was identified as well as the glutathione conjugate of M1 (M1-GSH; $n = 1$; Figure S1B). In the V3 samples of the Co group, only the M1-COOH was detected in one patient sample.

3.5. Pycnogenol® Constituents and Metabolites in Synovial Fluid Samples

In the present study, synovial fluid samples were obtained at the time of knee surgery. The analysis revealed the highest concentrations for caffeic acid, followed by ferulic acid, catechin, M1, and taxifolin (Table 2, panel A). With the exception of taxifolin, there were no vast differences in the concentrations of the other polyphenols.

3.6. Distribution of Pycnogenol® Constituents and Metabolites between Specimen

To exclude the chance that individual trends in distribution of the analytes were overlooked if only group mean concentrations were considered, the individual ratios of the analyte concentrations in the different specimen of single patients were calculated and summarized (Figure 3).

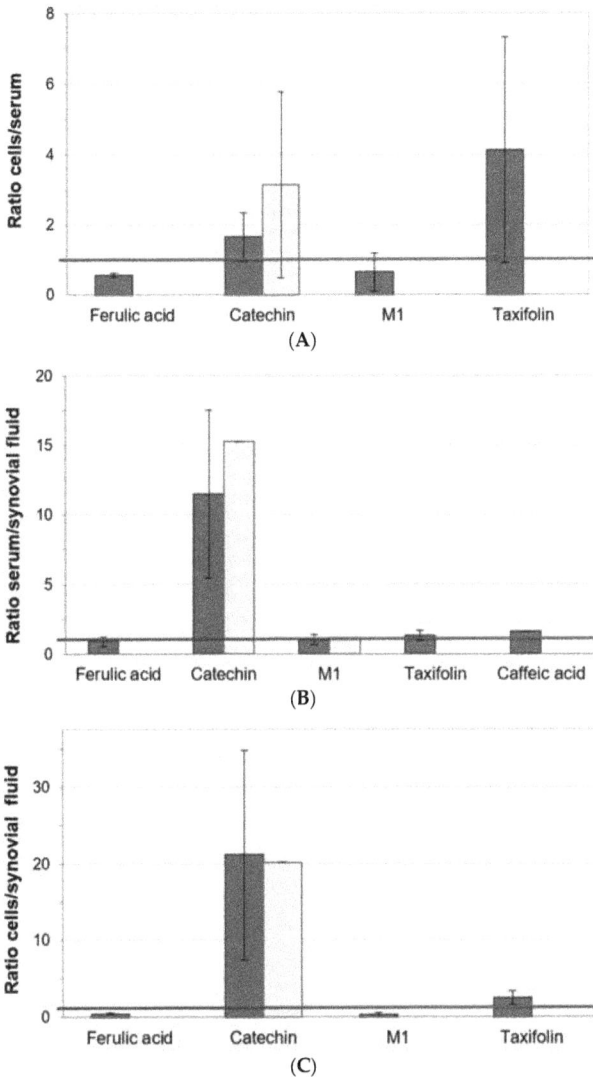

Figure 3. Summarized individual ratios of the analyte concentrations in different specimens of single study participants. Columns of the intervention (P+; dark gray) and control (Co; light grey) group represent the mean and standard deviation of the individual calculated ratios. (**A**) Ratio cells/serum. (**B**) Ratio serum/synovial fluid. (**C**) Ratio cells/synovial fluid.

The mean and standard deviations of the individual concentration ratios of the analytes in blood cells and serum (total concentrations, V3) showed that ferulic acid (0.56 ± 0.06; $n = 4$), M1 (0.64 ± 0.54; $n = 5$), and taxifolin (4.11 ± 3.21; $n = 5$) were detected in both matrices exclusively in the P+ group (Figure 3, panel A). With ratios above 1.0, taxifolin and catechin were clearly more present in blood cells compared to serum. In the patient group receiving 200 mg/day Pycnogenol®, the catechin distribution into blood cells (1.65 ± 0.69; $n = 11$) was less pronounced than in the control group (3.14 ± 2.65; $n = 7$).

The individual concentration ratios of analytes in serum and synovial fluid revealed that in both patient groups catechin was primarily distributed into serum compared to the synovial fluid

(P+: 11.51 ± 6.04; n = 4 and Co: 15.27; n = 1; Figure 3, panel B). Caffeic acid (1.60; n = 1), taxifolin (1.33 ± 0.38; n = 2), and ferulic acid (0.89 ± 0.32; n = 4) were present in both matrices only after intake of Pycnogenol® and not in the control group. Ferulic acid preferentially resided in the synovial fluid, while taxifolin and caffeic acid showed the opposite tendency. The metabolite M1 was detected both in the P+ (1.01 ± 0.37; n = 3) and Co group (1.14; n = 1) and it appeared to be almost in equilibrium between serum and synovial fluid.

The individual analyte distribution between blood cells and synovial fluid revealed a strong tendency of catechin for localization within blood cells compared to the synovial fluid (Figure 3, panel C). This was observed in both groups of the study participants (P+: 21.11 ± 13.70; n = 2 and Co: 20.15; n = 1). Taxifolin (2.48 ± 0.90; n = 2), M1 (0.27 ± 0.27; n = 2), and ferulic acid (0.45 ± 0.15; n = 5)) were present in both matrices exclusively in the P+ group. With a distribution ratio higher than 1.0, taxifolin was more present in blood cells compared to synovial fluid, while M1 and ferulic acid preferentially resided in the synovial fluid.

4. Discussion

In the present study, the in vivo distribution of constituents and metabolites of the maritime pine extract Pycnogenol® between human serum, blood cells, and synovial fluid was investigated for the first time. A newly developed and validated highly sensitive LC-ESI/MS/MS method allowed for the detection and quantification of various polyphenolic compounds in synovial fluid and thereby facilitated the proof that polyphenols are actually distributed into joints.

Analysis of samples obtained before the start of the intervention (V1) revealed that catechin and other polyphenols were ubiquitously present in human serum samples at measurable basal levels. Similar observations have been reported by others [21]. Based on the fact that the most controlled condition (lifestyle/diet, timely intake of Pycnogenol® capsules) the patients were subjected to was after their hospitalization (V3) when they were under observation of a study nurse, data analysis focused on V3 samples comparing the intervention (P+) with the control group (Co).

As already observed in an earlier pharmacokinetic study [5], not all polyphenols were discovered in biofluid samples of all participants, which reflected the high interindividual variablity of absorption, distribution, metabolism, and/or elimination of plant constituents. The fact that the time between the last intake of Pycnogenol® and the collection of the specimen slightly varied around 12 h might have also contributed to the variability of measured compound concentrations. Although the mean polyphenol concentrations in serum, blood cells, and synovial fluid were similar in the P+ and Co group, due to non-adherence to the dietary restrictions, distinctive observations were made in the P+ group.

In serum samples, taxifolin and ferulic acid were only detectable in the P+, not in the Co group. In a previous pharmacokinetic study with healthy volunteers, taxifolin was not detectable under steady state conditions, which was most probably due to the less sensitive analytical method [5]. This is consistent with the very low concentrations of taxifolin found in the present study. Ferulic acid has been suggested to be a marker of consumption of maritime pine bark extract. In healthy volunteers adhering to a low polyphenol diet, both free and conjugated ferulic acid were determined in urine samples [22].

The conjugation degree of the investigated polyphenols in serum was high and ranged from 54.29% ± 26.77% for catechin to 98.34% ± 4.40% for M1. This is consistent with the data determined in a former investigation [5]. However, as observed before and reported by others [22], the interindividual variability of the conjugation degree of the analytes was high. Even in the individual person the degree of conjugation cannot be regarded as a constant since it apparently also depends on the current analyte concentration in the specimen [23].

Blood cells and erythrocytes represent a significant pharmacological compartment for distribution of xenobiotics [24,25]. Individual polyphenols have been shown to accumulate in human blood cells, macrophage-derived foam, or endothelial cells [15,16,25,26]. Notably, only low concentrations of

M1 were found in the cellular fraction of the blood samples. This apparently contradicts previous results showing an enhanced cellular uptake of M1, possibly via the GLUT-1 transporter, into human erythrocytes [16]. However, M1 is subsequently subjected to an extensive intracellular metabolism [17] which would explain the low remaining intracellular levels of M1 under steady state conditions. Consequently, the blood cells samples of the present study were also screened for the presence of any of the previously detected cellular M1 metabolites [17]. Indeed, in the P+ group, the open-chained ester form of M1 (M1-COOH) and the glutathione conjugate of M1 (M1-GSH) were identified, though not quantified. In the Co group, only M1-COOH was detected.

Sampling of synovial fluid is typically practiced for diagnostic reasons (e.g., for detection of a septic arthritis). In research, there is great interest in osteoarthritis biomarkers such as cytokines that might assist diagnosis or prognosis [27]. In contrast, drug concentrations are rarely reported for synovial fluid samples. To the best of our knowledge, this is the first study investigating polyphenol concentrations in human synovial fluid samples of patients with osteoarthritis. Similar to the results of serum analysis, mean polyphenol concentrations were similar in the P+ and Co groups, but taxifolin was only detectable in the P+ group. Thus, it might be a marker of Pycnogenol® consumption.

Comparing mean concentrations of the constituents and metabolites in serum, blood cells, and synovial fluid revealed that the individual compounds did not distribute equally between the specimen. Notably, the highest concentrations of the polyphenols were not detected in serum. Catechin and taxifolin primarily resided within the blood cells, while M1, ferulic, and caffeic acid were mainly present in synovial fluid samples. Generally, data on distribution of polyphenols in humans is scarce. Although numerous investigations focus on absorption, metabolism, and elimination of polyphenols [1,28], only a few studies investigate the distribution, for example, into human tissues [29,30]. Distribution into or accumulation in certain body compartments might help with understanding the effects of polyphenols despite the typically low plasma/serum concentrations that are usually observed [1,29].

Although there were some trends towards higher analyte concentrations in the specimen of the patients who received Pycnogenol® in the present study, the mean concentrations were similar for both groups and were subject to high interindividual variability. It was possible that individual trends in distribution of the analytes could have been overlooked if only group mean concentrations were considered. Therefore, the individual ratios of the analyte concentrations in the different specimens of single patients were calculated and summarized. Since ratios higher than 1 indicate that the analyte is primarily distributed into, for example, blood cells compared to serum, it can be concluded that higher concentrations of taxifolin and catechin were present in blood cells while ferulic acid and M1 preferentially resided in serum. This observation confirms the differential distribution of polyphenolic compounds between serum, blood cells, and synovial fluid that was already seen when mean concentrations were examined. On an individual level, a simultaneous presence of ferulic acid, M1, and taxifolin in blood cells and serum or cells and synovial fluid was only observed after intake of the pine bark extract. Also, ferulic acid, taxifolin, and caffeic acid were only detected in both serum and synovial fluid in the P+ group.

The fact that the control group received no placebo capsules to conceal the allocation to the intervention group could be seen as a potential study limitation. However, the primary interest was the bioanalysis of polyphenols in different specimens, and it is highly unlikely that any of the analyte concentrations were deliberately influenced by the patients' knowledge of group allocation. All analytical procedures were fully validated and left no room for subjective data interpretation. A study limitation was the small group size. Since not all polyphenols were present in the biofluid samples of all patients due to interindividual pharmacokinetic differences and also as a result of the non-adherence of the participants to the dietary restrictions, a statistical differentiation between the groups was not feasible. However, the results of the present study provide a basis for sample size calculations in future studies. Those studies would then be sufficiently powered for statistical analysis and could reliably uncover significant differences between treatment and control groups. The fact that the study participants of the present study did not follow the dietary suggestions improves the generalizability of the results since they mirror real life conditions under which foods or beverages rich in polyphenols are occasionally or regularly consumed.

5. Conclusion

The results of this study provide the first evidence that polyphenols distribute into the synovial fluid of patients with osteoarthritis, which supports rationalizing the results of clinical efficacy studies.

Supplementary Materials: The following are available online at http://www.mdpi.com/2072-6643/9/5/443/s1, Figure S1: Example chromatograms for identification of intracellular metabolites of M1 in blood cells of study participants after multiple dosing of 200 mg/day Pycnogenol® over the course of three weeks (P+, V3), Table S1: Additional optimized transitions and parameters in dynamic multiple reaction monitoring (DMRM) mode for identification of compounds in human blood cells, Table S2: Optimized transitions and parameters in dynamic multiple reaction monitoring (DMRM) employing negative ESI ionization mode for LC-MS/MS analysis of prepared synovial fluid samples, Table S3: Calibration range, calibration function and correlation coefficients of the five analytes extracted from human pooled synovial fluid, Table S4: Intraday accuracy and precision of the analytes in human pooled synovial fluid, Table S5: Interday accuracy and precision of the analytes in human pooled synovial fluid, Table S6: Robustness of the developed method at two concentrations with human pooled synovial fluid which was intentionally contaminated with 1% human whole blood, Table S7: Post-preparative stability: autosampler stability of the analytes after 6 h and 12 h at room temperature after previous LC/MS/MS analysis, Table S8: Post-preparative stability: stability of the analytes after one freeze-thaw cycle, Table S9: Lower limit of quantification (LLOQ) and related accuracy of the five analytes extracted from human pooled synovial fluid, Table S10: Recovery, matrix effects and process efficiency of the five analytes extracted from human pooled synovial fluid at three concentrations, Table S11: Recovery, matrix effects and process efficiency of the five analytes extracted from three lots of synovial fluid at two concentrations, Table S12: Internal standard (hydrocaffeic acid) normalized matrix factor at human pooled synovial fluid in three concentrations and in three lots of synovial fluid at two concentrations.

Acknowledgments: We gratefully acknowledge the excellent assistance of Jasmin Bauman and Ursula Hellwich (Orthopedic Center for Musculoskeletal Research, Würzburg) in patient management. We would like to thank Bruno Pasurka, Würzburg, for help with the collection of synovial fluid samples used for calibration standard preparation. We are grateful for an unrestricted educational grant from Horphag Research Ltd. The study sponsor was not involved in the study design, collection, analysis and interpretation of data, in writing the manuscript or in the decision to submit the manuscript for publication. This publication was funded by the German Research Foundation (DFG) and the University of Würzburg in the funding program Open Access Publishing.

Author Contributions: M.M. planned and performed the experiments and contributed to drafting of the manuscript; L.S. and F.G. were involved in patient management, recording of clinical data, and contributed to drafting of the manuscript; P.H. conceived of and planned the study and contributed to drafting of the manuscript.

Conflicts of Interest: M.M. declares no conflict of interests. P.H., L.S., and F.G. received research grants from Horphag Research, the producer of Pycnogenol®, within the past five years.

References

1. Manach, C.; Williamson, G.; Morand, C.; Scalbert, A.; Remesy, C. Bioavailability and bioefficacy of polyphenols in humans. I. Review of 97 bioavailability studies. *Am. J. Clin. Nutr.* **2005**, *81*, 230S–242S. [PubMed]
2. Monagas, M.; Urpi-Sarda, M.; Sanchez-Patan, F.; Llorach, R.; Garrido, I.; Gomez-Cordoves, C.; Andres-Lacueva, C.; Bartolome, B. Insights into the metabolism and microbial biotransformation of dietary flavan-3-ols and the bioactivity of their metabolites. *Food Funct.* **2010**, *1*, 233–253. [CrossRef] [PubMed]
3. Högger, P. Nutrition-derived bioactive metabolites produced by gut microbiota and their potential impact on human health. *Nutr. Med. (NUME)* **2013**, *1*, 1.
4. Düweler, K.G.; Rohdewald, P. Urinary metabolites of French maritime pine bark extract in humans. *Pharmazie* **2000**, *55*, 364–368. [PubMed]
5. Grimm, T.; Skrabala, R.; Chovanova, Z.; Muchova, J.; Sumegova, K.; Liptakova, A.; Durackova, Z.; Högger, P. Single and multiple dose pharmacokinetics of maritime pine bark extract (Pycnogenol) after oral administration to healthy volunteers. *BMC Clin. Pharmacol.* **2006**, *6*, 4. [CrossRef] [PubMed]
6. Rohdewald, P. A review of the French maritime pine bark extract (Pycnogenol), a herbal medication with a diverse clinical pharmacology. *Int. J. Clin. Pharmacol. Ther.* **2002**, *40*, 158–168. [CrossRef] [PubMed]

7. Maimoona, A.; Naeem, I.; Saddiqe, Z.; Jameel, K. A review on biological, nutraceutical and clinical aspects of French maritime pine bark extract. *J. Ethnopharmacol.* **2011**, *133*, 261–277. [CrossRef] [PubMed]
8. Silverwood, V.; Blagojevic-Bucknall, M.; Jinks, C.; Jordan, J.L.; Protheroe, J.; Jordan, K.P. Current evidence on risk factors for knee osteoarthritis in older adults: A systematic review and meta-analysis. *Osteoarthr Cartil.* **2015**, *23*, 507–515. [CrossRef] [PubMed]
9. McAlindon, T.E.; Bannuru, R.R.; Sullivan, M.C.; Arden, N.K.; Berenbaum, F.; Bierma-Zeinstra, S.M.; Hawker, G.A.; Henrotin, Y.; Hunter, D.J.; Kawaguchi, H.; et al. Oarsi guidelines for the non-surgical management of knee osteoarthritis. *Osteoarthr Cartil.* **2014**, *22*, 363–388. [CrossRef] [PubMed]
10. Green, J.A.; Hirst-Jones, K.L.; Davidson, R.K.; Jupp, O.; Bao, Y.; MacGregor, A.J.; Donell, S.T.; Cassidy, A.; Clark, I.M. The potential for dietary factors to prevent or treat osteoarthritis. *Proc. Nutr. Soc.* **2014**, *73*, 278–288. [CrossRef] [PubMed]
11. Belcaro, G.; Cesarone, M.R.; Errichi, S.; Zulli, C.; Errichi, B.M.; Vinciguerra, G.; Ledda, A.; Di Renzo, A.; Stuard, S.; Dugall, M.; et al. Treatment of osteoarthritis with Pycnogenol. The SVOS (San Valentino Osteo-arthrosis Study). Evaluation of signs, symptoms, physical performance and vascular aspects. *Phytother. Res.* **2008**, *22*, 518–523. [CrossRef] [PubMed]
12. Cisar, P.; Jany, R.; Waczulikova, I.; Sumegova, K.; Muchova, J.; Vojtassak, J.; Durackova, Z.; Lisy, M.; Rohdewald, P. Effect of pine bark extract (Pycnogenol) on symptoms of knee osteoarthritis. *Phytother. Res.* **2008**, *22*, 1087–1092. [CrossRef] [PubMed]
13. Grimm, T.; Schäfer, A.; Högger, P. Antioxidant activity and inhibition of matrix metalloproteinases by metabolites of maritime pine bark extract (Pycnogenol). *Free Radic. Biol. Med.* **2004**, *36*, 811–822. [CrossRef] [PubMed]
14. Grimm, T.; Chovanova, Z.; Muchova, J.; Sumegova, K.; Liptakova, A.; Durackova, Z.; Högger, P. Inhibition of NF-κb activation and MMP-9 secretion by plasma of human volunteers after ingestion of maritime pine bark extract (Pycnogenol). *J. Inflamm. (Lond.)* **2006**, *3*, 1. [CrossRef] [PubMed]
15. Uhlenhut, K.; Högger, P. Facilitated cellular uptake and suppression of inducible nitric oxide synthase by a metabolite of maritime pine bark extract (Pycnogenol). *Free Radic. Biol. Med.* **2012**, *53*, 305–313. [CrossRef] [PubMed]
16. Kurlbaum, M.; Mülek, M.; Högger, P. Facilitated uptake of a bioactive metabolite of maritime pine bark extract (Pycnogenol) into human erythrocytes. *PLoS ONE* **2013**, *8*, e63197. [CrossRef] [PubMed]
17. Mülek, M.; Fekete, A.; Wiest, J.; Holzgrabe, U.; Mueller, M.J.; Högger, P. Profiling a gut microbiota-generated catechin metabolite's fate in human blood cells using a metabolomic approach. *J. Pharm. Biomed. Anal.* **2015**, *114*, 71–81. [CrossRef] [PubMed]
18. Mülek, M.; Högger, P. Highly sensitive analysis of polyphenols and their metabolites in human blood cells using dispersive SPE extraction and LC-MS/MS. *Anal. Bioanal. Chem.* **2015**, *407*, 1885–1899. [CrossRef] [PubMed]
19. Mülek, M. Distribution and Metabolism of Constituents and Metabolites of a Standardized Maritime Pine Bark Extract (Pycnogenol®) in Human Serum, Blood Cells and Synovial Fluid of Patients with Severe Osteoarthritis. Ph.D. Thesis, Julius Maximilians-Universität, Würzburg, Germany, 2015.
20. Cavaliere, C.; Foglia, P.; Gubbiotti, R.; Sacchetti, P.; Samperi, R.; Lagana, A. Rapid-resolution liquid chromatography/mass spectrometry for determination and quantitation of polyphenols in grape berries. *Rapid Commun. Mass Spectrom.* **2008**, *22*, 3089–3099. [CrossRef] [PubMed]
21. Henning, S.M.; Wang, P.; Abgaryan, N.; Vicinanza, R.; de Oliveira, D.M.; Zhang, Y.; Lee, R.P.; Carpenter, C.L.; Aronson, W.J.; Heber, D. Phenolic acid concentrations in plasma and urine from men consuming green or black tea and potential chemopreventive properties for colon cancer. *Mol. Nutr. Food Res.* **2013**, *57*, 483–493. [CrossRef] [PubMed]
22. Virgili, F.; Pagana, G.; Bourne, L.; Rimbach, G.; Natella, F.; Rice-Evans, C.; Packer, L. Ferulic acid excretion as a marker of consumption of a French maritime pine (*Pinus maritima*) bark extract. *Free Radic. Biol. Med.* **2000**, *28*, 1249–1256. [CrossRef]
23. Soleas, G.J.; Yan, J.; Goldberg, D.M. Ultrasensitive assay for three polyphenols (catechin, quercetin and resveratrol) and their conjugates in biological fluids utilizing gas chromatography with mass selective detection. *J. Chromatogr. B Biomed. Sci. Appl.* **2001**, *757*, 161–172. [CrossRef]
24. Highley, M.S.; de Bruijn, E.A. Erythrocytes and the transport of drugs and endogenous compounds. *Pharm. Res.* **1996**, *13*, 186–195. [CrossRef] [PubMed]

25. Biasutto, L.; Marotta, E.; Hgarbisa, S.; Zoratti, M.; Paradisi, C. Determination of quercetin and resveratrol in whole blood—Implications for bioavailability studies. *Molecules* **2010**, *15*, 6570–6579. [CrossRef] [PubMed]
26. Kawai, Y.; Tanaka, H.; Murota, K.; Naito, M.; Terao, J. (−)-epicatechin gallate accumulates in foamy macrophages in human atherosclerotic aorta: Implication in the anti-atherosclerotic actions of tea catechins. *Biochem. Biophys. Res. Commun.* **2008**, *374*, 527–532. [CrossRef] [PubMed]
27. Mabey, T.; Honsawek, S. Cytokines as biochemical markers for knee osteoarthritis. *World J. Orthop.* **2015**, *6*, 95–105. [CrossRef] [PubMed]
28. Clifford, M.N.; van der Hooft, J.J.; Crozier, A. Human studies on the absorption, distribution, metabolism, and excretion of tea polyphenols. *Am. J. Clin. Nutr.* **2013**, *98*, 1619S–1630S. [CrossRef] [PubMed]
29. Henning, S.M.; Aronson, W.; Niu, Y.; Conde, F.; Lee, N.H.; Seeram, N.P.; Lee, R.P.; Lu, J.; Harris, D.M.; Moro, A.; et al. Tea polyphenols and theaflavins are present in prostate tissue of humans and mice after green and black tea consumption. *J. Nutr.* **2006**, *136*, 1839–1843. [PubMed]
30. Del Rio, D.; Borges, G.; Crozier, A. Berry flavonoids and phenolics: Bioavailability and evidence of protective effects. *Br. J. Nutr.* **2010**, *104* (Suppl. 3), S67–S90. [CrossRef] [PubMed]

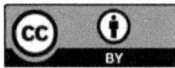

nutrients

MDPI

Review

Bone-Protective Effects of Dried Plum in Postmenopausal Women: Efficacy and Possible Mechanisms

Bahram H. Arjmandi [1,2,*], Sarah A. Johnson [3], Shirin Pourafshar [1,2], Negin Navaei [1,2,4], Kelli S. George [1,2], Shirin Hooshmand [5], Sheau C. Chai [6] and Neda S. Akhavan [1,2]

[1]   Department of Nutrition, Food and Exercise Sciences, College of Human Sciences, Florida State University, Tallahassee, FL 32306, USA; sp12r@my.fsu.edu (S.P.); negin.navaei@life.edu (N.N.); ksg15c@my.fsu.edu (K.S.G.); nsa08@my.fsu.edu (N.S.A.)
[2]   Center for Advancing Exercise and Nutrition Research on Aging (CAENRA), College of Human Sciences, Florida State University, Tallahassee, FL 32306, USA
[3]   Department of Food Science and Human Nutrition, College of Health and Human Sciences, Colorado State University, Fort Collins, CO 80523, USA; Sarah.Johnson@colostate.edu
[4]   Department of Nutrition, College of Graduate and Undergraduate Studies, Life University, Marietta, GA 30060, USA
[5]   School of Exercise and Nutritional Sciences, College of Health & Human Services, San Diego State University, San Diego, CA 92182, USA; shooshmand@mail.sdsu.edu
[6]   Department of Behavioral Health and Nutrition, College of Health Sciences, University of Delaware, Newark, DE 19716, USA; scchai@udel.edu
*   Correspondence: barjmandi@fsu.edu; Tel.: +1-850-645-1517

Received: 15 April 2017; Accepted: 12 May 2017; Published: 14 May 2017

Abstract: Osteoporosis is an age-related chronic disease characterized by a loss of bone mass and quality, and is associated with an increased risk of fragility fractures. Postmenopausal women are at the greatest risk of developing osteoporosis due to the cessation in ovarian hormone production, which causes accelerated bone loss. As the demographic shifts to a more aged population, a growing number of postmenopausal women will be afflicted with osteoporosis. Certain lifestyle factors, including nutrition and exercise, are known to reduce the risk of developing osteoporosis and therefore play an important role in bone health. In terms of nutrition, accumulating evidence suggests that dried plum (*Prunus domestica* L.) is potentially an efficacious intervention for preventing and reversing bone mass and structural loss in an ovariectomized rat model of osteoporosis, as well as in osteopenic postmenopausal women. Here, we provide evidence supporting the efficacy of dried plum in preventing and reversing bone loss associated with ovarian hormone deficiency in rodent models and in humans. We end with the results of a recent follow-up study demonstrating that postmenopausal women who previously consumed 100 g dried plum per day during our one-year clinical trial conducted five years earlier retained bone mineral density to a greater extent than those receiving a comparative control. Additionally, we highlight the possible mechanisms of action by which bioactive compounds in dried plum exert bone-protective effects. Overall, the findings of our studies and others strongly suggest that dried plum in its whole form is a promising and efficacious functional food therapy for preventing bone loss in postmenopausal women, with the potential for long-lasting bone-protective effects.

Keywords: bioactive compounds; functional foods; menopause; nutrition; polyphenols; (poly)phenols; prune; osteopenia; osteoporosis

1. Introduction

The postmenopausal period typically occupies one-third of a woman's life [1], and it is estimated that by the year 2020, more than 46 million women in the United States (U.S.) will be postmenopausal [2]. Menopause is associated with the development of numerous chronic diseases [3], due to an abrupt cessation of ovarian hormone production, namely estrogen. Osteoporosis is a chronic and debilitating age-related skeletal disease characterized by the loss of bone mass and a deterioration of the microstructural properties of bone, resulting in an increased propensity for fragility fractures [4]. Osteoporosis is responsible for more than 1.5 million fractures per year in the U.S., with most occurring in postmenopausal women [5]. Osteoporosis and its related bone fractures are a major public health concern as they are associated with increased morbidity and mortality, a poor quality of life, and a large economic burden [6,7]. Approximately 44 million men and women over the age of 50 have osteoporosis or low bone mass in the U.S. [3]. Diminished estrogen levels associated with menopause result in an initial phase of rapid bone loss, followed by a period of a slower deterioration of the skeleton [8]. This rapid phase of bone loss occurs within the first five to 10 years following the cessation of menses or the surgical removal of the ovaries [9]. As the demographic shifts to a more aged population, the prevalence and incidence of osteoporosis are likely to continue to increase, with affected individuals being at a greater risk of falls, fragility fractures, and therefore morbidity and mortality [3]. As such, therapeutic strategies that can delay, slow down, or prevent bone loss in aging individuals, and particularly in postmenopausal women, are critically needed.

Hormone replacement therapy is a logical therapeutic strategy for postmenopausal women since age-related chronic disease development typically begins after the cessation of ovarian hormone production. However, evidence from the Women's Health Initiative indicates that the risks associated with hormone replacement therapy outweigh its benefits, making the exploration of alternative therapies necessary [10]. Although the Food and Drug Administration has approved several anti-resorptive pharmacological agents such as bisphosphonates and denosumab, as well as the bone-forming pharmacological agent teriparatide, these drugs are associated with adverse side effects, are costly, and often have low compliance [11]. Therefore, it is imperative that safe and cost-effective therapeutic strategies, aside from medications, that can delay, slow down, or prevent bone loss in postmenopausal women be identified, investigated for efficacy, and disseminated for public use.

It is well-known that certain lifestyle factors, including diet and nutrition, play an important role in bone health. In fact, research has demonstrated that certain foods (i.e., functional foods) and their bioactive compounds, including nutrient and non-nutrient compounds, have bone-protective effects [12]. Of the functional foods investigated for their bone-protective properties, the most efficacious have typically been in the form of fruits and vegetables. The findings from our studies [13–15] and others [16,17] suggest that dried plum (*Prunus domestica* L.) is the most effective in preventing and reversing bone loss among the fruits and vegetables investigated. This has also been demonstrated by Mühlbauer et al. [18,19], who examined the effects of 60 fruits and vegetables on bone. Their findings indicated that onion and dried plum had the most potent bone-protective effects. Though the consumption of fruits and vegetables for general health and well-being is encouraged, in terms of bone health, not all fruits and vegetables offer the same benefits. For instance, while certain fruits such as dried plum and to some extent blueberries exert bone-protective effects [20], in our observations [14], the same may not be true for other fruits such as raisins and dates. We are using a conditional term for the effectiveness of blueberry on bone, because our findings [20], as well as those of Zhang et al. [21,22], are preliminary at this point and await confirmation in human studies. The reasons for these discrepancies in the efficacy among fruits and vegetables remain unknown.

Due to the bioactive compound content and composition of dried plum, as well as promising preclinical and clinical research findings, dried plum has been and continues to be investigated as a potential functional food with respect to bone health. Numerous studies in cells, rodent models of postmenopausal osteoporosis, and postmenopausal women have demonstrated its efficacy and have identified possible mechanisms of action. Studies have aimed to identify specific bioactive compounds in dried plum responsible for its bone-protective properties. The present review provides an overview of dried plum, including its nutritional and bioactive compound composition, and provides evidence from preclinical and clinical studies supporting the efficacy of dried plum in preventing and reversing bone loss in postmenopausal women, as well as evidence to support possible mechanisms of action, and bioactive compounds in dried plum responsible for its efficacy. Additionally, gaps in the research and promising new areas of investigation are discussed.

A literature search was performed using the PubMed database and Google Scholar. The following keywords, alone and in combination, were used: bone, dried plum, menopause, osteopenia, osteoporosis, ovariectomy, ovariectomized, plum, postmenopausal, and prune. Preclinical studies using rodent models of postmenopausal osteoporosis and clinical trials with postmenopausal women were included in this review.

2. Dried Plum: A Promising Functional Food for Bone Health

The U.S., primarily California, is a major producer of dried plum, with approximately 99% of the U.S. and 40% of the world supply grown in California. Dried plum was previously referred to as prunes until a formal name change was requested and approved by the Food and Drug Administration in 2001 [23]. It is most commonly known for its effects on gastrointestinal motility and research has been and continues to be conducted with respect to gastrointestinal health to support these observations. In addition, dried plum has been investigated for its antimicrobial, cancer-preventive, cardiometabolic, neurological, and bone-protective effects [24,25].

To date, the most notable research has been in the area of bone metabolism and health. The unique ability of dried plum to promote bone health is likely related to its bioactive compound composition. Dried plum is rich in nutrient bioactive compounds including dietary fiber, vitamin K, boron, copper, magnesium, manganese, among others, many of which are known to positively influence bone [23–25]. It is also rich in non-nutrient bioactive compounds including (poly)phenols such as chlorogenic acids (e.g., chlorogenic acid, neochlorogenic acid, cryptochlorogenic acid) and proanthocyanidins [24,25]. Dried plum has been ranked as having one of the highest oxygen radical absorbance capacities among the commonly consumed fruits and vegetables. It has been suggested that this is likely to be primarily due to its (poly)phenolic compound composition and content, as dried plum is low in ascorbic acid, carotenoids, and vitamin E [23]. In addition, previous research has demonstrated that phenolic compounds, including those found in dried plum, exert bone-protective effects and profoundly affect bone metabolism [25]. For instance, rutin, a flavonoid commonly found in plums and various berries, has been reported to inhibit ovariectomy-induced bone loss in a rat model of osteoporosis [26]. Nonetheless, the question still remains as to which bioactive component(s) of dried plum are responsible for its bone-protective effects. The answer may simply be that the whole fruit is more efficacious than its isolated components due to the additive and/or synergistic effects of these components within the food matrix.

3. Dried Plum and Bone Health: Rodent Models of Postmenopausal Osteoporosis

Previous studies investigating the role of dried plum on bone health in rodent models of postmenopausal osteoporosis are summarized in Table 1. Our laboratory [27] was the first to report the bone-protective effects of dried plum both in general, and specifically in an established rat model of postmenopausal osteoporosis [28]. We showed that ovariectomy led to significant declines in the bone mineral density (BMD) of the 4th lumbar vertebrae and femurs, as well as a decrease in the tibial trabecular bone area compared to sham-operated (Sham) rats. However, ovariectomized (Ovx) rats that received 25% of the diet as dried plum for 45 days did not lose bone, while those receiving 5% of the diet as dried plum lost bone similarly to Ovx rats not receiving dried plum (Figure 1). Despite this, we also found that dried plum dose-dependently increased circulating insulin-like growth factor-I (IGF-I) levels, while having no effect on tartrate-resistant acid phosphatase-5b (TRAP-5b) levels. At that time, TRAP-5b was considered to be a biomarker of bone resorption. Therefore, these results suggested that dried plum prevented bone loss, in part, by increasing the rate of bone formation, but not through inhibiting bone resorption.

(A)   (B)

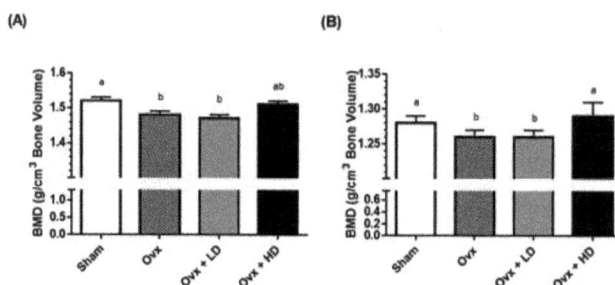

Figure 1. (**A**) Effects of ovariectomy and dried plum on bone density of right femur; (**B**) Effects of ovariectomy and dried plum on bone density of 4th lumbar spine. Bars represent mean ± standard error of the mean. Bars that do not share the same letters are significantly ($p < 0.05$) different from each other. BMD, bone mineral density; HD, high dose (25%) dried plum; LD, low dose (5%) dried plum; Ovx, ovariectomized; Sham, sham-operated.

We next asked the question: could the addition of dried plum to the diet restore bone mass after bone loss has occurred? Toward this end, our laboratory [27] used an Ovx rat model of postmenopausal osteoporosis to evaluate the ability of dried plum at different doses to reverse bone loss. In this study, 90-day-old female Sprague-Dawley rats were divided into six groups: Sham control, Ovx control, Ovx + 17β-estradiol (E$_2$), Ovx + 5% of the diet as dried plum, Ovx + 15% of the diet as dried plum, and Ovx + 25% of the diet as dried plum for 60 days. Interestingly, the consumption of all doses of dried plum (5%, 15%, and 25%) effectively restored femoral and tibial BMD to the same extent as E$_2$, while only the group receiving 25% dried plum showed the restoration of 4th lumbar BMD (Figure 2). At the time in which this study was conducted, the loss of bone volume accompanied by the loss of trabecular connectivity was generally believed to be an irreversible process [29]. To our knowledge, our study was the first to demonstrate that an agent of any kind could reverse the loss of trabecular microstructures including the bone volume/total volume, connectivity density, trabecular number, trabecular separation, and structure model index (Figure 3).

(A)   (B)

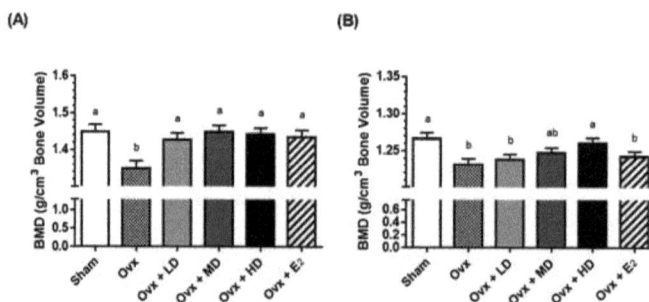

Figure 2. (**A**) Effects of ovariectomy, dried plum, and estrogen on bone density of right femur; (**B**) Effects ovariectomy, dried plum, and estrogen on bone density of 4th lumbar spine. Bars represent mean ± standard error of the mean. Bars that do not share the same letters are significantly ($p < 0.05$) different from each other. BMD, bone mineral density; E$_2$, 17β-estradiol, LD, low dose (5%) dried plum; high dose (25%) dried plum; MD, medium dose (15%) dried plum; Ovx, ovariectomized; Sham, sham-operated.

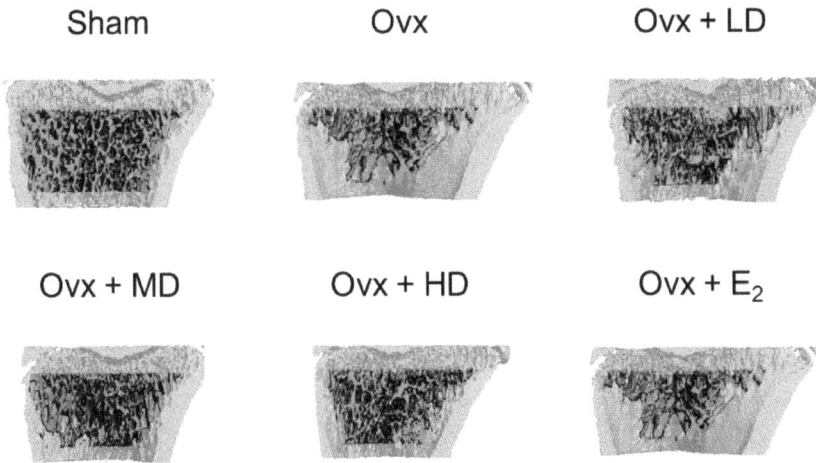

Figure 3. Representative images of proximal tibia demonstrating the effect of ovariectomy, dried plum, and estrogen on trabecular bone structure. E_2, 17β-estradiol; LD, high dose (25%) dried plum; low dose (5%) dried plum; MD, medium dose (15%) dried plum, Ovx, ovariectomized; Sham, sham-operated.

We next sought to evaluate the efficacy of several potentially bone-protective functional foods and bioactive compounds (i.e., dried plum, figs, dates, raisins, blueberries, dried plum (poly)phenols, fructooligosaccharides (FOS), and β-hydroxy-β-methylbutyrate, alone and in combination, on the bone mass and quality in Ovx rats after bone loss had already occurred [14]. Our findings revealed that the group receiving 5% FOS + 7.5% dried plum in their diet had the greatest reversal of BMD loss in the right femur and 4th lumbar spine, 4th lumbar spine calcium loss, and trabecular separation. Interestingly, none of the treatments altered the serum or urinary markers of bone turnover. The findings of this study suggest that the addition of prebiotic FOS to dried plum improves its efficacy in restoring bone mass and quality after bone loss has occurred. Although the mechanisms remain unknown, FOS has been demonstrated to increase the absorption of minerals, including calcium and magnesium, in the colon [30]. Additionally, considering that FOS is a prebiotic, it is likely that the combination of FOS and dried plum worked through gut microbiota-related mechanisms including an increase in mineral absorption. Importantly, the dose of dried plum (i.e., 7.5% of the diet) that was efficacious in combination with FOS was lower than what was previously found to be effective. This suggests that the addition of FOS to dried plum may improve the efficacy of dried plum and should be further investigated. These findings will be particularly important if they can be translated to humans, as it could be a novel strategy for reducing the amount of dried plum an individual would need to consume on a daily basis to achieve the same outcomes.

In addition to demonstrating the bone-protective effects of dried plum alone and in combination with FOS, we have also demonstrated in numerous studies that soy is a potentially efficacious functional food for promoting bone health [31–35]. We therefore sought to determine the efficacy of a soy-based diet in combination with 7.5% dried plum, 5% FOS, or 7.5% dried plum + 5% FOS on reversing bone loss in a rat model of postmenopausal osteoporosis. We found that the combination of a soy-based diet with dried plum, FOS, or both, significantly improved the whole body BMD and femoral BMD, while the combination of all components (i.e., soy, dried plum, and FOS) had the most pronounced effect on lumbar BMD [15]. All interventions were noted to improve the biomechanical properties of bone, as demonstrated by the increased ultimate load. The serum biomarker results suggest that these improvements may have been due, in part, to their ability to enhance bone formation and reduce bone resorption, as shown by increases in blood alkaline phosphatase (ALP) and decreased urinary deoxypyridinoline (Dpd).

Other investigators have also demonstrated the bone-protective effects of dried plum in rodent models postmenopausal osteoporosis. Rendina et al. [16] showed that feeding 25% of the diet as dried plum for four weeks to female Ovx C57BL/6J mice prevented the loss of BMD and bone mineral content (BMC) of the spine, and trabecular microarchitectural properties of the vertebrae and proximal tibiae, resulting in greater bone strength and stiffness in the vertebrae. Additionally, feeding dried plum in the diet at 15% and 25% doses restored myeloid and lymphoid levels to that of the sham-operated mice and suppressed ex vivo concanavalin A stimulated lymphocyte tumor necrosis factor-α production in splenocytes.

In another study, Rendina et al. [36] reported the results of a study comparing the bone-protective effects of dried plum with other fruits (i.e., dried apple, apricot, grape, and mango) in Ovx C57BL/6 mice over an eight-week period. They demonstrated that dried plum had superior anabolic effects on the trabecular bone microarchitectural properties of the vertebrae, was able to prevent tibial bone loss, and restored the trabecular biomechanical properties of the spine when compared with the other fruits. In addition, dried plum was more efficacious than the other fruits in enhancing plasma glutathione peroxidase activity, downregulating osteoclast differentiation, upregulating osteoblast activity, and suppressing Ovx-induced apoptosis.

Smith et al. [37] reported the findings of a study out of the same laboratory in which they compared the effects of six weeks of dried plum supplementation to treatment with parathyroid hormone (PTH). Treatment with dried plum at doses of 15% and 25% in the diet restored the whole body and femoral BMD to that of the Sham group and improved the trabecular bone volume and cortical thickness. Systemic blood biomarkers of bone metabolism (i.e., N-terminal procollagen type 1 and Dpd) were reduced, indicating a reduction in bone turnover. Dynamic bone histomorphometric analysis of the tibial metaphysis revealed that dried plum restored the Ovx-induced increase in the cancellous bone formation rate and mineralizing surface to that of the Sham group. Dried plum also upregulated the gene expression of *bone morphogenetic protein 2*, a regulator of osteogenesis, and *IGF-I* while downregulating the *nuclear factor T cell activator 1*, a transcription factor involved in the regulation of osteoclast differentiation. Compared with that of the effects of PTH on bone, dried plum reduced the rate of bone turnover, rather than increasing the rate of bone formation.

In summary, our data and others strongly suggest that dried plum is an efficacious functional food for preventing and reversing the loss of bone mass and structural properties in a rat model of postmenopausal osteoporosis. We have also shown that dried plum dose-dependently increases systemic and local indices of bone formation, e.g., serum and mRNA levels of ALP. These findings suggest that dried plum prevents and reverses bone loss, primarily through enhanced bone formation.

Table 1. Preclinical studies investigating the role of dried plum on bone health in rodent models of postmenopausal osteoporosis.

Reference	Model	Number	Groups	Duration	Primary Outcomes	Primary Findings
Arjmandi et al., 2001 [27]	Sham and Ovx female 90-day old Sprague–Dawley rats	48	(1) Sham control, (2) Ovx control, (3) Ovx + 5% dried plum, or (4) Ovx + 25% dried plum	45 days	BMD and % mineral content of right femur and 4th lumbar vertebrae; trabecular total area and bone area; cortical total area, bone area, marrow space, endosteal perimeter, and periosteal perimeter; serum ALP, TRAP, and IGF-1	Compared to Ovx control: 4th lumbar vertebrae and femur BMD and trabecular bone area were significantly ↑ in the 25% dried plum group
Deyhim et al., 2005 [38]	Sham and Ovx female 90-day old Sprague–Dawley rats	80	(1) Sham control, (2) Ovx control, (3) Ovx + 17β-estradiol, (4) Ovx + 5% dried plum, (5) Ovx + 15% dried plum, (6) Ovx + 25% dried plum	60 days	BMD of femur, left tibiae, and 4th lumbar; biomechanical properties (length, cortical area, unit yield force, and unit ultimate force); trabecular microarchitectural properties (BV/TV), Tb N, Tb S, Tb Th, ConnDens, SMI); serum IGF-1, ALP, and TRAP; urinary Dpd	Compared to Ovx control: Femur and tibia BMD were ↑ in all dried plum groups, 4th lumbar BMD tended to be significantly and was significantly ↑ in the 15% and 25% dried plum groups, respectively; unit yield force tended to be significantly ↑ in all dried plum groups; Tb S was significantly ↑ in all dried plum groups while Tb N and Tb Th were significantly ↑ in 15% and 25% dried plum groups and BV/TV and ConnDens were significantly ↑ in 25% dried plum group; urinary Dpd tended to be significantly ↓ in all dried plum groups
Arjmandi et al., 2010 [14]	Sham and Ovx female 90-day old Sprague–Dawley rats	180	(1) Sham control, (2) Ovx control, (3) Ovx + 2% FOS, (4) Ovx + 5% FOS + 7.5% dried plum, (5) Ovx + 2% FOS + 5% dried plum, (6) Ovx + 2% FOS + dried plum polyphenols, (7) Ovx + 2% FOS + dried plum juice, (8) Ovx + 2% FOS + dried plum puree, or (9) Ovx + 2% FOS + dried plum pulp/skins	60 days	BMD and BMC of whole body, right femur, and 4th lumbar vertebrae; bone histomorphometric parameters (BV/TV, Tb N, Tb S, Tb Th, ConnDens, and SMI); 4th lumbar calcium content; serum osteocalcin and IGF-1; serum and urinary calcium, magnesium, and phosphorus; urinary Dpd	Compared to Ovx control: 4th lumbar vertebrae and femur BMD were significantly ↑ in 5% FOS + 7.5% dried plum group with tendency to significantly ↓ loss of lumbar vertebrae calcium, and significantly ↓ trabecular separation
Johnson et al., 2011 [15]	Sham and Ovx female 90-day old Sprague–Dawley rats	72	(1) Sham control, (2) Ovx control, (3) Ovx + soy, (4) Ovx + soy + dried plum, Ovx + soy + FOS, or (5) Ovx + soy + dried plum + FOS	60 days	BMD and BMC of the whole body, right femur, and 4th lumbar vertebrae; femoral strength; bone histomorphometric parameters (BV/TV, Tb N, Tb S, Tb Th, and MS/BS); serum total ALP; urinary creatinine and Dpd	Compared to Ovx control: Whole body and 4th lumbar BMD tended to be significantly ↑ in Ovx + soy + dried plum group and was significantly increased in Ovx + soy + dried plum + FOS group, and right femur BMD was significantly ↑; Tb Th tended to be significantly ↑ and Tb Sp, and MS/BS tended to be significantly ↓ in Ovx + soy + dried plum + FOS group; serum ALP and urinary Dpd tended to be significantly ↓ in Ovx + soy + dried plum group and urinary Dpd was significantly ↓ in Ovx + soy + dried plum + FOS group
Rendina et al., 2012 [16]	Sham and Ovx female 90-day old C57BL/6J mice	59	(1) Sham control, (2) Ovx control, (3) Ovx + 5% dried plum, (4) Ovx + 15% dried plum, (5) Ovx + 25% dried plum	4 weeks	BMA, BMC, and BMD of the 4th to 5th lumbar vertebrae; bone microarchitecture parameters of tibia and 4th lumbar vertebrae (BV/TV, Tb N, Tb S, Tb Th, ConnDens, and SMI); biomechanical properties of trabecular bone (total force, stiffness, size-independent stiffness, and Von Mises stresses); plasma PINP and IGF-1; Runx2, osteocalcin, and NFATc1 bone gene expression	Compared to Ovx control: BMC and BMD were significantly ↑ in 25% dried plum group; BV/TV and vertebra Tb N were significantly ↑ in 15% and 25% dried plum groups, tibia Tb N was increased in 25% dried plum group, tibia Tb S was significantly ↓ in 15% and 25% dried plum groups while vertebra Tb S was significantly decreased in 25% dried plum group; vertebra ConnDens and SMI were significantly ↑ and ↓, respectively, in 15% and 25% dried plum groups while vertebra apparent mean/density tended to be ↑ in 15% dried plum group and was significantly ↑ in 25% dried plum group; tibia ConnDens and SMI, were significantly ↑ and ↓, respectively, in 15% and 25% dried plum groups while apparent mean density was increased in 25% dried plum group; vertebra total force, stiffness, and size-independent stiffness were significantly ↑ and Von Mises stresses was significantly ↓ in 15% and 25% dried plum groups; PINP, NFATc1, and Runx2 were significantly ↑ in all dried plum groups while IGF-1 was significantly ↑ in 15% dried plum group and osteocalcin was significantly decreased in 15% and 25% dried plum groups

Table 1. *Cont.*

Reference	Model	Number	Groups	Duration	Primary Outcomes	Primary Findings
Rendina et al., 2013 [36]	Sham and Ovx female 90-day old C57BL/6J mice	68	(1) Sham control, (2) Ovx control, (3) Ovx + 25% dried plum, (4) Ovx + 25% dried apple, (5) Ovx + 25% dried apricot, (6) Ovx + 25% dried grape, (7) Ovx + 25% dried mango	8 weeks	BMA, BMC, and BMD of the whole body and 4th and 5th lumbar vertebrae; bone microarchitecture parameters of tibia and 4th lumbar vertebrae (BV/TV, Tb N, Tb S, Tb Th, ConnDens, SMI, and trabecular density); biomechanical properties of trabecular bone (total force, stiffness, size-independent stiffness); plasma GPx; bone marrow gene expression of NFATc1, Col1a1, ALP, osteocalcin, Bak1; flushed femur expression of Bak1, Casp3, Casp9	25% dried plum compared to Ovx control: Whole body and vertebra BMA, BMD, and BMC were significantly ↑, vertebra and tibia BV/TV were significantly ↑; vertebra Tb N, Tb Th, Tb Sp, ConnDens and trabecular density were significantly ↑ and SMI was significantly ↓; proximal tibia Tb N and trabecular density were significantly ↑; vertebra total force, stiffness, and size independent stiffness and tibia size independent stiffness were significantly ↑; plasma GPx was significantly ↑; NFATc1 was significantly ↓ and Col1a1 tended to be ↑, bone marrow Bak1 was significantly ↑, and Casp9 was significantly ↓
Smith et al., 2014 [37]	Sham and Ovx female 6-month old Sprague-Dawley rats	84	(1) Sham control, (2) Ovx control, (3) Ovx + 5% dried plum, (4) Ovx + 15% dried plum, (5) Ovx + 25% dried plum, (6) Ovx + PTH	6 weeks	BMA, BMC, and BMD of the whole body, femur, and 4th and 5th lumbar vertebrae; bone microarchitecture parameters of tibia and 4th lumbar vertebrae (BV/TV, Tb N, Tb S, Tb Th, ConnDens, and SMI); dynamic bone histomorphometry (proximal tibia metaphysis BFR, MS/BS, and MAR; tibial cancellous MS/bone area, and BFR/BV; tibial cortical bone periosteal BFR, periosteal MS, periosteal MAR, endocortical BFR, endocortical MS, and endocortical MAR), plasma PINP; urinary Dpd; bone gene expression of NFATc1, Col1a1, ALP, osteocalcin, Runx2, BMP 2 and 4, IFG-1, RANKL, OPG	Compared to Ovx control: Whole body and femur BMD was significantly ↑ in all dried plum groups; vertebral BMD was significantly ↑ in 15% and 25% dried plum groups and tended to be significantly increased in 5% dried plum group; vertebral BV/TV and Tb N significantly ↑ and Tb S and ConnDens significantly ↓ in all dried plum groups, whereas Tb Th and SMI ↑ and ↑, respectively, in 15% and 25% dried plum groups; proximal tibia metaphysis Tb Sp ↓ in 15% and 25% dried plum groups; tibial mid-diaphysis cortical thickness ↑ in all dried plum groups while cortical area tended to be significantly ↑ in 5% dried plum group; plasma PINP was significantly ↓ in all dried plum groups; urinary Dpd tended to be significantly decreased and was significantly decreased in 5% and 15% dried plum groups, respectively; proximal tibial metaphysis BFR tended to be significantly ↓ in 5% dried plum group and was significantly ↓ in 15% and 25% dried plum groups, MS/BS was significantly ↓ in 15% and 25% dried plum groups, and MAR was significantly ↓ in 15% dried plum group and tended to be significantly ↓ in 5% and 25% dried plum groups; tibial cancellous MS/bone area and BFR/BV were significantly ↓ in all dried plum groups; tibial endocortical MAR was significantly ↓ in the 5% dried plum group and tended to be significantly reduced in the 15% and 25% dried plum groups; tibial endocortical MAR was significantly ↓ and BMP4 was significantly ↑ in all dried plum groups, while Col1a1 tended to be significantly reduced in all dried plum groups and IGF-1 was significantly ↑ in 25% dried plum group and tended to be significantly ↑ in 15% dried plum group
Pawlowski et al., 2014 [39]	Ovx female 3-month old Sprague-Dawley rats	44	(1) Control, (2) grape seed extract-high, (3) grape seed extract-low, (4) blueberry-high, (5) blueberry-low, (6) dried plum-high, (7) dried plum-low, (8) grape-high, (9) grape-low, (10) resveratrol-high, (11) resveratrol-low, (12) soy isoflavone-glycosylated, (13) soy isoflavone-genistein aglycone	10 days	Urine calcium (⁴⁵Ca and total calcium); serum BALP; urinary NTx	Bone calcium retention was significantly ↑ in dried plum-high group compared to baseline

Table 1. Cont.

Reference	Model	Number	Groups	Duration	Primary Outcomes	Primary Findings
Léotoing et al., 2016 [40]	Ovx female 5-month old Wistar rats	84	(1) Sham control, (2) Ovx control, (3) high chlorogenic acid dried plum, (4) low chlorogenic acid dried plum, (5) high chlorogenic acid dried plum juice, (6) low chlorogenic acid dried plum juice, (7) low chlorogenic acid dried plum + fiber	90 days	Total femoral BMD, metaphyseal BMD, and diaphyseal BMD; total BMC; blood osteocalcin, CPII, CTX-II, and CRI; urinary Dpd and calcium; BRI	Compared to Ovx control: Total femoral BMD and metaphyseal BMD were significantly ↑ in low chlorogenic acid dried plum + fiber and low chlorogenic acid dried plum juice group and tended to be significantly ↑ in all other dried plum groups; diaphyseal BMD was significantly ↑ in high chlorogenic acid dried plum, low chlorogenic acid dried plum + fiber and the low chlorogenic acid dried plum juice groups; total BMC was significantly ↑ in all low chlorogenic acid dried plum groups and tended to be significantly ↑ in high chlorogenic acid dried plum groups; blood osteocalcin was significantly ↓ in high chlorogenic acid dried plum, low chlorogenic acid dried plum + fiber, and low chlorogenic acid dried plum groups; urinary Dpd was significantly ↓ in low chlorogenic acid dried plum + fiber and low chlorogenic acid dried plum juice groups and tended to be significantly ↓ in the other dried plum groups; BRI tended to be ↓ in all high chlorogenic acid dried plum groups and tended to be ↑ in all low chlorogenic acid dried plum groups; all groups had significantly ↑ calciurea; CPII and CRI were significantly ↑ in high chlorogenic acid dried plum group

BALP, bone alkaline phosphatase; BMA, bone mineral area; BMC, bone mineral content; BMD, bone mineral density; BFR, bone formation rate; BMP, bone morphogenetic proteins; BRI, bone remodeling index; BSAP, bone-specific alkaline phosphatase; BV/TV, bone volume to total volume ratio; ^{45}Ca, calcium-45; Col1a1, type 1 collagen; ConnDens, connectivity density; CPII, C-propeptide of type II collagen; CRI, cartilage remodeling index; CTX-II, C-terminal telopeptides of type II collagen; Dpd, deoxypyridinoline; HP, helical peptide; IGF-1, insulin-like growth factor-1, IGFBP-3, insulin-like growth factor binding protein-3; IL-6, interleukin-6; MAR, mineral apposition rate; MS, mineralizing surface; MS/BS, mineral surface as percent of bone surface; NFATc1, nuclear factor of activated T cells; NTx, cross-linked N-telopeptides of type 1 collagen; OPG, osteoprotegerin; PINP, N-terminal propeptide of type 1 procollagen; PTH, parathyroid hormone; RANKL, receptor activator of nuclear factor kappa-B ligand; Runx2, runt-related protein 2; Tb N, trabecular number; Tb Sp, trabecular separation; Tb Th, trabecular thickness; TRAP, tartrate-resistant acid phosphatase; TNF-α, tumor necrosis factor-alpha; Ovx, ovariectomized; Sham, sham-operated; SMI, structural model index.

4. Dried Plum and Bone Health: Clinical Trials in Postmenopausal Women

Previously conducted clinical trials investigating the role of dried plum on bone health in postmenopausal women are summarized in Table 2. To our knowledge, our laboratory was the first to evaluate the bone-protective properties of dried plum in humans. Initially, we reported the findings of a three-month clinical trial evaluating the efficacy of dried plum versus dried apple (comparative control) on the biomarkers of bone formation in postmenopausal women [41]. Here, we showed that the consumption of 100 g/day dried plum significantly increased the serum markers of bone formation, namely total ALP, bone-specific ALP (BALP), and IGF-1 by 12, 6, and 17%, respectively. The increase in BALP is important as studies have shown that clinically relevant doses of bone-forming agents such as sodium fluoride, growth hormone, and PTH take several months to moderately increase the serum levels of BALP [42]. Interestingly, the serum and urinary biomarkers of bone resorption were not affected by either intervention. These observations further support our hypothesis that dried plum prevents and reverses bone loss through enhanced bone formation.

To evaluate whether a longer treatment period would lead to an improvement in bone mass, we conducted a one-year clinical trial comparing the effects of the daily consumption of 100 g dried plum to 75 g dried apple (comparative control) on BMD and the biomarkers of bone turnover in 100 osteopenic postmenopausal women. We found that dried plum consumption significantly improved the BMD of the ulna and lumbar spine compared with the dried apple control (Figure 4) [13]. Additionally, dried plum consumption led to significantly decreased serum TRAP-5b and BALP levels. Osteocalcin and C-reactive protein levels were significantly lower in the dried plum group than in the apple group. Although the findings of our initial three-month clinical trial indicated that BALP levels increased following dried plum consumption, this was not observed in our one-year clinical trial. We cannot offer a definitive reason for this discrepancy. However, variation is inherent in bone biomarkers due to intra- and inter-individual variability, analytical reasons, and sample stability. For these reasons, BMD remains the gold-standard for evaluating bone health [43].

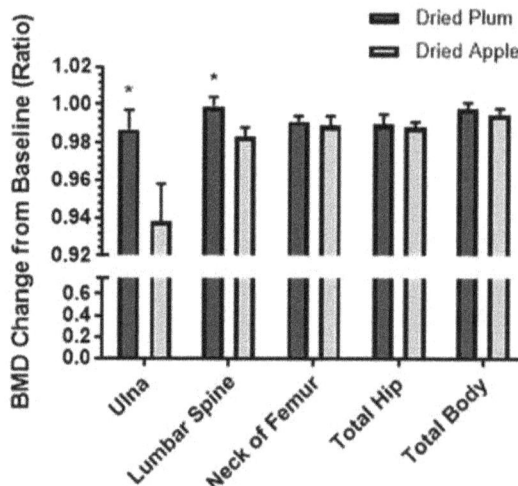

Figure 4. Change from baseline (ratio) in bone mineral density (BMD) from baseline to one-year following daily consumption of 100 g dried plum or 75 g dried apple. Bars represent mean ± standard error of the mean. * Denotes significant ($p < 0.05$) difference between groups.

We later investigated the potential mechanisms of action by which dried plum exerted these effects. We showed that compared to the baseline, dried plum increased receptor activator of nuclear factor kappa-B ligand levels by +1.99% versus +18.33% in the control group, increased the osteoprotegerin levels by +4.87% versus −2.15% in the control group, and decreased serum sclerostin levels by −1.12% in the dried plum group versus +3.78% in the control group [44]. While these percent changes did not reach statistical significance, they are clearly promising preliminary findings. Collectively, these findings suggest that dried plum prevents bone loss in postmenopausal women through the suppression of bone turnover.

Next, we [45] reported the findings of a six-month clinical trial evaluating the effects of resistance training with and without dried plum at a dose of 90 g in postmenopausal breast cancer survivors. While both groups were found to increase upper and lower body strength, no improvements were observed in the body composition or BMD. Interestingly, both groups displayed improvements in the blood biomarkers of bone turnover, with no added effect of dried plum observed.

Our successive six-month clinical trial evaluated the efficacy of two doses of dried plum (50 g versus 100 g) in preventing bone loss in older postmenopausal women [46]. Our findings confirmed dried plums' ability to prevent the loss of total body BMD and indicated that a lower dose of dried plum (i.e., 50 g) may be as effective as 100 g of dried plum. This study also demonstrated a reduction in serum TRAP-5b in both dried plum groups.

Most recently, we evaluated whether or not individuals who received the dried plum intervention in our previous one-year clinical trial conducted five years prior were able to retain BMD to a greater extent than those who received the dried apple intervention. Of the 100 women who completed the initial clinical trial, 20 came back for a follow-up visit. All participants, irrespective of group assignment, reported that they did not regularly consume dried plums. We found that individuals that received the dried plum intervention ($n = 8$) in our previous one-year clinical trial retained BMD of the ulna and lumbar spine to a greater extent than those who received the dried apple intervention ($n = 12$) (unpublished data, Figure 5). Although these findings are preliminary, they suggest that women in the dried plum group retained bone density in the lumbar spine and ulna to a greater extent than those in the dried apple group over the course of five years, even in the absence of regular dried plum consumption. These findings should be interpreted with caution as the influence of other factors including diet, physical activity, and medications have not been evaluated. Nonetheless, these findings are promising and further research is needed to evaluate the extent to which bone density is retained following the cessation of an intervention with dried plum.

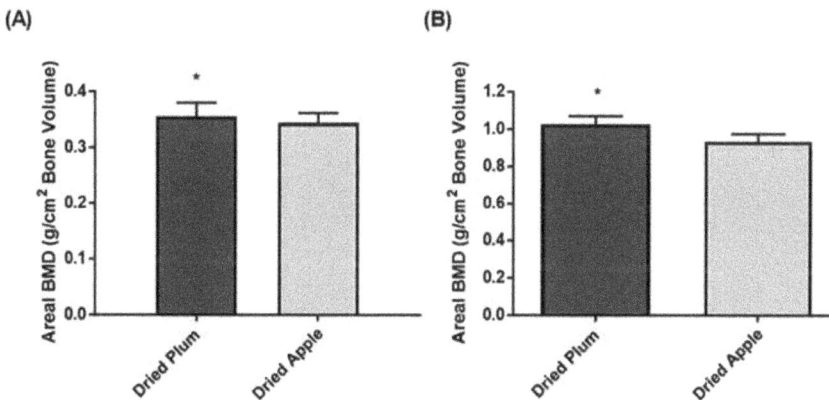

Figure 5. Bone mineral density (BMD) of the (**A**) ulna and (**B**) lumbar spine five years following one-year intervention study with daily consumption of 100 g dried plum or 75 g dried apple. Bars represent mean ± standard error of the mean. * Values were significantly ($p < 0.05$) different between groups.

Table 2. Clinical trials investigating the role of dried plum on bone health in postmenopausal women.

Reference	Design	Population	Number	Intervention	Duration	Primary Outcomes	Primary Findings
Arjmandi et al., 2002 [41]	RCT	Postmenopausal women	58	100 g/day dried plum or 75 g/day dried apple (comparative control)	3 months	Serum IGF-1, IGFBP-3, AP, TRAP, BSAP, calcium, phosphorus, and magnesium, urinary Dpd, HP, and creatinine	↑IGF-1, AP, and BSAP compared to baseline in dried plum group
Hooshmand et al., 2011 [13]	RCT	Postmenopausal women with osteopenia	160	100 g/day dried plum or 75 g/day dried apple (comparative control)	12 months	Whole body, lumbar spine, hip, and forearm BMD; serum BALP, osteocalcin, TRAP-5b, and CRP	↑ulna and lumbar spine BMD in dried plum group compared to dried apple (*p* < 0.05), ↓BALP in dried plum group compared to baseline
Hooshmand et al., 2014 [44]	RCT	Postmenopausal women with osteopenia	160	100 g/day dried plum or 75 g/day dried apple (comparative control)	12 months	Serum Dpd, RANKL, OPG, and sclerostin	Non-significant ↑ in RANKL, RANKL/OPG ratio, and sclerostin, and ↓ in OPG compared to baseline in dried apple group, non-significant ↑ in OPG and RANKL and ↓ in sclerostin in dried plum group compared to baseline
Simonavice et al., 2014 [45]	Non-randomized intervention trial	Postmenopausal breast cancer survivors	23	Resistance exercise with/without 90 g/day dried plum	6 months	Whole body, lumbar spine, femur, and forearm BMD; serum BAP, TRAP-5b, and CRP	No significant effects
Hooshmand et al., 2016 [46]	RCT	Older postmenopausal women	48	0, 50, or 100 g/day dried plum	6 months	Whole body, lumbar spine, hip, and forearm BMD: serum hs-CRP, IGF-1, BAP, TRAP-5b, BAP/TRAP-5b ratio, sclerostin, 25-OH vitamin D, RANKL, OPG, calcium, and phosphorus	↑whole body BMD in both dried plum groups compared to control, ↓TRAP-5b at 3 and 6 months in dried plum groups compared to control, ↑ BAP/TRAP-5b ratio at 6 months in both dried plum groups compared to baseline

BMD, bone mineral density; BSAP, bone-specific alkaline phosphatase; CRP, C-reactive protein; Dpd, deoxypyridinoline; HP, helical peptide; hs-CRP, high-sensitivity CRP; IGF-1, insulin-like growth factor-1, IGFBP-3, insulin-like growth factor binding protein-3; OPG, osteoprotegerin; RANKL, receptor activator of nuclear factor kappa-B ligand; RCT, randomized controlled trial; TRAP, tartrate-resistant acid phosphatase.

5. Bioactive Compounds and Possible Mechanisms of Action

Dried plum is known to contain several bioactive compounds including dietary fiber, vitamins (e.g., vitamin K), minerals (e.g., boron, copper), and (poly)phenolic compounds such as chlorogenic acids (i.e., chlorogenic acid, neochlorogenic acid, and cryptochlorogenic acid) and proanthocyanidins [24,25]. The exact nutrients and/or components contributing to the bone-protective effects of dried plum are unknown. However, many of these compounds are known to exert bone-protective effects and therefore likely work additively and/or synergistically.

Among the compounds found in dried plum is boron, which is a trace element critical for bone health as a deficiency or excess in consumption of boron can be harmful to bone. Dried plum contains a higher amount of boron than most fruits. In fact, the content of boron in 47.7 g dried plum (~5 dried plums) is about 1.1 mg [23]. The average daily intake of boron is about 1–2 mg/day, depending on sex and age, among other factors [47]. Boron has been shown to stimulate bone growth and bone metabolism [48], and play an important role in preserving BMD, bone microarchitecture, and bone strength [49–51]. A study by Chapin et al. [52] showed that rats fed diets containing 20 or more mg boron/100 g diet had a significantly improved vertebral strength. These authors also demonstrated that rats fed a boric acid diet of 200 ppm or more for nine weeks not only had a significant increase in the boron content of their bone, but retained their bone boron content three-fold greater than the controls 32 weeks after exposure to the diet ended. This suggests that boron has the ability to accumulate in bone, and though the half-life of boron in bone is uncertain, it may be similar to that of calcium, where the half-life is significantly longer than in tissue. This action of boron may play a role in the maintenance of bone density over long periods of time, even without regular consumption.

Another mineral abundant in dried plum important for bone health is potassium [53,54]. One hundred grams of dried plum contains 732 mg. Tucker et al. [55] investigated both the cross-sectional and longitudinal relationships between potassium and BMD using a Framingham Heart Study database and concluded that potassium contributes to the maintenance of BMD in men and women. Additionally, higher intakes of potassium have been shown to reduce bone resorption, particularly in the face of high protein intake [56].

Dried plum is also a good source of copper. A 47.7 g serving of dried plum provides 0.13 mg, which is 31.2% of the dietary reference intake. Copper is a cofactor for lysyl oxidase, which is involved in the cross-linking of collagen and elastin [24,57]. In an in vivo study by Yee et al. [57], Ovx Sprague-Dawley rats placed on a copper deficient diet had more severe osteopenia than the copper adequate diet. Copper may in part contribute to the beneficial properties of dried plum on bone, giving an additive effect.

Dried plum is rich in vitamin K and a 47.7 g serving of dried plum provides 348 mg vitamin K, or 15.6% of the dietary reference intake [53]. Vitamin K is important for bone health as it promotes a calcium balance [58]. Additionally, it is a cofactor for the γ-carboxylation of osteocalcin, a bone matrix protein secreted by osteoblasts that promotes normal bone mineralization by regulating the growth of hydroxyapatite crystals [58]. A study by Braam et al. [59] demonstrated that supplementation with vitamin K at the level of 1 mg daily for three years attenuated the loss of BMD in the lumbar spine.

Among the (poly)phenols found in dried plum, chlorogenic acids (e.g., neochlorogenic acid, cryptochlorigenic acid, and chlorogenic acid) are the most abundant. In fact, 100 g of dried plum is estimated to contain between 108 and 153 mg chlorogenic acids. Previous research has demonstrated that chlorogenic acids are bone-protective. For instance, Zhou et al. [60] demonstrated that supplementing Ovx rats with chlorogenic acid led to improved BMD and microarchitecture, and an increased proliferation of osteoblast precursors and osteoblast differentiation, as well as increases in bone formation biomarkers. Despite this, Léotoing et al. [40] demonstrated that the bone-protective effects of dried plum is not dependent on the content of chlorogenic acids. As the authors pointed out, it is important to consider that dried plum contains other (poly)phenols such as quercetin, rutin, proanthocyanidins, among others, as well as dietary fiber in the form of soluble and insoluble fiber including pectin, fructans, hemicelluloses, and cellulose [23,40], which may be responsible for the effects of dried plum on bone. (Poly)phenols and their metabolites are known to not only act as antioxidants themselves [53,61,62], but to also activate endogenous antioxidant and inhibit inflammatory signaling pathways [63,64]. Considering that bone loss has been linked to oxygen-derived free radicals in the bone microenvironment, an imbalance in antioxidant defenses, and oxidative stress [65,66], as well as a pro-inflammatory state [67], it is possible that other dried plum (poly)phenols and their metabolites work through this mechanism. In fact, we and others have demonstrated the antioxidant and anti-inflammatory properties of dried plum [68,69]. Dried plum has a high oxygen radical absorbance capacity (ORAC) compared with many commonly consumed fruits and vegetables [70]. More recently, Kayano et al. [61], have isolated several ortho-diphenolic and mono hydroxyl phenolic compounds with ORAC values as high as 4.68 units of Trolox equivalent per mg of dried plum. Therefore, the beneficial effects of dried plum on bone may be partly mediated through its antioxidant properties.

Importantly, dried plum is rich in soluble and insoluble fibers, including pectin, fructans, hemicelluloses, and cellulose [23,40], which are known to increase mineral absorption (e.g., calcium) [71]. For instance, fibers are fermented by colonic bacteria, resulting in the production of short-chain fatty acids (SCFA). SCFAs enhance calcium absorption through reductions in the pH of the intestinal lumen and increasing the solubility of calcium, thereby facilitating passive diffusion through exchanges of luminal calcium with cellular hydrogen, and increasing the permeability of gut epithelial cells and paracellular transport [40,71,72]. Dietary fiber, including prebiotic dietary fibers, as well as (poly)phenolic compounds, have been shown to alter the microbial composition in the gut [71,73,74]. As such, it is possible that chronic dried plum consumption induces changes in the gut microbiome, thereby increasing SCFA production. It is also possible that these changes in the gut microbiome promote bone health through other mechanisms including those involving the immune system. However, this has yet to be investigated and is therefore speculative.

Lastly, previous research has shown that dried plum rich in chlorogenic acid increases bone calcium retention in an Ovx rodent model of postmenopausal osteoporosis [39]. Although changes in biomarkers of bone turnover were not noted, the observation that bone calcium retention was greater is consistent with the notion that dried plum reduces bone turnover. This is an interesting finding that warrants further investigation.

6. Conclusions

The bone-protective effects of dried plum in postmenopausal women have been supported by several animal studies and confirmed in randomized controlled trials. The exact mechanisms by which dried plum exerts these effects remains unknown. Additionally, it is unclear as to which bioactive compound(s) in dried plum is/are responsible for its bone-protective properties. Considering that many of the bioactive compounds present in dried plum have been shown to modulate bone metabolism, it is likely that there are additive and/or synergistic effects among these compounds. In addition to preventing bone loss in postmenopausal women, our recent findings suggest that the bone-protective effects of dried plum may be long-lasting, thereby contributing to the maintenance of bone density after regular consumption has ceased.

The findings of our previously conducted clinical trials indicate that dried plum is most efficacious in preventing bone loss in the ulna and lumbar spine. Although the reason for this is not currently known, both vertebra and ulna contain more trabecular bone than other sites (e.g., femur). In fact, vertebra and ulna contain more than 60% and up to 50% trabecular bone, respectively. Bone turnover is known to be greater in trabecular bone than cortical bone [75,76]. The body of literature suggests that dried plum slows the rate of bone turnover. As such, it is likely that dried plum has a more pronounced effect of reducing bone loss at these sites through reductions in trabecular bone turnover.

An important point to consider with any nutritional intervention, including functional foods, is caloric intake. The addition of dried plum to the diet contributes approximately 120 kcal and 240 kcal for 50 g and 100 g doses, respectively [23]. In our previous clinical trials, study participants were advised to maintain their usual diet and physical activity patterns throughout the duration of the study. We did not observe significant changes in nutritional intake, including calories, nor in body weight. Considering that self-reported dietary intake and physical activity are known to have limitations, including measurement error, it is therefore unknown as to whether our study participants made alterations in their diets or physical activity to maintain their body weight. Dried plum is high in dietary fiber which alters the transit time and may increase satiety, thereby reducing the overall caloric intake. Logically, one would assume that the addition of dried plum to the diet would displace other calories. However, this is speculative and needs future confirmation.

Future research should aim not only to better understand the mechanisms by which dried plum consumption contributes to bone health, including the involvement of the gut microbiome, but also to elucidate the long-term maintenance of such effects, including their role in fracture prevention. With respect to feasibility, we have observed good study participant treatment compliance and retention with long-term dried plum consumption at doses of 50 g (six months) and 100 g (one year). Study participants were generally willing to commit to the regular consumption of dried plum in order to improve their bone health and avoid taking osteoporosis medications. Our study participants were educated on ways to incorporate dried plum into their diets (e.g., in their meals) in an effort to promote compliance. Nonetheless, there are challenges with any long-term dietary intervention. For this reason, it is important that future studies aim to establish the lowest dose of dried plum or alternative dosing methods (e.g., intermittent dosing regimens) that provide the same efficacy as 100 g/day. Additionally, the combination of other foods and/or bioactive compounds that show promise for bone health, such as FOS, with dried plum should be further investigated, as this may enhance its efficacy. Finally, many of the previously conducted clinical trials evaluating the bone-protective effects of dried plum had small sample sizes, which may have contributed to null findings. Therefore, future large-scale clinical trials are needed to further establish the bone-protective effects of dried plum in postmenopausal women.

Acknowledgments: This work was funded in part by the California Dried Plum Board and the United States Department of Agriculture.

Conflicts of Interest: The authors declare no conflict of interest.

References

1. Barrett-Connor, E. Epidemiology and the Menopause: A Global Overview. *Int. J. Fertil. Menopausal. Stud.* **1993**, *38* (Suppl. 1), 6–14. [PubMed]
2. American Congress of Obstetricians and Gynecologists. 2011 Women's Health Stats and Facts. Available online: https://www.acog.org/-/media/NewsRoom/MediaKit.pdf (accessed on 14 April 2017).
3. Facts and Statistics. International Osteoporosis Foundation. Available online: https://www.iofbonehealth.org/facts-statistics (accessed on 14 April 2017).
4. Raisz, L.G. Pathogenesis of Osteoporosis: Concepts, Conflicts, and Prospects. *J. Clin. Investig.* **2005**, *115*, 3318–3325. [CrossRef] [PubMed]
5. Kamienski, M.; Tate, D.; Vega, M. The Silent Thief: Diagnosis and Management of Osteoporosis. *Orthop. Nurs.* **2011**, *30*, 162–171. [CrossRef] [PubMed]
6. Burge, R.; Dawson-Hughes, B.; Solomon, D.H.; Wong, J.B.; King, A.; Tosteson, A. Incidence and Economic Burden of Osteoporosis-Related Fractures in the United States, 2005–2025. *J. Bone Miner. Res.* **2007**, *22*, 465–475. [CrossRef] [PubMed]
7. Looker, A.C.; Borrud, L.G.; Dawson-Hughes, B.; Shepherd, J.A.; Wright, N.C. Osteoporosis or Low Bone Mass at the Femur Neck or Lumbar Spine in Older Adults: United States, 2005–2008. *NCHS Data Brief* **2012**, *93*, 1–8.
8. Demontiero, O.; Vidal, C.; Duque, G. Aging and Bone Loss: New Insights for the Clinician. *Ther. Adv. Musculoskelet. Dis.* **2012**, *4*, 61–76. [CrossRef] [PubMed]

9.   Almeida, M.; Laurent, M.R.; Dubois, V.; Claessens, F.; O'Brien, C.A.; Bouillon, R.; Vanderschueren, D.; Manolagas, S.C. Estrogens and Androgens in Skeletal Physiology and Pathophysiology. *Physiol. Rev.* **2017**, *97*, 135–187. [CrossRef] [PubMed]

10.   Rossouw, J.E.; Anderson, G.L.; Prentice, R.L.; LaCroix, A.Z.; Kooperberg, C.; Stefanick, M.L.; Jackson, R.D.; Beresford, S.A.; Howard, B.V.; Johnson, K.C.; et al. Risks and Benefits of Estrogen Plus Progestin in Healthy Postmenopausal Women: Principal Results from the Women's Health Initiative Randomized Controlled Trial. *JAMA* **2002**, *288*, 321–333. [CrossRef] [PubMed]

11.   Kayser, J.; Ettinger, B.; Pressman, A. Postmenopausal Hormonal Support: Discontinuation of Raloxifene Versus Estrogen. *Menopause* **2001**, *8*, 328–332. [CrossRef] [PubMed]

12.   Cashman, K.D. Diet, Nutrition, and Bone Health. *J. Nutr.* **2007**, *137*, 2507S–2512S. [PubMed]

13.   Hooshmand, S.; Chai, S.C.; Saadat, R.L.; Payton, M.E.; Brummel-Smith, K.; Arjmandi, B.H. Comparative Effects of Dried Plum and Dried Apple on Bone in Postmenopausal Women. *Br. J. Nutr.* **2011**, *106*, 923–930. [CrossRef] [PubMed]

14.   Arjmandi, B.H.; Johnson, C.D.; Campbell, S.C.; Hooshmand, S.; Chai, S.C.; Akhter, M.P. Combining Fructooligosaccharide and Dried Plum Has the Greatest Effect on Restoring Bone Mineral Density among Select Functional Foods and Bioactive Compounds. *J. Med. Food* **2010**, *13*, 312–319. [CrossRef] [PubMed]

15.   Johnson, C.D.; Lucas, E.A.; Hooshmand, S.; Campbell, S.; Akhter, M.P.; Arjmandi, B.H. Addition of Fructooligosaccharides and Dried Plum to Soy-Based Diets Reverses Bone Loss in the Ovariectomized Rat. *Evid. Based Complement. Alternat. Med.* **2011**, *2011*, 836267. [CrossRef] [PubMed]

16.   Rendina, E.; Lim, Y.F.; Marlow, D.; Wang, Y.; Clarke, S.L.; Kuvibidila, S.; Lucas, E.A.; Smith, B.J. Dietary Supplementation with Dried Plum Prevents Ovariectomy-Induced Bone Loss While Modulating the Immune Response in C57bl/6j Mice. *J. Nutr. Biochem.* **2012**, *23*, 60–68. [CrossRef] [PubMed]

17.   Halloran, B.P.; Wronski, T.J.; VonHerzen, D.C.; Chu, V.; Xia, X.; Pingel, J.E.; Williams, A.A.; Smith, B.J. Dietary Dried Plum Increases Bone Mass in Adult and Aged Male Mice. *J. Nutr.* **2010**, *140*, 1781–1787. [CrossRef] [PubMed]

18.   Mühlbauer, R.C.; Lozano, A.; Reinli, A. Onion and a Mixture of Vegetables, Salads, and Herbs Affect Bone Resorption in the Rat by a Mechanism Independent of Their Base Excess. *J. Bone Miner. Res.* **2002**, *17*, 1230–1236. [CrossRef] [PubMed]

19.   Mühlbauer, R.C.; Lozano, A.; Reinli, A.; Wetli, H. Various Selected Vegetables, Fruits, Mushrooms and Red Wine Residue Inhibit Bone Resorption in Rats. *J. Nutr.* **2003**, *133*, 3592–3597. [PubMed]

20.   Devareddy, L.; Hooshmand, S.; Collins, J.K.; Lucas, E.A.; Chai, S.C.; Arjmandi, B.H. Blueberry Prevents Bone Loss in Ovariectomized Rat Model of Postmenopausal Osteoporosis. *J. Nutr. Biochem.* **2008**, *19*, 694–699. [CrossRef] [PubMed]

21.   Zhang, J.; Lazarenko, O.P.; Blackburn, M.L.; Shankar, K.; Badger, T.M.; Ronis, M.J.; Chen, J.R. Feeding Blueberry Diets in Early Life Prevent Senescence of Osteoblasts and Bone Loss in Ovariectomized Adult Female Rats. *PLoS ONE* **2011**, *6*, e24486. [CrossRef] [PubMed]

22.   Zhang, J.; Lazarenko, O.P.; Blackburn, M.L.; Badger, T.M.; Ronis, M.J.; Chen, J.R. Blueberry Consumption Prevents Loss of Collagen in Bone Matrix and Inhibits Senescence Pathways in Osteoblastic Cells. *Age (Dordr)* **2013**, *35*, 807–820. [CrossRef] [PubMed]

23.   Bowen, P.E. Role of Commodity Boards in Advancing the Understanding of the Health Benefits of Whole Foods: California Dried Plums. *Nutr. Today* **2017**, *52*, 19–25. [CrossRef] [PubMed]

24.   Stacewicz-Sapuntzakis, M. Dried Plums and Their Products: Composition and Health Effects—An Updated Review. *Crit. Rev. Food Sci. Nutr.* **2013**, *53*, 1277–1302. [CrossRef] [PubMed]

25.   Hooshmand, S.; Arjmandi, B.H. Viewpoint: Dried Plum, an Emerging Functional Food That May Effectively Improve Bone Health. *Ageing Res. Rev.* **2009**, *8*, 122–127. [CrossRef] [PubMed]

26.   Horcajada-Molteni, M.N.; Crespy, V.; Coxam, V.; Davicco, M.J.; Rémésy, C.; Barlet, J.P. Rutin Inhibits Ovariectomy-Induced Osteopenia in Rats. *J. Bone Miner. Res.* **2000**, *15*, 2251–2258. [CrossRef] [PubMed]

27.   Arjmandi, B.H.; Lucas, E.A.; Juma, S.; Soliman, A.; Stoecker, B.J.; Khalil, D.A.; Smith, B.J.; Wang, C. Prune Prevents Ovariectomy-Induced Bone Loss in Rats. *J. Am. Nutraceutical Assoc.* **2001**, *4*, 50–56.

28.   Kalu, D.N. The Ovariectomized Rat Model of Postmenopausal Bone Loss. *Bone Miner.* **1991**, *15*, 175–191. [CrossRef]

29. Lane, N.E.; Haupt, D.; Kimmel, D.B.; Modin, G.; Kinney, J.H. Early Estrogen Replacement Therapy Reverses the Rapid Loss of Trabecular Bone Volume and Prevents Further Deterioration of Connectivity in the Rat. *J. Bone Miner. Res.* **1999**, *14*, 206–214. [CrossRef] [PubMed]

30. Tokunaga, T. Novel Physiological Function of Fructooligosaccharides. *Biofactors* **2004**, *21*, 89–94. [CrossRef] [PubMed]

31. Devareddy, L.; Khalil, D.A.; Korlagunta, K.; Hooshmand, S.; Bellmer, D.D.; Arjmandi, B.H. The Effects of Fructo-Oligosaccharides in Combination with Soy Protein on Bone in Osteopenic Ovariectomized Rats. *Menopause* **2006**, *13*, 692–699. [CrossRef] [PubMed]

32. Devareddy, L.; Khalil, D.A.; Smith, B.J.; Lucas, E.A.; Soung, D.Y.; Marlow, D.D.; Arjmandi, B.H. Soy Moderately Improves Microstructural Properties without Affecting Bone Mass in an Ovariectomized Rat Model of Osteoporosis. *Bone* **2006**, *38*, 686–693. [CrossRef] [PubMed]

33. Arjmandi, B.H.; Lucas, E.A.; Khalil, D.A.; Devareddy, L.; Smith, B.J.; McDonald, J.; Arquitt, A.B.; Payton, M.E.; Mason, C. One Year Soy Protein Supplementation Has Positive Effects on Bone Formation Markers but Not Bone Density in Postmenopausal Women. *Nutr. J.* **2005**, *4*, 8. [CrossRef] [PubMed]

34. Arjmandi, B.H.; Khalil, D.A.; Smith, B.J.; Lucas, E.A.; Juma, S.; Payton, M.E.; Wild, R.A. Soy Protein Has a Greater Effect on Bone in Postmenopausal Women Not on Hormone Replacement Therapy, as Evidenced by Reducing Bone Resorption and Urinary Calcium Excretion. *J. Clin. Endocrinol. Metab.* **2003**, *88*, 1048–1054. [CrossRef] [PubMed]

35. Arjmandi, B.H.; Birnbaum, R.; Goyal, N.V.; Getlinger, M.J.; Juma, S.; Alekel, L.; Hasler, C.M.; Drum, M.L.; Hollis, B.W.; Kukreja, S.C. Bone-Sparing Effect of Soy Protein in Ovarian Hormone-Deficient Rats Is Related to Its Isoflavone Content. *Am. J. Clin. Nutr.* **1998**, *68*, 1364S–1368S. [PubMed]

36. Rendina, E.; Hembree, K.D.; Davis, M.R.; Marlow, D.; Clarke, S.L.; Halloran, B.P.; Lucas, E.A.; Smith, B.J. Dried Plum's Unique Capacity to Reverse Bone Loss and Alter Bone Metabolism in Postmenopausal Osteoporosis Model. *PLoS ONE* **2013**, *8*, e60569. [CrossRef] [PubMed]

37. Smith, B.J.; Bu, S.Y.; Wang, Y.; Rendina, E.; Lim, Y.F.; Marlow, D.; Clarke, S.L.; Cullen, D.M.; Lucas, E.A. A Comparative Study of the Bone Metabolic Response to Dried Plum Supplementation and Pth Treatment in Adult, Osteopenic Ovariectomized Rat. *Bone* **2014**, *58*, 151–159. [CrossRef] [PubMed]

38. Deyhim, F.; Stoecker, B.J.; Brusewitz, G.H.; Devareddy, L.; Arjmandi, B.H. Dried Plum Reverses Bone Loss in an Osteopenic Rat Model of Osteoporosis. *Menopause* **2005**, *12*, 755–762. [CrossRef] [PubMed]

39. Pawlowski, J.W.; Martin, B.R.; McCabe, G.P.; Ferruzzi, M.G.; Weaver, C.M. Plum and Soy Aglycon Extracts Superior at Increasing Bone Calcium Retention in Ovariectomized Sprague Dawley Rats. *J. Agric. Food Chem.* **2014**, *62*, 6108–6117. [CrossRef] [PubMed]

40. Leotoing, L.; Wauquier, F.; Davicco, M.J.; Lebecque, P.; Gaudout, D.; Rey, S.; Vitrac, X.; Massenat, L.; Rashidi, S.; Wittrant, Y.; et al. The Phenolic Acids of Agen Prunes (Dried Plums) or Agen Prune Juice Concentrates Do Not Account for the Protective Action on Bone in a Rat Model of Postmenopausal Osteoporosis. *Nutr. Res.* **2016**, *36*, 161–173. [CrossRef] [PubMed]

41. Arjmandi, B.H.; Khalil, D.A.; Lucas, E.A.; Georgis, A.; Stoecker, B.J.; Hardin, C.; Payton, M.E.; Wild, R.A. Dried Plums Improve Indices of Bone Formation in Postmenopausal Women. *J. Womens Health Gend. Based Med.* **2002**, *11*, 61–68. [CrossRef] [PubMed]

42. Hodsman, A.B.; Fraher, L.J.; Watson, P.H.; Ostbye, T.; Stitt, L.W.; Adachi, J.D.; Taves, D.H.; Drost, D. A Randomized Controlled Trial to Compare the Efficacy of Cyclical Parathyroid Hormone Versus Cyclical Parathyroid Hormone and Sequential Calcitonin to Improve Bone Mass in Postmenopausal Women with Osteoporosis. *J. Clin. Endocrinol. Metab.* **1997**, *82*, 620–628. [CrossRef] [PubMed]

43. Wheater, G.; Elshahaly, M.; Tuck, S.P.; Datta, H.K.; van Laar, J.M. The Clinical Utility of Bone Marker Measurements in Osteoporosis. *J. Transl. Med.* **2013**, *11*, 201. [CrossRef] [PubMed]

44. Hooshmand, S.; Brisco, J.R.; Arjmandi, B.H. The Effect of Dried Plum on Serum Levels of Receptor Activator of Nf-Kappab Ligand, Osteoprotegerin and Sclerostin in Osteopenic Postmenopausal Women: A Randomised Controlled Trial. *Br. J. Nutr.* **2014**, *112*, 55–60. [CrossRef] [PubMed]

45. Simonavice, E.; Liu, P.Y.; Ilich, J.Z.; Kim, J.S.; Arjmandi, B.; Panton, L.B. The Effects of a 6-Month Resistance Training and Dried Plum Consumption Intervention on Strength, Body Composition, Blood Markers of Bone Turnover, and Inflammation in Breast Cancer Survivors. *Appl. Physiol. Nutr. Metab.* **2014**, *39*, 730–739. [CrossRef] [PubMed]

46. Hooshmand, S.; Kern, M.; Metti, D.; Shamloufard, P.; Chai, S.C.; Johnson, S.A.; Payton, M.E.; Arjmandi, B.H. The Effect of Two Doses of Dried Plum on Bone Density and Bone Biomarkers in Osteopenic Postmenopausal Women: A Randomized, Controlled Trial. *Osteoporos. Int.* **2016**, *27*, 2271–2279. [CrossRef] [PubMed]

47. Trumbo, P.; Yates, A.A.; Schlicker, S.; Poos, M. Dietary Reference Intakes: Vitamin A, Vitamin K, Arsenic, Boron, Chromium, Copper, Iodine, Iron, Manganese, Molybdenum, Nickel, Silicon, Vanadium, and Zinc. *J. Am. Diet. Assoc.* **2001**, *101*, 294–301. [CrossRef]

48. Nielsen, F.H.; Hunt, C.D.; Mullen, L.M.; Hunt, J.R. Effect of Dietary Boron on Mineral, Estrogen, and Testosterone Metabolism in Postmenopausal Women. *FASEB J.* **1987**, *1*, 394–397. [CrossRef]

49. Nielsen, F.H. Biochemical and Physiologic Consequences of Boron Deprivation in Humans. *Environ. Health Perspect.* **1994**, *102* (Suppl. 7), 59–63. [CrossRef] [PubMed]

50. Nielsen, F.H. Is Boron Nutritionally Relevant? *Nutr. Rev.* **2008**, *66*, 183–191. [CrossRef] [PubMed]

51. Zofkova, I.; Davis, M.; Blahos, J. Trace Elements Have Beneficial, as Well as Detrimental Effects on Bone Homeostasis. In *Physiol. Res.*; 2017. Available online: https://www.ncbi.nlm.nih.gov/pubmed/28248532 (accessed on 14 April 2017).

52. Chapin, R.E.; Ku, W.W.; Kenney, M.A.; McCoy, H. The Effects of Dietary Boric Acid on Bone Strength in Rats. *Biol. Trace Elem. Res.* **1998**, *66*, 395–399. [CrossRef] [PubMed]

53. Dismore, M.L.; Haytowitz, D.B.; Gebhardt, S.E.; Peterson, J.W.; Booth, S.L. Vitamin K Content of Nuts and Fruits in the US Diet. *J. Am. Diet. Assoc.* **2003**, *103*, 1650–1652. [CrossRef] [PubMed]

54. Stacewicz-Sapuntzakis, M.; Bowen, P.E.; Hussain, E.A.; Damayanti-Wood, B.I.; Farnsworth, N.R. Chemical Composition and Potential Health Effects of Prunes: A Functional Food? *Crit. Rev. Food Sci. Nutr.* **2001**, *41*, 251–286. [CrossRef] [PubMed]

55. Tucker, K.L.; Hannan, M.T.; Chen, H.; Cupples, L.A.; Wilson, P.W.; Kiel, D.P. Potassium, Magnesium, and Fruit and Vegetable Intakes Are Associated with Greater Bone Mineral Density in Elderly Men and Women. *Am. J. Clin. Nutr.* **1999**, *69*, 727–736. [PubMed]

56. Zwart, S.R.; Hargens, A.R.; Smith, S.M. The Ratio of Animal Protein Intake to Potassium Intake Is a Predictor of Bone Resorption in Space Flight Analogues and in Ambulatory Subjects. *Am. J. Clin. Nutr.* **2004**, *80*, 1058–1065. [PubMed]

57. Yee, C.D.; Kubena, K.S.; Walker, M.; Champney, T.H.; Sampson, H.W. The Relationship of Nutritional Copper to the Development of Postmenopausal Osteoporosis in Rats. *Biol. Trace Elem. Res.* **1995**, *48*, 1–11. [CrossRef] [PubMed]

58. Iwamoto, J.; Takeda, T.; Sato, Y. Effects of Vitamin K2 on Osteoporosis. *Curr. Pharm. Des.* **2004**, *10*, 2557–2576. [CrossRef] [PubMed]

59. Braam, L.A.; Knapen, M.H.; Geusens, P.; Brouns, F.; Hamulyák, K.; Gerichhausen, M.J.; Vermeer, C. Vitamin K1 Supplementation Retards Bone Loss in Postmenopausal Women between 50 and 60 Years of Age. *Calcif. Tissue Int.* **2003**, *73*, 21–26. [CrossRef] [PubMed]

60. Zhou, R.P.; Lin, S.J.; Wan, W.B.; Zuo, H.L.; Yao, F.F.; Ruan, H.B.; Xu, J.; Song, W.; Zhou, Y.C.; Wen, S.Y.; et al. Chlorogenic Acid Prevents Osteoporosis by Shp2/Pi3k/Akt Pathway in Ovariectomized Rats. *PLoS ONE* **2016**, *11*, e0166751. [CrossRef] [PubMed]

61. Kayano, S.; Kikuzaki, H.; Fukutsuka, N.; Mitani, T.; Nakatani, N. Antioxidant Activity of Prune (*Prunus domestica* L.) Constituents and a New Synergist. *J. Agric. Food Chem.* **2002**, *50*, 3708–3712. [CrossRef] [PubMed]

62. Nakatani, N.; Kayano, S.; Kikuzaki, H.; Sumino, K.; Katagiri, K.; Mitani, T. Identification, Quantitative Determination, and Antioxidative Activities of Chlorogenic Acid Isomers in Prune (*Prunus domestica* L.). *J. Agric. Food Chem.* **2000**, *48*, 5512–5516. [CrossRef] [PubMed]

63. Rahman, I.; Biswas, S.K.; Kirkham, P.A. Regulation of Inflammation and Redox Signaling by Dietary Polyphenols. *Biochem. Pharmacol.* **2006**, *72*, 1439–1452. [CrossRef] [PubMed]

64. Stevenson, D.E.; Hurst, R.D. Polyphenolic Phytochemicals—Just Antioxidants or Much More? *Cell Mol. Life Sci.* **2007**, *64*, 2900–2916. [CrossRef] [PubMed]

65. Garrett, I.R.; Boyce, B.F.; Oreffo, R.O.; Bonewald, L.; Poser, J.; Mundy, G.R. Oxygen-Derived Free Radicals Stimulate Osteoclastic Bone Resorption in Rodent Bone in Vitro and in Vivo. *J. Clin. Investig.* **1990**, *85*, 632–639. [CrossRef] [PubMed]

66. Callaway, D.A.; Jiang, J.X. Reactive Oxygen Species and Oxidative Stress in Osteoclastogenesis, Skeletal Aging and Bone Diseases. *J. Bone Miner. Metab.* **2015**, *33*, 359–370. [CrossRef] [PubMed]

Nutrients **2017**, *9*, 496

67. Mundy, G.R. Osteoporosis and Inflammation. *Nutr. Rev.* **2007**, *65*, S147–S151. [CrossRef] [PubMed]

68. Igwe, E.O.; Charlton, K.E. A Systematic Review on the Health Effects of Plums (Prunus Domestica and Prunus Salicina). *Phytother. Res.* **2016**, *30*, 701–731. [CrossRef] [PubMed]

69. Hooshmand, S.; Kumar, A.; Zhang, J.Y.; Johnson, S.A.; Chai, S.C.; Arjmandi, B.H. Evidence for Anti-Inflammatory and Antioxidative Properties of Dried Plum Polyphenols in Macrophage Raw 264.7 Cells. *Food Funct.* **2015**, *6*, 1719–1725. [CrossRef] [PubMed]

70. McBride, J. Can Foods Forestall Aging? *Agric. Res.* **1999**, *47*, 14–17.

71. McCabe, L.; Britton, R.A.; Parameswaran, N. Prebiotic and Probiotic Regulation of Bone Health: Role of the Intestine and Its Microbiome. *Curr. Osteoporos. Rep.* **2015**, *13*, 363–371. [CrossRef] [PubMed]

72. Steves, C.J.; Bird, S.; Williams, F.M.; Spector, T.D. The Microbiome and Musculoskeletal Conditions of Aging: A Review of Evidence for Impact and Potential Therapeutics. *J. Bone Miner. Res.* **2016**, *31*, 261–269. [CrossRef] [PubMed]

73. Duda-Chodak, A.; Tarko, T.; Satora, P.; Sroka, P. Interaction of Dietary Compounds, Especially Polyphenols, with the Intestinal Microbiota: A Review. *Eur. J. Nutr.* **2015**, *54*, 325–341. [CrossRef] [PubMed]

74. Tuohy, K.M.; Conterno, L.; Gasperotti, M.; Viola, R. Up-Regulating the Human Intestinal Microbiome Using Whole Plant Foods, Polyphenols, and/or Fiber. *J. Agric. Food Chem.* **2012**, *60*, 8776–8782. [CrossRef] [PubMed]

75. Clarke, B. Normal Bone Anatomy and Physiology. *Clin. J. Am. Soc. Nephrol.* **2008**, *3* (Suppl. 3), S131–S139. [CrossRef] [PubMed]

76. Lespessailles, E.; Hambli, R.; Ferrari, S. Osteoporosis Drug Effects on Cortical and Trabecular Bone Microstructure: A Review of Hr-Pqct Analyses. *Bonekey Rep.* **2016**, *5*, 836. [CrossRef] [PubMed]

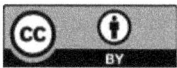

nutrients

MDPI

Article

Vegetable and Fruit Intake and Fracture-Related Hospitalisations: A Prospective Study of Older Women

Lauren C. Blekkenhorst [1,*], Jonathan M. Hodgson [1,2], Joshua R. Lewis [3,4], Amanda Devine [2], Richard J. Woodman [5], Wai H. Lim [6], Germaine Wong [3], Kun Zhu [6,7], Catherine P. Bondonno [1,2], Natalie C. Ward [1,8] and Richard L. Prince [6,7]

[1]   School of Medicine and Pharmacology, Royal Perth Hospital Unit, University of Western Australia, Perth, WA 6000, Australia; jonathan.hodgson@ecu.edu.au (J.M.H.); c.bondonno@ecu.edu.au (C.P.B.); natalie.ward@uwa.edu.au (N.C.W.)
[2]   School of Medical and Health Sciences, Edith Cowan University, Joondalup, WA 6027, Australia; a.devine@ecu.edu.au
[3]   Centre for Kidney Research, Children's Hospital at Westmead, Sydney, NSW 2145, Australia; joshua.lewis@sydney.edu.au (J.R.L.); germaine.wong@health.nsw.gov.au (G.W.)
[4]   School of Public Health, Sydney Medical School, University of Sydney, Sydney, NSW 2006, Australia
[5]   Centre for Epidemiology and Biostatistics, School of Public Health, Flinders University of South Australia, Adelaide, SA 5042, Australia; richard.woodman@flinders.edu.au
[6]   School of Medicine and Pharmacology, QEII Medical Centre Unit, University of Western Australia, Perth, WA 6009, Australia; wai.lim@health.wa.gov.au (W.H.L.); kun.zhu@uwa.edu.au (K.Z.); richard.prince@uwa.edu.au (R.L.P.)
[7]   Department of Endocrinology and Diabetes, and Department of Renal Medicine, Sir Charles Gairdner Hospital, Perth, WA 6009, Australia
[8]   School of Biomedical Sciences & Curtin Health Innovation Research Institute, Curtin University, Perth, WA 6102, Australia
*   Correspondence: lauren.blekkenhorst@research.uwa.edu.au; Tel.: +61-8-9224-0381

Received: 13 April 2017; Accepted: 15 May 2017; Published: 18 May 2017

Abstract: The importance of vegetable and fruit intakes for the prevention of fracture in older women is not well understood. Few studies have explored vegetable and fruit intakes separately, or the associations of specific types of vegetables and fruits with fracture hospitalisations. The objective of this study was to examine the associations of vegetable and fruit intakes, separately, and specific types of vegetables and fruits with fracture-related hospitalisations in a prospective cohort of women aged ≥70 years. Vegetable and fruit intakes were assessed at baseline (1998) in 1468 women using a food frequency questionnaire. The incidence of fracture-related hospitalisations over 14.5 years of follow-up was determined using the Hospital Morbidity Data Collection, linked via the Western Australian Data Linkage System. Fractures were identified in 415 (28.3%) women, of which 158 (10.8%) were hip fractures. Higher intakes of vegetables, but not fruits, were associated with lower fracture incidence. In multivariable-adjusted models for vegetable types, cruciferous and allium vegetables were inversely associated with all fractures, with a hazard ratio (HR) (95% confidence interval) of 0.72 (0.54, 0.95) and 0.66 (0.49, 0.88), respectively, for the highest vs. lowest quartiles. Increasing vegetable intake, with an emphasis on cruciferous and allium vegetables, may prevent fractures in older postmenopausal women.

Keywords: vegetables; fruit; cruciferous; allium; fracture; bone; postmenopausal women

1. Introduction

Dietary patterns rich in vegetables and fruits may provide benefits to bone health [1–5]. A number of studies have explored the relationships of defined dietary patterns with fracture risk. Although the results of these studies are inconsistent [1,4–7], they do suggest that certain components of these diets may contribute to lower fracture risk [8–10]. A major contribution may be the high intake of vegetables and fruits which are a key attribute of all healthy dietary patterns. This concept is supported by the results of prospective studies in a variety of populations finding that higher vegetable and fruit intakes are associated with lower risk of fracture [2,3,9,11]. However, there is little data on the effects of specific vegetable or fruit types on fracture outcomes. It is possible that some vegetables and fruits may be more protective than others due to specific nutrients and bioactive compounds such as phytochemicals.

In this study, we explored the associations of vegetable and fruit intakes, separately, with 14.5 years fracture-related hospitalisations in a prospective cohort of postmenopausal women aged ≥70 years. We then examined the associations of specific types of vegetables and fruits with fracture outcomes.

2. Materials and Methods

2.1. Study Population

The population included women in the Perth Longitudinal Study of Aging in Women (PLSAW). The women were originally recruited to a 5-year, double-blind, randomised controlled trial of daily calcium supplementation to prevent fracture, the Calcium Intake Fracture Outcome Study (CAIFOS). The women were included on the basis of an expected survival beyond 5 years and not receiving any medication (including hormone replacement therapy) known to affect bone metabolism. This trial has been previously described [12]. The women ($n = 1500$) were recruited from the Western Australian general population of women aged ≥70 years by mail using the electoral roll, which is a requirement of Australian citizenship. At the completion of the 5-year trial, women were invited to participate in two follow-up observational studies. Total follow-up was 14.5 years. A total of 1485 women completed a food frequency questionnaire at baseline in 1998. Participants ($n = 17/1485$, 1.1%) with implausible energy intakes (<2100 kJ (500 kcal) or >14,700 kJ (3500 kcal)) were not included in the analysis. The current study then included 1468 women. All participants provided written informed consent. Ethics approval was granted by the Human Ethics Committee of the University of Western Australia. Both studies were retrospectively registered on the Australian New Zealand Clinical Trials Registry (CAIFOS trial registration number #ACTRN12615000750583 and PLSAW trial registration number #ACTRN12617000640303), and complied with the Declaration of Helsinki. Human ethics approval for the use of linked data was provided by the Human Research Ethics Committee of the Western Australian Department of Health (project number #2009/24).

2.2. Dietary Assessment

Dietary intake was assessed at baseline (1998), 5 years (2003), and 7 years (2005) using a self-administered, semiquantitative food frequency questionnaire developed and validated by the Cancer Council of Victoria [13–15]. The women were supported when completing the questionnaire by a research assistant. Food models and food charts as well as measuring cups and measuring spoons were provided to ensure the accuracy of reported food consumption. The Cancer Council of Victoria calculated energy (kJ/day) and nutrient intakes by using the NUTTAB95 food composition database [16] and other sources where necessary. Intakes of individual food items were calculated in g/day. This included 24 vegetables and 11 fruits. The diet assessment analysis also provided estimates of protein, calcium, and alcohol intakes.

2.2.1. Vegetable and Fruit Intake

Vegetable and fruit intake were calculated in serves per day. This was based on the 2013 Australian Dietary Guidelines of 1 serve of vegetables equivalent to 75 g and 1 serve of fruit equivalent to 150 g [17]. Serves per day were calculated as continuous variables and then categorised as discrete variables (vegetables: <2 serves, 2 to <3 serves, ≥3 serves; fruit: <1 serve, 1 to <2 serves, ≥2 serves). Estimations of vegetable intake did not include 'Potatoes, roasted or fried, including hot chips' as hot chips are not recommended as part of a healthy diet [17]. 'Potatoes cooked without fat' were included. Estimations of fruit intake did not include 'Tinned or frozen fruit (any kind)' or 'Fruit juice' as foods and drinks containing added sugars are not recommended as part of a healthy diet [17].

2.2.2. Vegetable and Fruit Type

Vegetables were grouped into five types. These vegetable types were based on the 2013 Australian Dietary Guidelines [17] and modified slightly to include cruciferous vegetables (cabbage, brussel sprouts, cauliflower, and broccoli); allium vegetables (onion, leek, and garlic); yellow/orange/red vegetables (tomato, capsicum, beetroot, carrot, and pumpkin); leafy green vegetables (lettuce and other salad greens, celery, silverbeet, and spinach); and legumes (peas, greens beans, bean sprouts and alfalfa sprouts, baked beans, soy beans, soy bean curd, and tofu, and other beans). For fruit, classification of type included: apples and pears (pome fruit); oranges and other citrus (citrus); bananas; and other fruits (melon, pineapple, strawberries, apricots, peaches, mango and avocado). Intakes of vegetable and fruit types were calculated in g/day as continuous variables. Intakes of vegetable types were also categorised as discrete variables into quartiles of intake.

2.2.3. Nutrient-Rich Foods Index

Overall diet quality was assessed using the Nutrient-Rich Foods Index by calculating nutrient density scores [18]. This index was adapted using the Nutrient Reference Values (NRVs) for Australia and New Zealand based on adult females aged >70 years [19]. The calculation of the Nutrient-Rich Foods Index in this cohort of older women has been described previously [20].

2.3. Fracture Outcome Assessment

Fracture-related hospitalisations were retrieved from linked data via the Western Australian Data Linkage System (Department of Health Western Australia, East Perth, Australia) for each participant from their baseline visit until 14.5 years after their baseline visit. Fracture-related hospitalisations were identified from the Hospital Morbidity Data Collection which provides a complete record of participants' primary diagnosis at hospital discharge using coded data from all hospitals in Western Australia. Fracture-related hospitalisations were defined using the International Statistical Classification of Diseases and Related Health Problems, 10th Revision [21]. Codes used for identification included S02–S92, M80, T02, T08, T10, T12, and T14.2. Fractures of the face (S02.2–S02.6), fingers (S62.5–S62.7), and toes (S92.4–S92.5), and fractures caused by motor vehicle injuries were excluded (external cause of injury codes V00–V99).

2.4. Baseline Characteristic Assessment

Questionnaires completed at baseline were used to assess values for potential confounding variables including age, physical activity, and smoking history. Participants were asked about participation in sport, recreation, and/or regular physical activities undertaken in the three months prior to their baseline visit [22,23]. The level of activity, expressed in kilojoules per day, was then calculated using a validated method applying the type of activity, time engaged in the activity, and the participant's body weight [24,25]. Smoking history was coded as non-smoker or ex-smoker/current smoker if they had consumed >1 cigarette per day for more than 3 months at any time in their life. Body weight was measured using digital scales to the nearest 0.1 kg and height was assessed using a wall-mounted stadiometer to the nearest 0.1 cm, both whilst participants were wearing light clothes and without socks and shoes. Body mass index (BMI) (kg/m^2) was then calculated. Treatment (placebo or calcium) over the 5 years of the CAIFOS trial was included as a covariate. Current medication use at baseline was used to assess prevalent diabetes mellitus. Medications were verified by participants' general practitioner where possible and were coded (T89001–T90009) using the International Classification of Primary Care-Plus (ICPC-Plus) method which allows aggregation of different terms for similar pathologic entities as defined by the ICD-10 coding system [26]. Socioeconomic status (SES) was calculated using the Socioeconomic Indexes for Areas developed by the Australian Bureau of Statistics which ranked residential postcodes according to relative socio-economic advantage and disadvantage [27]. Participants were then coded into six groups from the top 10% most highly disadvantaged to the top 10% least disadvantaged [27]. Prevalent fractures were determined by self-reported fractures that had occurred after the age of 50 and prior to the participants' baseline visit. Self-reported fractures were defined as a fracture due to a minimal trauma fall from less than 1 m that did not include fractures of the face, skull, and phalanges.

2.5. Statistical Analysis

Statistical analysis was performed using IBM SPSS Statistics for Windows, version 21.0 (IBM Corp., Armonk, NY, USA) and SAS software, version 9.4 (SAS Institute Inc., Cary, NC, USA). Statistical significance was set at a 2-sided Type 1 error rate of $p < 0.05$ for all tests. Descriptive statistics of normally distributed continuous variables were expressed as mean $\pm$ standard deviation (SD). Non-normally distributed continuous variables (physical activity, alcohol intake, allium vegetable intake, and all fruit types) were expressed as median and interquartile range. Categorical variables were expressed as number and proportion (%). Baseline characteristics were tested for differences across categories using one-way analysis of variance (ANOVA) for normally distributed continuous variables, the Kruskal-Wallis test for non-normally distributed variables, and the Chi-squared test for categorical variables.

The primary outcome of the study was first hospitalisation for fracture, with further analysis of hip fracture which accounted for more than one-third of all events. Complete follow-up was available for all participants that remained in Western Australia, which was likely to be almost all participants given their age. The follow-up time period for each participant commenced from their baseline visit date until the first fracture-related hospitalisation or loss to follow-up due to death or 174 months of complete follow-up. Cox proportional hazards modelling was used to assess the associations of vegetable and fruit intake variables with fracture outcomes. Two models of adjustment were used: age-adjusted and multivariable-adjusted. The multivariable-adjusted models included age, BMI, treatment code, prevalent diabetes mellitus, SES, physical activity, smoking history, and intakes of energy, protein, calcium, and alcohol. Associations were explored using continuous variables and then as discrete variables. We also tested for evidence of linear trends across categories of discrete variables using the median value for each category as continuous variables in separate Cox proportional hazards models. Cox proportional hazards assumptions were tested using log-log plots, which were shown to be parallel indicating that proportional hazards assumptions were not violated. For the primary analysis, we treated deaths as censored. This cause-specific approach meant that the hazard ratios could be interpreted as the risk of fracture for any time during follow-up assuming that the participant stayed alive for that duration of time. The calculated risk of fracture, therefore, assumed that the risk of fracture would have remained the same during the remainder of the follow-up period in those that died. This model was chosen as we have previously demonstrated that fruit intakes are associated with mortality risk in this cohort [28]. Based on the given data with 16,458 years of follow up and fracture event rates of 28.3% and 10.8%, respectively, for "all fractures" and "hip fractures", the study had 80% power to detect a hazard ratio of 0.79 for all fractures and a hazard ratio of 0.69 for hip fractures, assuming a two-tailed type 1 error rate of alpha = 0.05.

Sensitivity Analyses

The relationships between cruciferous, allium, and total vegetables were investigated using Spearman Rank Order Correlation (rho). To examine whether the independent associations of cruciferous and allium vegetables were not due to collinearity with each other, a forward stepwise Cox proportional hazards model with all multivariable-adjusted variables as well as cruciferous (per 10 g/day) and allium (per 5 g/day) vegetables was analysed for all fractures. To examine whether the associations of cruciferous and allium vegetables were independent of total vegetable intake (per serve, 75 g/day), a forward stepwise Cox proportional hazards model with all multivariable-adjusted variables as well as intakes of cruciferous (per 10 g/day) and allium (per 5 g/day) vegetables, and total vegetable intake (per serve) was tested for all fractures. Intakes of cruciferous, allium, and total vegetables at baseline (1998), 5 years (2003), and 7 years (2005) were tested for differences using one-way repeated measures ANOVA. To account for change in cruciferous, allium, and total vegetable intakes, the average of the three time points (baseline, 5 years, and 7 years) for each vegetable variable were used in the multivariable-adjusted Cox proportional hazards model for all fractures. Since vegetable intake may be considered a surrogate marker of a healthier diet, we adjusted for diet quality using the Nutrient-Rich Foods Index in the multivariable-adjusted Cox proportional hazards model for all fractures. This was separately completed for cruciferous, allium, and total vegetable intakes. Lastly, since previous fractures can increase the risk of subsequent fracture [29], an interaction term between total vegetable intake and prevalent fracture was tested in the multivariable-adjusted Cox proportional hazards model. This was completed to evaluate if prevalent fracture had an impact on the relationship between total vegetable intake and all fractures. This test was repeated for intakes of cruciferous vegetables as well as intakes of allium vegetables. Lastly, as women may have commenced calcium or calcium plus vitamin D supplementation after the completion of the CAIFOS, we assessed whether the proportion of women who re-enrolled in the 5-year extension study (2003–2008) and commenced these supplements were different across vegetable serve categories. Furthermore, we analysed differences amongst women who commenced taking bisphosphonates from 1998–2003. It should be noted that data on calcium, calcium plus vitamin D, and bisphosphonate use were only available for $n = 1007/1456$ (69%) participants.

3. Results

3.1. Baseline Characteristics

Baseline characteristics of participants are presented according to all participants and categories of vegetable (Table 1) and fruit (Table 2) intakes. The mean age of participants at baseline was 75.2 years (SD 2.7 years). Significant differences were observed across vegetable intake categories for energy, protein, and calcium intakes ($p < 0.001$) (Table 1). Significant differences were observed across fruit intake categories for energy, protein, calcium, and alcohol intakes, physical activity, and smoking status ($p < 0.01$) (Table 2).

Mean (SD) intake for vegetables was 196.4 (79.1) g/day and 2.6 (1.0) serves per day, and for fruit it was 245.1 (128.6) g/day and 1.6 (0.9) serves per day. Mean (SD) intake (from highest to lowest) of vegetable types were: yellow/orange/red vegetables 51.8 (27.5) g/day; cruciferous vegetables 32.1 (21.9) g/day; legume vegetables 27.5 (18.7) g/day; and leafy green vegetables 18.6 (12.0) g/day. Median (interquartile range (IQR)) intake for allium vegetables was 6.2 (2.9–10.7) g/day. Median (IQR) intake (from highest to lowest) for fruit types were: apple and pears 54.4 (22.2–103.6) g/day; other fruits 49.5 (22.0–95.4) g/day; bananas 44.5 (18.5–72.6) g/day; and orange and other citrus fruits 35.5 (5.6–85.9) g/day.

3.2. Fracture-Related Hospitalisation

Over 14.5 years (16,458 person-years) of follow-up, 415/1468 (28.3%) participants were hospitalised with a fracture, of which 158/1468 (10.8%) were hip fractures.

Table 1. Baseline characteristics according to all participants and vegetable intake categories [1].

	All Participants	Vegetable Serve Intake [2]			p Value [3]
		<2 Serves/Day	2 to <3 Serves/Day	≥3 Serves/Day	
Number	1468	424	584	460	
Age, years	75.2 ± 2.7	75.2 ± 2.7	75.2 ± 2.7	75.0 ± 2.7	0.455
Body mass index (BMI) [4], kg/m²	27.2 ± 4.7	27.0 ± 4.8	27.2 ± 4.6	27.5 ± 5.0	0.233
Treatment (calcium) [5]	755 (51.4)	202 (47.6)	309 (53.0)	244 (53.0)	0.175
Prevalent fracture [5]	397 (27.0)	112 (26.4)	156 (26.8)	129 (28.0)	0.843
Prevalent diabetes mellitus	90 (6.1)	28 (6.6)	34 (5.8)	28 (6.1)	0.877
Physical activity [4], kJ/day	467.1 (0.0–855.4)	455.0 (0.0–886.3)	443.5 (159.4–836.9)	491.4 (157.7–852.0)	0.743
Smoked ever [6]	546 (37.2)	156 (36.9)	224 (38.7)	166 (36.2)	0.698
Socioeconomic status [7]					0.659
Top 10% most highly disadvantaged	63 (4.3)	16 (3.8)	24 (4.1)	23 (5.1)	-
Highly disadvantaged	174 (11.9)	51 (12.1)	66 (11.4)	57 (12.6)	-
Moderate–highly disadvantaged	237 (16.1)	67 (15.9)	94 (16.2)	76 (16.7)	-
Low–moderately disadvantaged	222 (15.1)	73 (17.3)	77 (13.3)	72 (15.9)	-
Low disadvantaged	309 (21.0)	84 (19.9)	124 (21.4)	101 (22.2)	-
Top 10% least disadvantaged	451 (30.7)	131 (31.0)	195 (33.6)	125 (27.5)	-
Dietary intakes					
Energy, kJ/day	7097.4 ± 2077.6	6232.8 ± 1811.3	6945.4 ± 1924.6	8087.4 ± 2089.2	<0.001
Protein, g/day	79.5 ± 26.6	67.3 ± 22.0	78.1 ± 25.4	92.5 ± 26.1	<0.001
Calcium, mg/day	952.9 ± 345.4	869.7 ± 327.6	950.5 ± 342.7	1032.8 ± 347.2	<0.001
Alcohol, g/day	1.8 (0.3–9.8)	1.8 (0.3–9.3)	1.7 (0.3–9.3)	2.0 (0.3–10.4)	0.905

[1] Data presented as mean ± SD, median (interquartile range) or number (n) and (%); [2] Vegetable serves were calculated based on the 2013 Australian Dietary Guidelines of a vegetable serve equal to 75 g/day; [3] p values are a comparison between groups using ANOVA, Kruskal-Wallis test, and Chi-square test where appropriate; [4] n = 1466; [5] n = 1467; [6] n = 1460; [7] n = 1456.

Table 2. Baseline characteristics according to fruit intake categories [1].

	Fruit Serve Intake [2]			
	<1 Serves/Day	1 to <2 Serves/Day	≥2 Serves/Day	*p* Value [3]
Number	417	560	491	
Age, years	74.9 ± 2.7	75.2 ± 2.7	75.3 ± 2.7	0.140
BMI [4], kg/m^2	26.9 ± 4.6	27.3 ± 4.7	27.4 ± 4.9	0.257
Treatment (calcium) [5]	210 (50.4)	279 (49.9)	266 (54.2)	0.335
Prevalent fracture [5]	109 (26.2)	154 (27.5)	134 (27.3)	0.894
Prevalent diabetes mellitus	19 (4.6)	32 (5.7)	39 (7.9)	0.092
Physical activity [4], kJ/day	399.2 (0.0–806.6)	451.7 (70.6–811.6)	532.7 (210.2–928.8)	0.002
Smoked ever [6]	178 (42.9)	175 (31.5)	193 (39.5)	0.001
Socioeconomic status [7]				
Top 10% most highly disadvantaged	18 (4.4)	24 (4.3)	21 (4.3)	0.998
Highly disadvantaged	54 (13.1)	65 (11.7)	55 (11.3)	-
Moderate-highly disadvantaged	70 (16.9)	90 (16.2)	77 (15.8)	-
Low-moderately disadvantaged	63 (15.3)	82 (14.7)	77 (15.8)	-
Low disadvantaged	85 (20.6)	123 (22.1)	101 (20.7)	-
Top 10% least disadvantaged	123 (29.8)	172 (30.9)	156 (32.0)	-
Dietary intakes				
Energy, kJ/day	6829.9 ± 1948.7	6812.5 ± 2003.7	7649.7 ± 2158.5	<0.001
Protein, g/day	75.5 ± 24.9	76.2 ± 24.7	86.6 ± 28.5	<0.001
Calcium, mg/day	854.9 ± 306.2	952.1 ± 338.8	1037.2 ± 362.5	<0.001
Alcohol, g/day	2.6 (0.3–11.9)	1.8 (0.4–9.3)	1.2 (0.1–7.9)	0.008

[1] Data presented as mean ± SD, median [interquartile range] or number (*n*) and (%); [2] Fruit serves were calculated based on the 2013 Australian Dietary Guidelines of a fruit serve equal to 150 g/day; [3] *p* values are a comparison between groups using ANOVA, Kruskal-Wallis test, and Chi-square test where appropriate; [4] *n* = 1466; [5] *n* = 1467; [6] *n* = 1460; [7] *n* = 1456.

3.2.1. Vegetable Intake

Vegetable intake (per serve) was inversely associated with all fractures and hip fractures in age-adjusted and multivariable-adjusted models ($p < 0.05$) (Table 3). Compared with low intakes of vegetables (<2 serves/day), intakes of ≥3 serves/day were associated with a 27% lower hazard for all fractures (multivariable-adjusted p_{trend} = 0.023) and a 39% lower hazard for hip fractures (multivariable-adjusted p_{trend} = 0.037) (Table 3).

The associations between intakes of vegetable types and fracture-related hospitalisations in multivariable-adjusted models are presented in Table 4. Intakes of cruciferous and allium vegetables were inversely associated with all fractures ($p < 0.05$) (Table 4). The highest quartiles of cruciferous (multivariable-adjusted p_{trend} = 0.030) and allium (multivariable-adjusted p_{trend} = 0.003) vegetables in comparison to the lowest quartiles were associated with a 28% and 34%, respectively, lower hazard for all fractures. After additional adjustment for total vegetable intake, the hazard for all fractures was reduced and became non-significant for the highest quartile of cruciferous vegetables (multivariable-adjusted hazard ratio (HR): 0.80, 95% confidence interval (CI) 0.58, 1.10, p_{trend} = 0.160) compared to the lowest quartile. Allium vegetables, however, remained statistically significant (multivariable-adjusted HR: 0.70, 95% CI 0.52, 0.95, p_{trend} = 0.019).

For hip fractures, the association of allium vegetables was borderline significant ($p = 0.050$), but did not reach significance for cruciferous vegetables ($p = 0.157$). Intakes of yellow/orange/red, leafy green, and legumes were not associated with all fractures ($p > 0.05$ for all) or hip fractures ($p > 0.05$ for all) (Table 4).

3.2.2. Fruit Intake

Fruit intake (per serve) was not associated with all fractures ($p > 0.05$) and hip fractures ($p > 0.05$) (Table 5). The associations between intakes of fruit types and fracture-related hospitalisations in multivariable-adjusted models are presented in Table 6. All fruit types were not associated with all fractures ($p > 0.05$ for all) and hip fractures ($p > 0.05$ for all).

Table 3. Hazard ratios for fracture-related hospitalisation by vegetable serve intake [1].

	All Participants	p Value	Vegetable Serve Intake			
			<2 Serves/Day	2 to <3 Serves/Day	≥3 Serves/Day	p for Trend [2]
All fractures						
Number	1468		424	584	460	
Events, n (%)	415 (28.3)		133 (31.4)	172 (29.5)	110 (23.9)	
Age-adjusted	0.85 (0.77, 0.94)	0.002	1.00 (Referent)	0.87 (0.69, 1.09)	0.67 (0.52, 0.87)	0.002
Multivariable-adjusted [3]	0.88 (0.79, 0.98)	0.024	1.00 (Referent)	0.88 (0.70, 1.11)	0.73 (0.55, 0.96)	0.023
Hip fractures						
Events, n (%)	158 (10.8)		57 (13.4)	66 (11.3)	35 (7.6)	
Age-adjusted	0.77 (0.65, 0.90)	0.002	1.00 (Referent)	0.78 (0.55, 1.12)	0.52 (0.34, 0.79)	0.002
Multivariable-adjusted	0.82 (0.69, 0.98)	0.033	1.00 (Referent)	0.88 (0.61, 1.27)	0.61 (0.39, 0.97)	0.037

[1] Hazard ratios (95% CI) for fracture-related hospitalisation by vegetable serve intake analysed using Cox proportional hazard models. Vegetable serves were calculated based on the 2013 Australian Dietary Guidelines of a vegetable serve equal to 75 g/day; [2] Test for trend conducted using median value for each vegetable serve category (1.6, 2.5, and 3.6 serves/day); [3] Multivariable-adjusted model included age, BMI, treatment code, prevalent diabetes mellitus, socioeconomic status, physical activity, smoking history, and energy, protein, calcium, and alcohol intake.

Table 4. Multivariable-adjusted hazard ratios for fracture-related hospitalisation by vegetable type [1].

	All Participants [2]	p Value	Quartiles of Vegetable Types [3]				
			Q1	Q2	Q3	Q4	p For Trend [4]
All fractures							
Cruciferous	0.90 (0.81, 0.99)	0.026	1.00 (Referent)	0.79 (0.61, 1.04)	0.80 (0.61, 1.05)	0.72 (0.54, 0.95)	0.030
Allium	0.81 (0.68, 0.96)	0.013	1.00 (Referent)	0.89 (0.68, 1.16)	0.77 (0.59, 1.01)	0.66 (0.49, 0.88)	0.003
Yellow/orange/red	0.95 (0.88, 1.03)	0.184	1.00 (Referent)	0.83 (0.64, 1.09)	0.71 (0.54, 0.94)	0.80 (0.61, 1.06)	0.118
Leafy green	0.97 (0.82, 1.15)	0.772	1.00 (Referent)	0.80 (0.61, 1.05)	0.73 (0.55, 0.96)	0.84 (0.64, 1.10)	0.229
Legumes	0.94 (0.84, 1.05)	0.264	1.00 (Referent)	0.91 (0.70, 1.20)	0.82 (0.62, 1.08)	0.87 (0.66, 1.16)	0.332
Hip fractures							
Cruciferous	0.89 (0.76, 1.05)	0.157	1.00 (Referent)	0.80 (0.53, 1.22)	0.79 (0.51, 1.22)	0.65 (0.41, 1.04)	0.083
Allium	0.75 (0.56, 1.00)	0.050	1.00 (Referent)	0.74 (0.48, 1.14)	0.85 (0.56, 1.31)	0.61 (0.38, 0.99)	0.086
Yellow/orange/red	0.90 (0.79, 1.03)	0.130	1.00 (Referent)	1.05 (0.69, 1.61)	0.89 (0.57, 1.40)	0.75 (0.47, 1.22)	0.181
Leafy green	0.91 (0.69, 1.19)	0.484	1.00 (Referent)	1.09 (0.71, 1.67)	0.75 (0.47, 1.20)	0.94 (0.60, 1.47)	0.531
Legumes	0.87 (0.72, 1.05)	0.152	1.00 (Referent)	1.15 (0.75, 1.77)	0.88 (0.56, 1.37)	0.79 (0.49, 1.27)	0.188

[1] Multivariable-adjusted hazard ratios (95% CI) for fracture-related hospitalisation by vegetable type analysed using Cox proportional hazard models, adjusted for age, BMI, treatment code, prevalent diabetes mellitus, socioeconomic status, physical activity, smoking history, and energy, protein, calcium, and alcohol intake; [2] Results are presented per 10 g/day for allium vegetables and per 20 g/day for all other types of vegetables; [3] Quartiles for cruciferous vegetables were Q1 (<15 g/day), Q2 (15–28 g/day), Q3 (29–44 g/day), Q4 (>44 g/day); allium vegetables were Q1 (<3 g/day), Q2 (3–6 g/day), Q3 (7–11 g/day), Q4 (>11 g/day); yellow/orange/red vegetables were Q1 (<32 g/day), Q2 (32–47 g/day), Q3 (48–68 g/day), Q4 (>68 g/day); leafy green vegetables were Q1 (<9 g/day), Q2 (9–16 g/day), Q3 (17–25 g/day), Q4 (>25 g/day); and legumes were Q1 (<15 g/day), Q2 (15–23 g/day), Q3 (24–36 g/day), Q4 (>36 g/day); [4] Test for trend conducted using median values of each quartile of vegetable type.

Table 5. Hazard ratios for fracture-related hospitalisation by fruit serve intake [1].

| | | All Participants | p Value | Fruit Serve Intake | | | |
				<1 Serves/Day	1 to <2 Serves/Day	≥2 Serves/Day	p for Trend [2]
All fractures	Number	1468		417	560	491	
	Events, *n* (%)	415 (28.3)		119 (28.5)	159 (28.4)	137 (27.9)	
	Age-adjusted	0.94 (0.84, 1.06)	0.333	1.00 (Referent)	0.93 (0.73, 1.18)	0.90 (0.70, 1.15)	0.412
	Multivariable-adjusted [3]	0.99 (0.88, 1.12)	0.855	1.00 (Referent)	0.94 (0.74, 1.21)	0.97 (0.75, 1.25)	0.825
Hip fractures	Events, *n* (%)	158 (10.8)		50 (12.0)	60 (10.7)	48 (9.8)	
	Age-adjusted	0.86 (0.71, 1.03)	0.109	1.00 (Referent)	0.82 (0.46, 1.19)	0.73 (0.49, 1.09)	0.129
	Multivariable-adjusted	0.89 (0.73, 1.08)	0.242	1.00 (Referent)	0.81 (0.55, 1.19)	0.76 (0.50, 1.15)	0.207

[1] Hazard ratios (95% CI) for fracture-related hospitalisation by fruit serve intake analysed using Cox proportional hazard models. Fruit serves were calculated based on the 2013 Australian Dietary Guidelines of a fruit serve equal to 150 g/day; [2] Test for trend conducted using median value for each fruit serve category (0.7, 1.5 and 2.5 serves/day); [3] Multivariable-adjusted model included age, BMI, treatment code, prevalent diabetes mellitus, socioeconomic status, physical activity, smoking history, and energy, protein, calcium, and alcohol intake.

3.3. Sensitivity Analyses

There was a weak positive correlation between intakes of cruciferous and allium vegetables (Spearman's rho = 0.11, $p < 0.001$) and a moderate positive correlation between intakes of allium and total vegetables (Spearman's rho = 0.43, $p < 0.001$) and between intakes of cruciferous and total vegetables (Spearman's rho = 0.52, $p < 0.001$). In a forward stepwise Cox proportional hazards model, which included all multivariable-adjusted variables and both cruciferous and allium vegetable intakes separately, age (per year increase, HR: 1.10, 95% CI: 1.06, 1.14, $p < 0.001$), BMI (per kg/m^2 increase, HR: 0.98, 95% CI: 0.95, 1.00, $p = 0.034$), cruciferous vegetables (per 20 g/day increase, HR: 0.89, 95% CI: 0.81, 0.98, $p = 0.019$), and allium vegetables (per 10 g/day increase, HR: 0.82, 95% CI: 0.70, 0.97, $p = 0.018$) were associated with all fractures. In a forward stepwise Cox proportional hazards model, which included all multivariable-adjusted variables and total vegetable intakes as well as intakes of cruciferous and allium vegetables, age (per year increase, HR: 1.10, 95% CI: 1.06, 1.14, $p < 0.001$), BMI (per kg/m^2 increase, HR: 0.98, 95% CI: 0.95, 1.00, $p = 0.036$), and total vegetable intake (per 75 g/day increase, HR: 0.87, 95% CI: 0.79, 0.96, $p = 0.007$) were associated with all fractures.

Intakes of cruciferous, allium, and total vegetables were compared at baseline (1998), 5 years (2003), and 7 years (2005) in 986 participants. The mean (SD) at each time point for intakes of cruciferous, allium, and total vegetables are presented in Table S1. One-way repeated measures ANOVA were conducted for intakes of cruciferous, allium, and total vegetables and results confirmed a significant effect for time (Wilks' Lambda $p < 0.001$ for all). Intake of cruciferous vegetables was 2.5 g/day (7.8%) lower at 7 years compared to intake at baseline. Intake of allium vegetables was 1.5 g/day (18.5%) lower at 5 years and 2.2 g/day (27.2%) lower at 7 years compared to intake at baseline. Total vegetable intake was 22.3 g/day (11%) lower at 5 years and 31.5 g/day (16%) lower at 7 years compared to intake at baseline. To account for this change, the average across baseline, 5 years, and 7 years was calculated individually for cruciferous, allium, and total vegetable intakes. The average values for cruciferous, allium, and total vegetable intakes were then entered separately into multivariable-adjusted Cox proportional hazards models for all fractures. This did not substantively alter the hazard ratios observed for baseline values and fracture-related hospitalisations (Table S2).

Adjustment for the Nutrient-Rich Foods Index in multivariable-adjusted models attenuated the associations of all fractures with intakes of total vegetables and cruciferous vegetables ($p > 0.05$ for both), but not allium vegetables ($p = 0.027$). No effect modification by prevalent fracture was observed for intakes of total vegetables ($p_{interaction} = 0.617$), cruciferous vegetables ($p_{interaction} = 0.989$), or allium vegetables ($p_{interaction} = 0.482$). Lastly, there were no differences in calcium ($n = 12$), calcium plus vitamin D ($n = 393$), or bisphosphonate ($n = 80$) use across vegetables serve categories amongst the $n = 1007$ women with available data ($p > 0.05$ for all).

Table 6. Multivariable-adjusted hazard ratios for fracture-related hospitalisation by fruit type.

	All Participants	*p* Value
All fractures		
Apples and pears	0.99 (0.96, 1.02)	0.698
Oranges and other citrus fruits	1.01 (0.97, 1.04)	0.710
Bananas	1.02 (0.97, 1.07)	0.386
Other fruits	0.98 (0.95, 1.02)	0.378
Hip fractures		
Apples and pears	0.99 (0.94, 1.04)	0.604
Oranges and other citrus fruits	0.99 (0.94, 1.05)	0.828
Bananas	0.97 (0.89, 1.05)	0.432
Other fruits	0.97 (0.91, 1.03)	0.279

Multivariable-adjusted hazard ratios (95% CI) for fracture-related hospitalisation by fruit type (per 20 g/day) analysed using Cox proportional hazard models, adjusted for age, BMI, treatment code, prevalent diabetes mellitus, socioeconomic status, physical activity, smoking history, and energy, protein, calcium, and alcohol intake.

4. Discussion

In this prospective cohort study of older women, we identified vegetable intakes, but not fruit intakes, to be associated with a lower hazard of all fractures and hip fractures. We also identified cruciferous and allium vegetable intakes to be individually associated with a lower hazard of all fractures, but not hip fractures. This may be due to the relatively low prevalence of hip fractures in this study and, therefore, the insufficient power to detect an association. The study was only powered to detect relatively large reductions in risk between food intake categories of around 20% for all fractures and 30% for hip fractures. The associations were independent of dietary and lifestyle factors known to be related to fracture risk.

Habitual intakes of vegetables and fruits, combined, have been associated with lower risk of fracture outcomes [2,5,6,30]. In particular, vegetable and fruit intakes have also been individually associated with lower risk of fracture outcomes [2,5,30]. A meta-analysis has identified vegetables, but not fruits, to be associated with reduced risk of hip fracture [31]. Our study is consistent with this meta-analysis, having demonstrated vegetable intake, but not fruit intake, to be associated with lower risk of fracture outcomes.

There are two main explanations why higher vegetable intakes could contribute to a lower risk of fracture. These include effects on bone mineral density and risk of falling. A number of studies have explored the link between vegetable and fruit intake and bone mineral density with inconsistent results. Some observational studies have found associations of vegetable and fruit intakes with bone mineral density [2,3,5,8,30,32,33], whilst others have not observed an association [34]. In addition, results of randomised controlled trials have not found consistent effects on biomarkers of bone turnover [35–37]. Evidence on the relationship of vegetable and fruit intakes with risk of falling are scant. Therefore, although there is strong evidence supporting beneficial effects of vegetables on fracture risk, the pathways and mechanisms responsible remain unclear.

To our knowledge, this is one of the first studies to investigate the associations of different types of vegetables and fruits with fracture outcomes in a population of older postmenopausal women. We demonstrated both cruciferous and allium vegetable intakes to be inversely associated with fracture risk, both of which were independent of each other. Cruciferous and allium vegetables contain an abundance of specific nutrients and phytochemicals that may benefit bone biology and subsequent fracture outcomes. For example, intakes of vitamin K (rich in cruciferous vegetables) have been shown to be inversely associated with hip fractures [38]. However, other studies have shown conflicting results [39]. Intakes of allium vegetables, in particular onions, have been shown to be associated with increased bone density in perimenopausal and postmenopausal women [40].

One mechanism through which phytochemicals may benefit bone biology is by the reductions in oxidative stress. Oxidative stress has been demonstrated to inhibit in vitro osteoblastic differentiation [41], and in human studies, relationships between excessive reactive oxygen species and bone loss have been observed [42,43]. Particular phytochemicals of interest found in both cruciferous and allium vegetables are organosulfur compounds. Sulforaphane, an organosulfur compound found abundantly in cruciferous vegetables, has been shown to inhibit in vitro human osteoclast differentiation [44], possibly due to the activation of nuclear factor-erythroid 2-related factor 2 (Nrf2) [45]. Nrf2 is a redox-sensitive transcription factor that regulates the expression of antioxidant proteins protecting against oxidative stress. In addition, sulforaphane has been shown to epigenetically stimulate osteoblast activity and reduce osteoclast bone resorption [46]. Park et al. [47] have also shown the alliin-containing vegetable, allium hookeri, to have in vitro and in vivo anabolic effects on bone formation. Allium hookeri is a widely consumed allium vegetable in Southeast Asia and is a rich source of alliin, an organosulfur compound that is also found abundantly in other allium vegetables such as garlic.

Strengths to this current study include the prospective design and population-based setting with ascertainment of verified fracture-related hospitalisations with almost no loss to follow-up. Participants of this study were representative of older women of the Australian population. The average vegetable serves of the women in this study were 2.6 serves which is the same for older Australian women aged

≥75 years [48]. In addition, there was also relatively detailed information on a number of known confounders including alcohol intake and socioeconomic status. Dietary information was collected at different time points and was collected using a validated and reproducible method of assessment. Limitations, however, need to be acknowledged. Participants of this study may have commenced taking calcium supplements or medications known to affect bone metabolism after the completion of the CAIFOS. However, we have demonstrated the proportion of participants that commenced taking calcium or calcium plus vitamin D supplements at the completion of the CAIFOS were similar across vegetable serve categories. In addition, medications known to affect bone metabolism are most likely prescribed after an osteoporotic fracture. Therefore, it is unlikely this would have influenced the interpretation of our findings. In addition, the dietary information, including habitual intakes of vegetables and fruits, were self-reported which may lead to misclassification of these variables. In addition, even though we adjusted for potential confounders such as dietary and lifestyle factors known to be associated with fracture risk, higher vegetable intakes may be a marker of a healthier lifestyle not completely captured by the lifestyle variables that we included as potential confounders in the multivariable-adjusted analyses. For example, participants consuming ≥3 serves/day of vegetable intake versus participants consuming <2 serves/day reported a 30% higher energy intake despite similar BMI. This suggests that they were more physically active. Even though the relationships of cruciferous, allium, and total vegetable intakes with fracture-related hospitalisations persisted after adjustment for energy intake and physical activity, the reported physical activity is relatively imprecise in comparison with these lifestyle factors. Although physical activity has been associated with geometric indices of bone strength in this cohort [49], reported physical activity using questionnaires are somewhat unreliable with the likelihood of under adjustment. We attempted to further address the possibility of higher vegetable intakes being a marker of a healthier lifestyle by adjusting for diet quality. This did attenuate the relationship for total and cruciferous vegetables, but not allium vegetables. The attenuation of the relationship for total and cruciferous vegetables and fracture-related hospitalisations indicates other constituents of a healthy diet at least partially explain the observed associations. It should also be noted that moderate correlations did exist between cruciferous and allium vegetables and total vegetable intakes. In addition, the inverse association between intakes of cruciferous vegetables and fracture-related hospitalisations was attenuated when adjusting for total vegetable intake. It is, therefore, possible that some of the effects seen for cruciferous vegetables may be due to their contribution to the overall increase in vegetable intake. Lastly, the observational nature of this study cannot establish a causal relationship, and the results of this study cannot be applied to younger cohorts and cohorts of older men.

5. Conclusions

The findings of this prospective cohort study indicate that habitual intakes of vegetables, but not fruits, are associated with a lower hazard of hospitalisations relating to fracture. These results are consistent with a recent meta-analysis of earlier studies [31]. We also found that intakes of cruciferous and allium vegetables were independently associated with lower hazard of all fractures, but not hip fractures. Increasing vegetable intake with a focus on consuming cruciferous and allium vegetables may reduce the risk of fracture in older postmenopausal women.

Supplementary Materials: The following is available online at www.mdpi.com/2072-6643/9/5/511/s1: Table S1: Descriptive statistics for intakes of cruciferous, allium, and total vegetables at baseline, 5 years (2003), and 7 years (2005), Table S2: Multivariable-adjusted hazard ratios for fracture-related hospitalisation for mean intakes of cruciferous, allium, and total vegetables across baseline, 5 years, and 7 years.

Acknowledgments: The authors wish to thank the staff at the Western Australia Data Linkage Branch, Hospital Morbidity Data Collection and Registry of Births, Deaths and Marriages for their work on providing the data for this study. The study was supported by research grants from Healthway Health Promotion Foundation of Western Australia, Sir Charles Gairdner Hospital Research Advisory Committee, and by the project grants 254627, 303169, and 572604 from the National Health and Medical Research Council of Australia. The salary of J.M.H. is supported by a National Health and Medical Research Council of Australia Senior Research Fellowship. The salary of J.R.L.

Nutrients **2017**, *9*, 511

is supported by a National Health and Medical Research Council of Australia Career Development Fellowship (ID: 1107474). None of these funding agencies had any input into any aspect of the design and management of this study.

Author Contributions: L.C.B., J.M.H., N.C.W. and R.L.P. conceived and designed the study; J.R.L., A.D., W.H.L., G.W., K.Z. and R.L.P. collected the data; L.C.B., J.M.H. and R.J.W. analysed the data; L.C.B. and J.M.H. wrote the paper; all authors critically reviewed the manuscript; L.C.B. had the primary responsibility for the final content. All authors read and approved the final manuscript.

Conflicts of Interest: The authors declare no conflict of interest.

References

1. Bhupathiraju, S.N.; Lichtenstein, A.H.; Dawson-Hughes, B.; Hannan, M.T.; Tucker, K.L. Adherence to the 2006 American heart association diet and lifestyle recommendations for cardiovascular disease risk reduction is associated with bone health in older Puerto Ricans. *Am. J. Clin. Nutr.* **2013**, *98*, 1309–1316. [CrossRef] [PubMed]

2. Byberg, L.; Bellavia, A.; Orsini, N.; Wolk, A.; Michaëlsson, K. Fruit and vegetable intake and risk of hip fracture: A cohort study of Swedish men and women. *J. Bone Miner. Res.* **2015**, *30*, 976–984. [CrossRef] [PubMed]

3. Benetou, V.; Orfanos, P.; Feskanich, D.; Michaëlsson, K.; Pettersson-Kymmer, U.; Eriksson, S.; Grodstein, F.; Wolk, A.; Bellavia, A.; Ahmed, L.A.; et al. Fruit and vegetable intake and hip fracture incidence in older men and women: The chances project. *J. Bone Miner. Res.* **2016**, *31*, 1743–1752. [CrossRef] [PubMed]

4. Whittle, C.R.; Woodside, J.V.; Cardwell, C.R.; McCourt, H.J.; Young, I.S.; Murray, L.J.; Boreham, C.A.; Gallagher, A.M.; Neville, C.E.; McKinley, M.C. Dietary patterns and bone mineral status in young adults: The northern Ireland young hearts project. *Br. J. Nutr.* **2012**, *108*, 1494–1504. [CrossRef] [PubMed]

5. Benetou, V.; Orfanos, P.; Pettersson-Kymmer, U.; Bergström, U.; Svensson, O.; Johansson, I.; Berrino, F.; Tumino, R.; Borch, K.B.; Lund, E.; et al. Mediterranean diet and incidence of hip fractures in a European cohort. *Osteoporos. Int.* **2013**, *24*, 1587–1598. [CrossRef] [PubMed]

6. Feart, C.; Lorrain, S.; Ginder Coupez, V.; Samieri, C.; Letenneur, L.; Paineau, D.; Barberger-Gateau, P. Adherence to a Mediterranean diet and risk of fractures in French older persons. *Osteoporos. Int.* **2013**, *24*, 3031–3041. [CrossRef] [PubMed]

7. Dai, Z.; Butler, L.M.; van Dam, R.M.; Ang, L.-W.; Yuan, J.-M.; Koh, W.-P. Adherence to a vegetable-fruit-soy dietary pattern or the alternative healthy eating index is associated with lower hip fracture risk among Singapore Chinese. *J. Nutr.* **2014**, *144*, 511–518. [CrossRef] [PubMed]

8. Tucker, K.L.; Hannan, M.T.; Chen, H.; Cupples, L.A.; Wilson, P.W.F.; Kiel, D.P. Potassium, magnesium, and fruit and vegetable intakes are associated with greater bone mineral density in elderly men and women. *Am. J. Clin. Nutr.* **1999**, *69*, 727–736. [PubMed]

9. Dai, Z.; Wang, R.; Ang, L.-W.; Low, Y.-L.; Yuan, J.-M.; Koh, W.-P. Protective effects of dietary carotenoids on risk of hip fracture in men: The Singapore Chinese health study. *J. Bone Miner. Res.* **2014**, *29*, 408–417. [CrossRef] [PubMed]

10. Fujita, Y.; Iki, M.; Tamaki, J.; Kouda, K.; Yura, A.; Kadowaki, E.; Sato, Y.; Moon, J.S.; Tomioka, K.; Okamoto, N.; et al. Association between vitamin K intake from fermented soybeans, natto, and bone mineral density in elderly Japanese men: The fujiwara-kyo osteoporosis risk in men (formen) study. *Osteoporos. Int.* **2012**, *23*, 705–714. [CrossRef] [PubMed]

11. Xu, L.; Dibley, M.; D'Este, C.; Phillips, M.; Porteous, J.; Attia, J. Food groups and risk of forearm fractures in postmenopausal women in Chengdu, China. *Climacteric* **2009**, *12*, 222–229. [CrossRef] [PubMed]

12. Prince, R.L.; Devine, A.; Dhaliwal, S.S.; Dick, I.M. Effects of calcium supplementation on clinical fracture and bone structure: Results of a 5-year, double-blind, placebo-controlled trial in elderly women. *Arch. Intern. Med.* **2006**, *166*, 869–875. [CrossRef] [PubMed]

13. Ireland, P.; Jolley, D.; Giles, G.; O'Dea, K.; Powles, J.; Rutishauser, I.; Wahlqvist, M.L.; Williams, J. Development of the melbourne FFQ: A food frequency questionnaire for use in an Australian prospective study involving an ethnically diverse cohort. *Asia Pac. J. Clin. Nutr.* **1994**, *3*, 19–31. [PubMed]

14. Hodge, A.; Patterson, A.J.; Brown, W.J.; Ireland, P.; Giles, G. The anti cancer council of victoria FFQ: Relative validity of nutrient intakes compared with weighed food records in young to middle-aged women in a study of iron supplementation. *Aust. N. Z. J. Public Health* **2000**, *24*, 576–583. [CrossRef] [PubMed]

15. Woods, R.K.; Stoney, R.M.; Ireland, P.D.; Bailey, M.J.; Raven, J.M.; Thien, F.C.K.; Walters, E.H.; Abramson, M.J. A valid food frequency questionnaire for measuring dietary fish intake. *Asia Pac. J. Clin. Nutr.* **2002**, *11*, 56–61. [CrossRef] [PubMed]

16. Lewis, J.; Milligan, G.; Hunt, A. *Nuttab95 Nutrient Data Table for Use in Australia*; Australian Government Publishing Service: Canberra, Australia, 1995.

17. National Health and Medical Research Council. *Australian Dietary Guidelines*; National Health and Medical Research Council: Canberra, Australia, 2013.

18. Fulgoni, V.L.; Keast, D.R.; Drewnowski, A. Development and validation of the nutrient-rich foods index: A tool to measure nutritional quality of foods. *J. Nutr.* **2009**, *139*, 1549–1554. [CrossRef] [PubMed]

19. National Health and Medical Research Council. *Nutrient Reference Values for Australia and New Zealand*; National Health and Medical Research Council: Canberra, Australia, 2006.

20. Blekkenhorst, L.C.; Bondonno, C.P.; Lewis, J.R.; Devine, A.; Woodman, R.J.; Croft, K.D.; Lim, W.H.; Wong, G.; Beilin, L.J.; Prince, R.L.; et al. Association of dietary nitrate with atherosclerotic vascular disease mortality: A prospective cohort study of older adult women. *Am. J. Clin. Nutr.* **2017**, in press.

21. National Centre for Classification in Health. *International Statistical Classification of Diseases and Related Health Problems*, 10th ed.; National Centre for Classification in Health: Sydney, Australia, 1998.

22. Bruce, D.G.; Devine, A.; Prince, R.L. Recreational physical activity levels in healthy older women: The importance of fear of falling. *J. Am. Geriatr. Soc.* **2002**, *50*, 84–89. [CrossRef] [PubMed]

23. Devine, A.; Dhaliwal, S.S.; Dick, I.M.; Bollerslev, J.; Prince, R.L. Physical activity and calcium consumption are important determinants of lower limb bone mass in older women. *J. Bone Miner. Res.* **2004**, *19*, 1634–1639. [CrossRef] [PubMed]

24. McArdle, W.D.; Katch, F.I.; Katch, V.L. *Energy, Nutrition and Human Performance*; Lea & Febiger: Philadelphia, PA, USA, 1991.

25. Pollock, M.L.; Wilmore, J.H.; Fox, S.M. *Health and Fitness Through Physical Activity*; Wiley: New York, NY, USA, 1978.

26. Britt, H.; Scahill, S.; Miller, G. ICPC plus for community health? A feasibility study. *Health Inf. Manag.* **1997**, *27*, 171–175. [PubMed]

27. Australian Bureau of Statistics. *Socio-Economic Indexes for Areas*; Australian Government Publishing Service: Canberra, Australia, 1991.

28. Hodgson, J.M.; Prince, R.L.; Woodman, R.J.; Bondonno, C.P.; Ivey, K.L.; Bondonno, N.; Rimm, E.B.; Ward, N.C.; Croft, K.D.; Lewis, J.R. Apple intake is inversely associated with all-cause and disease-specific mortality in elderly women. *Br. J. Nutr.* **2016**, *115*, 860–867. [CrossRef] [PubMed]

29. Kanis, J.A.; Johnell, O.; De Laet, C.; Johansson, H.; Oden, A.; Delmas, P.; Eisman, J.; Fujiwara, S.; Garnero, P.; Kroger, H.; et al. A meta-analysis of previous fracture and subsequent fracture risk. *Bone* **2004**, *35*, 375–382. [CrossRef] [PubMed]

30. Xie, H.L.; Wu, B.H.; Xue, W.Q.; He, M.G.; Fan, F.; Ouyang, W.F.; Tu, S.L.; Zhu, H.L.; Chen, Y.M. Greater intake of fruit and vegetables is associated with a lower risk of osteoporotic hip fractures in elderly Chinese: A 1:1 matched case—Control study. *Osteoporos. Int.* **2013**, *24*, 2827–2836. [CrossRef] [PubMed]

31. Luo, S.Y.; Li, Y.; Luo, H.; Yin, X.H.; Lin, D.R.; Zhao, K.; Huang, G.L.; Song, J.K. Increased intake of vegetables, but not fruits, may be associated with reduced risk of hip fracture: A meta-analysis. *Sci. Rep.* **2016**, *6*, 19783. [CrossRef] [PubMed]

32. Li, J.-J.; Huang, Z.-W.; Wang, R.-Q.; Ma, X.-M.; Zhang, Z.-Q.; Liu, Z.; Chen, Y.-M.; Su, Y.-X. Fruit and vegetable intake and bone mass in Chinese adolescents, young and postmenopausal women. *Public Health Nutr.* **2013**, *16*, 78–86. [CrossRef] [PubMed]

33. Chen, Y.-M.; Ho, S.C.; Woo, J.L.F. Greater fruit and vegetable intake is associated with increased bone mass among postmenopausal Chinese women. *Br. J. Nutr.* **2006**, *96*, 745–751. [PubMed]

34. Kaptoge, S.; Welch, A.; McTaggart, A.; Mulligan, A.; Dalzell, N.; Day, N.E.; Bingham, S.; Khaw, K.T.; Reeve, J. Effects of dietary nutrients and food groups on bone loss from the proximal femur in men and women in the 7th and 8th decades of age. *Osteoporos. Int.* **2003**, *14*, 418–428. [PubMed]

35. Neville, C.E.; Young, I.S.; Gilchrist, S.E.C.M.; McKinley, M.C.; Gibson, A.; Edgar, J.D.; Woodside, J.V. Effect of increased fruit and vegetable consumption on bone turnover in older adults: A randomised controlled trial. *Osteoporos. Int.* **2014**, *25*, 223–233. [CrossRef] [PubMed]

36. Macdonald, H.M.; Black, A.J.; Aucott, L.; Duthie, G.; Duthie, S.; Sandison, R.; Hardcastle, A.C.; Lanham New, S.A.; Fraser, W.D.; Reid, D.M. Effect of potassium citrate supplementation or increased fruit and vegetable intake on bone metabolism in healthy postmenopausal women: A randomized controlled trial. *Am. J. Clin. Nutr.* **2008**, *88*, 465–474. [PubMed]

37. Ebrahimof, S.; Hoshiarrad, A.; Hossein-Nezhad, A.; Larijani, B.; Kimiagar, S.M. Effects of increasing fruit and vegetable intake on bone turnover in postmenopausal osteopenic women. *DARU J. Pharm. Sci.* **2015**, *17* (Suppl. 1), 30–37. [CrossRef]

38. Feskanich, D.; Weber, P.; Willett, W.C.; Rockett, H.; Booth, S.L.; Colditz, G.A. Vitamin K intake and hip fractures in women: A prospective study. *Am. J. Clin. Nutr.* **1999**, *69*, 74–79. [PubMed]

39. Rejnmark, L.; Vestergaard, P.; Charles, P.; Hermann, A.P.; Brot, C.; Eiken, P.; Mosekilde, L. No effect of vitamin K1 intake on bone mineral density and fracture risk in perimenopausal women. *Osteoporos. Int.* **2006**, *17*, 1122–1132. [CrossRef] [PubMed]

40. Matheson, E.M.; Mainous Iii, A.G.; Carnemolla, M.A. The association between onion consumption and bone density in perimenopausal and postmenopausal non-Hispanic white women 50 years and older. *Menopause* **2009**, *16*, 756–759. [CrossRef] [PubMed]

41. Mody, N.; Parhami, F.; Sarafian, T.A.; Demer, L.L. Oxidative stress modulates osteoblastic differentiation of vascular and bone cells. *Free Radic. Biol. Med.* **2001**, *31*, 509–519. [CrossRef]

42. Basu, S.; Michaëlsson, K.; Olofsson, H.; Johansson, S.; Melhus, H. Association between oxidative stress and bone mineral density. *Biochem. Biophys. Res. Commun.* **2001**, *288*, 275–279. [CrossRef] [PubMed]

43. Maggio, D.; Barabani, M.; Pierandrei, M.; Polidori, M.C.; Catani, M.; Mecocci, P.; Senin, U.; Pacifici, R.; Cherubini, A. Marked decrease in plasma antioxidants in aged osteoporotic women: Results of a cross-sectional study. *J. Clin. Endocrinol. Metab.* **2003**, *88*, 1523–1527. [CrossRef] [PubMed]

44. Gambari, L.; Lisignoli, G.; Cattini, L.; Manferdini, C.; Facchini, A.; Grassi, F. Sodium hydrosulfide inhibits the differentiation of osteoclast progenitor cells via NRF2-dependent mechanism. *Pharmacol. Res.* **2014**, *87*, 99–112. [CrossRef] [PubMed]

45. Hyeon, S.; Lee, H.; Yang, Y.; Jeong, W. NRF2 deficiency induces oxidative stress and promotes rankl-induced osteoclast differentiation. *Free Radic. Biol. Med.* **2013**, *65*, 789–799. [CrossRef] [PubMed]

46. Thaler, R.; Maurizi, A.; Roschger, P.; Sturmlechner, I.; Khani, F.; Spitzer, S.; Rumpler, M.; Zwerina, J.; Karlic, H.; Dudakovic, A.; et al. Anabolic and antiresorptive modulation of bone homeostasis by the epigenetic modulator sulforaphane, a naturally occurring isothiocyanate. *J. Biol. Chem.* **2016**, *291*, 6754–6771. [CrossRef] [PubMed]

47. Park, H.; Jeong, J.; Hyun, H.; Kim, J.; Kim, H.; Oh, H.I.; Choi, J.Y.; Hwang, H.S.; Oh, D.B.; Kim, J.I.; et al. Effects of a hot-water extract of *Allium hookeri* roots on bone formation in human osteoblast-like mg-63 cells in vitro and in rats in vivo. *Planta Med.* **2016**, *82*, 1410–1415. [CrossRef] [PubMed]

48. Australian Bureau of Statistics. *National Health Survey: First Results, 2014–2015*; Australian Bureau of Statistics: Belconnen, Australia, 2015.

49. Nurzenski, M.K.; Briffa, N.K.; Price, R.I.; Khoo, B.C.C.; Devine, A.; Beck, T.J.; Prince, R.L. Geometric indices of bone strength are associated with physical activity and dietary calcium intake in healthy older women. *J. Bone Miner. Res.* **2007**, *22*, 416–424. [CrossRef] [PubMed]

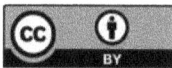

nutrients

MDPI

Article

Protective Effect of Chokeberry (*Aronia melanocarpa* L.) Extract against Cadmium Impact on the Biomechanical Properties of the Femur: A Study in a Rat Model of Low and Moderate Lifetime Women Exposure to This Heavy Metal

Małgorzata M. Brzóska *, Alicja Roszczenko, Joanna Rogalska, Małgorzata Gałażyn-Sidorczuk and Magdalena Mężyńska

Department of Toxicology, Medical University of Bialystok, Adama Mickiewicza 2C street,
15-222 Bialystok, Poland; alicja.roszczenko@umb.edu.pl (A.R.); joanna.rogalska@umb.edu.pl (J.R.);
malgorzata.galazyn-sidorczuk@umb.edu.pl (M.G.-S.); mmezynska1@student.umb.edu.pl (M.M.)
* Correspondence: malgorzata.brzoska@umb.edu.pl; Tel.: +48-85-748-5604; Fax: +48-85-748-5834

Received: 15 April 2017; Accepted: 23 May 2017; Published: 25 May 2017

Abstract: The hypothesis that the consumption of *Aronia melanocarpa* berries (chokeberries) extract, recently reported by us to improve bone metabolism in female rats at low-level and moderate chronic exposure to cadmium (1 and 5 mg Cd/kg diet for up to 24 months), may increase the bone resistance to fracture was investigated. Biomechanical properties of the neck (bending test with vertical head loading) and diaphysis (three-point bending test) of the femur of rats administered 0.1% aqueous chokeberry extract (65.74% of polyphenols) or/and Cd in the diet (1 and 5 mg Cd/kg) for 3, 10, 17, and 24 months were evaluated. Moreover, procollagen I was assayed in the bone tissue. The low-level and moderate exposure to Cd decreased the procollagen I concentration in the bone tissue and weakened the biomechanical properties of the femoral neck and diaphysis. Chokeberry extract administration under the exposure to Cd improved the bone collagen biosynthesis and femur biomechanical properties. The results allow for the conclusion that the consumption of chokeberry products under exposure to Cd may improve the bone biomechanical properties and protect from fracture. This study provides support for *Aronia melanocarpa* berries being a promising natural agent for skeletal protection under low-level and moderate chronic exposure to Cd.

Keywords: *Aronia melanocarpa* berries; bone biomechanical properties; cadmium; chokeberries; female rats; polyphenols; procollagen; protection

---

1. Introduction

The growing occurrence of osteoporosis with bone fracture in inhabitants of industrialized countries, which has generated an increasing amount of attention in recent years, has been focused on environmental risk factors for bone damage [1–3] and numerous efforts have been undertaken to find effective ways of protecting bone [4–6]. Among the factors that may be useful in this protection, a subject of special interest is dietary products that are rich in biologically active substances, characterized by a well-defined beneficial impact on bone metabolism, including polyphenolic compounds that occur in green tea and some fruit and vegetables [4–7].

More numerous epidemiological data provide evidence that important environmental risk factors for the increasing incidence of osteoporosis are toxic heavy metals, including cadmium (Cd) [1–3,8–10]. Due to the wide distribution of this metal in the environment and food pollution, as well as its presence in tobacco smoke, the whole population is exposed to this metal during their lifetime [8–12].

Bone damage is one of the main unfavourable health effects of long-term exposure to this xenobiotic in both human [1,8–12] and experimental animals [13–19]. We have reported, for a rat model with environmental human exposure to Cd, that this metal disturbs bone metabolism and weakens the biomechanical properties of long bones and lumbar spine vertebral bodies, which may even result in femoral neck and vertebral fractures [13–18]. In recent years, numerous epidemiological data have shown that even low-level lifetime exposure to this heavy metal may decrease the bone mineral density (BMD) and contribute to osteoporosis with an increased risk of bone fracture in the general population [1,8–10]. Moreover, the forecasts indicate that the exposure of the general population to this xenobiotic will increase in the future decades [11]. Thus, it seems very important to recognize effective ways of preventing these health effects due to exposure to Cd, including its impact on the skeleton.

The attention of researchers regarding effective agents that may play a role in protecting against the effects of Cd action has been focused on natural products, including those rich in polyphenolic compounds [20–22]. Due to the multidirectional favourable action of polyphenols (antioxidative, anti-inflammatory, anticoagulative, antiatherogenic, antidiabetic, antibacterial, and anticancer), products abundant in these compounds are recommended to be used as functional food in the case of cardiovascular diseases, diabetes, neurodegenerative disorders, urinary tract infection, non-alcoholic fatty liver disease, and chemotherapy [20,22,23]. Moreover, polyphenols are also known for their beneficial impact on the skeleton [4,6,7,24].

Available data, including our own findings, show that some plant products rich in polyphenolic compounds, including the berries of *Aronia melanocarpa* (chokeberries; [Michx.] Elliott, Rosaceae), possess the potential to protect from various unfavourable effects that result from the exposure to Cd [21,22,25–27]. Recently, using a rat model of lifetime low-level and moderate female exposure to Cd (1 and 5 mg Cd/kg diet), we have revealed that the consumption of an extract from the berries of *A. melanocarpa* (AE) protected against these heavy metal-induced disturbances in the bone turnover and bone mineral status (findings are summarized as Tables S1 and S2) [26,27]. Because the mineral status of the bone tissue determines its biomechanical properties and susceptibility to fracture [28], taking into account our recent findings [25–27], we have hypothesized that the consumption of AE under Cd exposure may also improve the bone biomechanical properties and, in this way, decrease the bone susceptibility to fracture. The aim of the present study was to investigate this hypothesis. For this purpose, the impact of AE administration under chronic low-level and moderate exposure to Cd on the biomechanical properties of the femoral neck and femoral diaphysis was estimated for the animals in which we have revealed the protective impact of the extract against the body burden of Cd and disorders in the bone tissue metabolism [25–27]. Moreover, because the bone biomechanical properties are determined not only by the bone mineral status, but also by the bone matrix composed mainly of collagen [29,30], the concentration of procollagen I (PC I) in the bone tissue, as a marker of collagen biosynthesis, was assayed.

2. Materials and Methods

2.1. Animals

One hundred and ninety-two young (aged three to four week) female Wistar rats [Crl: WI (Han)] purchased from the certified Laboratory Animal House (Brwinów, Poland) were used. The animals were housed in controlled conventional conditions (temperature $22 \pm 2\,^{\circ}\text{C}$, relative humidity $50 \pm 10\%$, 12-h light/dark cycle) and had free access to drinking water and feed (Labofeed B diet through the first three months and then a Labofeed H diet; Label Food 'Morawski', Kcynia, Poland) [25,26].

2.2. Cd Diets

The diets containing 1 and 5 mg Cd/kg were prepared by the addition, at the stage of production, of appropriate amounts of $CdCl_2 \times H_2O$ (POCh, Gliwice, Poland) into the ingredients of the standard feed (Labofeed B and Labofeed H diets). The mean Cd concentration determined by us (by atomic absorption spectrometry method) in the diets reached 1.09 ± 0.11 mg/kg and 4.92 ± 0.78 mg/kg (mean ± SE), respectively, whereas its mean concentration in the standard Labofeed diets was 0.0584 ± 0.0046 mg/kg.

2.3. A. melanocarpa Extract

Powdered aronia extract was received from Adamed Consumer Healthcare (Tuszyn, Poland). According to the producer, the extract contained 65.74% of polyphenols (including 18.65% of anthocyanins). Although the polyphenols content in the powdered *A. melanocarpa* extract was certified and is widely reported [22,23,31,32], the phytochemical profile of the extract was evaluated and the concentrations of total polyphenols, phenolic acids (including chlorogenic acid), flavonoids, proanthocyanidins, and anthocyanins (including cyanidin 3-*O*-β-galactoside, cyanidin 3-*O*-α-arabinoside, and cyanidin 3-*O*-β-glucoside) were quantified by us [26] (Table S3). According to the producer's declaration and literature data [22,31], the extract also contained other components such as pectins, sugar, sugar alcohols (sorbitol, parasorboside), triterpenes, carotenoids, and phytosterols, as well as minerals and vitamins.

2.4. Study Design

The study was approved by the Local Ethics Committee for Animal Experiments in Bialystok (Poland) and was performed following the ethical principles, institutional guidelines, and international Guide for the Use of Animals in Biomedical Research.

The rats were allowed to adjust to the experimental facility for five days before the study was started and were randomly divided into six groups, each containing 32 animals. One group received 0.1% aqueous solution of aronia extract alone as the only drinking fluid (AE group), two groups were intoxicated with Cd alone via the diets containing 1 and 5 mg Cd/kg (Cd$_1$ group and Cd$_5$ group), and the next two groups received the AE during the whole course of the exposure to Cd (Cd$_1$ + AE group and Cd$_5$ + AE group) for 3, 10, 17, and 24 months. The Cd$_1$ group and Cd$_5$ group, unlike the Cd$_1$ + AE group and Cd$_5$ + AE group, did not receive the AE. The last group, maintained on redistilled water (containing < 0.05 µg Cd/L and not completely deprived of bioelements necessary for the bone health) and standard Labofeed diet, served as a control.

The daily intake of Cd throughout the 24-month exposure to the 1 and 5 mg Cd/kg diets, irrespective of whether this xenobiotic was administered alone or in conjunction with the AE, reached 37.50–84.88 µg/kg b.w. and 196.69–404.76 µg/kg b.w., respectively. Cd intake in the control group and AE group was negligible compared to its intake in the Cd$_1$, Cd$_1$ + AE, Cd$_5$, and Cd$_5$ + AE groups (Table S4) [25,26].

The 0.1% AE was prepared daily by dissolving 1 g of the powdered aronia extract in 1 L of redistilled water. The total polyphenols concentration in the 0.1% aqueous AE reached 0.612 ± 0.003 mg/mL (mean ± SE) and was stable for 24 h after this solution preparation, while the Cd concentration was <0.05 µg/L [26]. The daily intake of polyphenolic compounds during the whole experiment, irrespective of the manner of their administration, reached 41.5–104.6 mg/kg b.w. and did not differ, regardless of whether the AE was administered alone or under the treatment with Cd (Table S5) [26].

At the end of the 3rd, 10th, 17th, and 24th month of the experiment, eight rats of each group (except for seven animals in the AE group, and the groups treated with 1 and 5 mg Cd/kg diet alone after 24 months), after overnight starvation, were subjected to anaesthesia with Morbital (pentobarbital sodium and pentobarbital 5:1, 30 mg/kg b.w., *i.p.*). The whole blood was taken by cardiac puncture with and without anticoagulant (heparin), and various organs and tissues, including the right femur used in the present study, were dissected.

The femur was immediately cleaned of all adherent soft tissues and weighed with an automatic balance (OHAUS, Switzerland, accuracy to 0.0001 g). Moreover, the bone length and the anterior–posterior (A–P) and medial–lateral (M–L) diameters at the midpoint of the diaphysis were measured with an electronic calliper (±0.02 mm). All the measurements were performed by the same investigator. The precision of these measurements (determined by three measurements of three bones), expressed as a coefficient of variation (CV) for the femur length and diameter, was <0.45% and 0.5%, respectively. The femur of each rat was stored in physiological saline (0.9% sodium chloride) at $-20\,°C$ until biomechanical testing was performed. After biomechanical testing, the bone slices collected from the distal epiphysis and diaphysis of the femur were subjected to a PC I measurement.

The experimental model has been described in detail in our previous reports [25–27].

2.5. Bone Biomechanical Testing

The femur was subjected to the mechanical study performed using a testing machine (Zwick 2.5; Zwick GmbH & Co. KG, Ulm, Germany) equipped with a load cell (range of forces up to 2.5 N) and a computer for data acquisition and storage (TestXpert II V3.31 software; Zwick GmbH & Co. KG, Ulm, Germany). A three-point bending test (Section 2.5.1) was performed to estimate the biomechanical properties of the femoral diaphysis (Figure 1A) [15]. Next, the proximal end of the broken femur was used for the measurement of the biomechanical properties of the femoral neck in a bending test (Section 2.5.1; Figure 1B) [15]. All of the tests were performed by the same operator. According to the producer, the measurement error of the method is 0.12% of the value recorded.

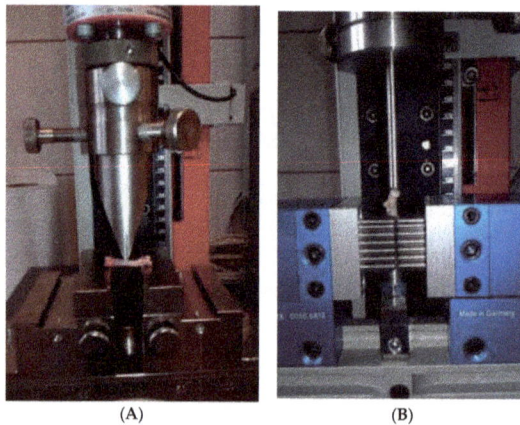

(A) (B)

Figure 1. Representation of the biomechanical testing of the femur (the photos originate from our private collection). (**A**) Three-point bending test of the femoral diaphysis; (**B**) Fracture test of the femoral neck.

The load-deformation curves were recorded during the testing (Sections 2.5.1 and 2.5.2). The yield load and fracture load were determined from the load-deformation curve and computer readings. The yield load is defined as the force causing the first bone damage visible in the load-deformation curve (the force at which the load-deformation curve broke from linearity), whereas the fracture load is the force causing bone fracture. These two forces (yield load and fracture load) describe the bone strength. The yield load (yield strength) reflects the maximum load-bearing capacity under elastic conditions, whereas the fracture load (fracture strength) is the force necessary to cause the bone fracture. Moreover, the bone stiffness was automatically calculated from the linear portion of the load-deformation curve as the ratio of the yield load and the bone deformation at the yield point. The area under the load-deformation curve, reflecting the total energy absorbed by the bone during the test, was measured as work to the bone fracture.

2.5.1. Three Point Bending Test of the Femoral Diaphysis

The femur placed horizontally on two rounded supporting bars, located at a distance of 18 mm, was loaded at the midpoint of the diaphysis in the A–P plane by lowering the third bar (stainless steel pin) at a rate of 2 mm/min, until the bone fracture (Figure 1A).

After finishing the three-point bending test, the vertical (A–P orientation) and horizontal (M–L) internal and external heights at the point of diaphysis fracture were measured. Based on the internal and external heights, geometric properties such as the wall thickness (WT), cross-sectional properties of the M–L axis like cross-sectional area (CSA), and cross-sectional moment of inertia (CSMI) at the point of diaphysis fracture were calculated [15].

The yield load, fracture load, and stiffness describe the "structural" properties of the femur as a whole anatomical unit. To better estimate the biomechanical properties of the femur, the "material" (intrinsic; independent of the tissue size) properties of the bone tissue at the femoral diaphysis were also evaluated. For this purpose, the structural properties of the femoral diaphysis, such as the yield load, fracture load, and stiffness, were normalized for their "geometric" properties, giving the yield stress, fracture stress, and elastic modulus (Young modulus of elasticity), respectively [15]. The yield stress and fracture stress reflect the strength of the bone tissue at the femoral diaphysis, and the values of these parameters were automatically calculated based on the recorded forces and the vertical and horizontal internal and external heights at the point of diaphysis fracture in the three-point bending test [15].

2.5.2. Fracture Test of the Femoral Neck

The proximal end of the broken femur was used for the measurement of the biomechanical properties of the femoral neck (Figure 1B) [15]. The proximal part of the femur was immobilized with special equipment of the Zwick 2.5 testing machine. Next, the bone head was vertically loaded at a displacement rate of 6 mm/min, until the neck fracture [15].

2.6. Determination of PC I

After the femur biomechanical testing, slices of the bone tissue collected from the femoral distal epiphysis (trabecular bone region) and diaphysis (cortical bone region) were separated, with the aim of determining the PC I concentration. The bone tissue was crumbled and washed in ice-cold physiological saline (0.9% sodium chloride), to eliminate the remove-available bone marrow. Next, known weight bone slices were homogenized in cold potassium phosphate buffer (50 mM, pH = 7.4) at 4 °C using a high-performance homogenizer (Ultra-Turrax T25; IKA®, Staufen, Germany) equipped with a stainless-steel dispersing element (S25N-8G; IKA®) to receive an appearing homogenous liquid. The prepared 10% homogenates were centrifuged (MPW-350R centrifugator, Medical Instruments, Warsaw, Poland) at $700 \times g$ for 20 min at 4 °C, and the aliquots were separated.

The concentration of PC I in the aliquots of the bone tissue was determined with the use of an Enzyme-linked Immunosorbent Assay Kit by Uscn Life Science Inc. (Wuhan, China). The precision of the measurement, expressed as the intra- and inter-assay CV, was <4.8% and 5.2%, respectively.

In order to adjust the bone tissue PC I for the protein concentration, the total protein was assayed in the bone aliquots with the use of a BioMaxima kit (Lublin, Poland).

2.7. Statistical Analysis

A one-way analysis of variance (Anova) was used to determine if there were statistically significant ($p < 0.05$) differences among the six experimental groups and then the Duncan's multiple range post hoc test was conducted for comparisons between individual groups and to determine which two means differed statistically significantly ($p < 0.05$). To discern whether the possible beneficial impact of the AE resulted from an independent action of the extract ingredients and/or their interaction with Cd, a two-way analysis of variance (Anova/Manova, test F) was performed. F values having $p < 0.05$ were considered statistically significant. With the aim of investigating the dependence between the impact of the AE consumption on the biomechanical properties and mineral status of the femur, Spearman rank correlation analysis between the variables describing the bone vulnerability to fracture in the females receiving the extract under the exposure to Cd and previously determined in these animals BMD of the femur [26], was conducted. Correlations were considered statistically significant at $p < 0.05$. All of the statistical calculations were performed using the Statistica package (StatSoft, Tulsa, OK, USA).

3. Results

3.1. Effect of AE on the Femur Weight in Rats Exposed to Cd

The mean absolute and relative weight of the femur in the control rats ranged from 0.6098 ± 0.014 g and 0.2006 ± 0.005 g/100 g b.w., respectively, after three months, up to 0.7703 ± 0.013 g and 0.1306 ± 0.002 g/100 g b.w., respectively, after 24 months of the experiment. The administration of the AE and Cd alone and together had no impact on the absolute and relative femur weight (Table S6).

3.2. Effect of AE on the Geometric Properties of the Femur in Rats Exposed to Cd

The femur length in the control rats ranged from 31.30 ± 0.42 mm after three months to 32.69 ± 0.29 mm after 24 months. The mid-diaphyseal femoral geometric properties such as the M–L and A–P within these animals reached 4.130 ± 0.057 mm and 2.791 ± 0.066 mm, respectively, after three months, and 4.618 ± 0.078 mm and 3.370 ± 0.170 mm, respectively, after 24 months. The administration of the AE and/or Cd for up to 24 months had no impact on the femur length and diameter at the mid-diaphysis (Table S7).

The administration of AE during the whole experiment had no impact on the geometric properties of the femoral diaphysis at the point of its fracture in the three-point bending test (WT, CSA, and CSMI; Table 1). The WT and CSA at the point of diaphysis fracture in the three-point bending test were lower in the animals exposed to the 1 and 5 mg Cd/kg diet for three months (by 14.6% and 15.6%, and 17.7% and 13.2%, respectively), whereas the CSMI was unaffected (Table 1). However, after the longer treatment with Cd, the WT and CSA at the point of diaphysis fracture did not differ compared to the control group, except for the increase (by 12.9%) in the CSA in the Cd_1 group (Table 1).

Table 1. Effect of the extract from the berries of *Aronia melanocarpa* (AE) on the geometric properties of the femur at the point of diaphysis fracture in the three-point bending test in rats exposed to cadmium (Cd).

Group	Experiment Duration			
	3 Months	10 Months	17 Months	24 Months
	WT (mm)			
Control	0.718 ± 0.047	0.691 ± 0.010	0.786 ± 0.036	0.799 ± 0.018
AE	0.636 ± 0.021	0.693 ± 0.017	0.860 ± 0.034	0.798 ± 0.019
Cd_1	0.613 ± 0.019 *	0.678 ± 0.018	0.848 ± 0.021	0.899 ± 0.038
$Cd_1 + AE$	0.636 ± 0.032 *	0.744 ± 0.023 †	0.756 ± 0.158	0.826 ± 0.051
Cd_5	0.591 ± 0.020 **	0.721 ± 0.020	0.753 ± 0.023	0.819 ± 0.043
$Cd_5 + AE$	0.633 ± 0.015	0.651 ± 0.020 †,‡‡	0.821 ± 0.054	0.869 ± 0.028
	CSA (mm^2)			
Control	7.610 ± 0.386	7.650 ± 0.083	9.114 ± 0.428	9.571 ± 0.247
AE	6.937 ± 0.365	7.642 ± 0.299	10.011 ± 0.478	9.082 ± 0.214
Cd_1	6.419 ± 0.274 *	7.871 ± 0.235	9.788 ± 0.246	10.810 ± 0.275 *
$Cd_1 + AE$	6.902 ± 0.335	8.362 ± 0.440	8.999 ± 0.250	9.926 ± 0.407
Cd_5	6.602 ± 0.221 *	8.122 ± 0.286	8.485 ± 0.449	9.616 ± 0.457 ‡
$Cd_5 + AE$	6.775 ± 0.278	7.277 ± 0.396 ‡	9.178 ± 0.584	10.039 ± 0.433
	CSMI			
Control	3.681 ± 0.208	4.342 ± 0.274	6.338 ± 0.382	8.615 ± 1.682
AE	4.080 ± 0.414	4.980 ± 0.472	7.660 ± 0.612	7.442 ± 0.175
Cd_1	3.606 ± 0.168	4.882 ± 0.200	6.963 ± 0.609	9.850 ± 0.524
$Cd_1 + AE$	3.778 ± 0.205	5.201 ± 0.381	7.061 ± 0.442	9.271 ± 0.200
Cd_5	4.395 ± 0.390	4.793 ± 0.188	5.239 ± 0.516 ‡	8.943 ± 0.726
$Cd_5 + AE$	3.721 ± 0.185	4.772 ± 0.356	5.801 ± 0.613	7.762 ± 0.670

Data are represented as mean $\pm$ SE for eight rats (except for seven animals in the AE, Cd_1, and Cd_5 groups after 24 months). Statistically significant differences (Anova, Duncan's multiple range test) compared to the control group (* $p < 0.05$, ** $p < 0.01$), respective group receiving Cd alone († $p < 0.05$), and respective group receiving 1 mg Cd/kg diet alone or with the AE (‡ $p < 0.05$, ‡‡ $p < 0.01$) are marked. WT, cortical width; CSA, cross-sectional area; CSMI, cross-sectional moment of inertia.

3.3. Effect of AE on the Biomechanical Properties of the Femoral Neck in Rats Exposed to Cd

The administration of the AE alone for three months increased the yield and fracture strength of the femoral neck (Figure 2), as well as the work to the neck fracture (Figure 3), but had no impact on its stiffness (Figure 3). After a longer administration of the extract, all evaluated biomechanical properties of the femoral neck were unchanged compared to the control, except for an increase in the work to the neck fracture after 17 months (Figures 2 and 3).

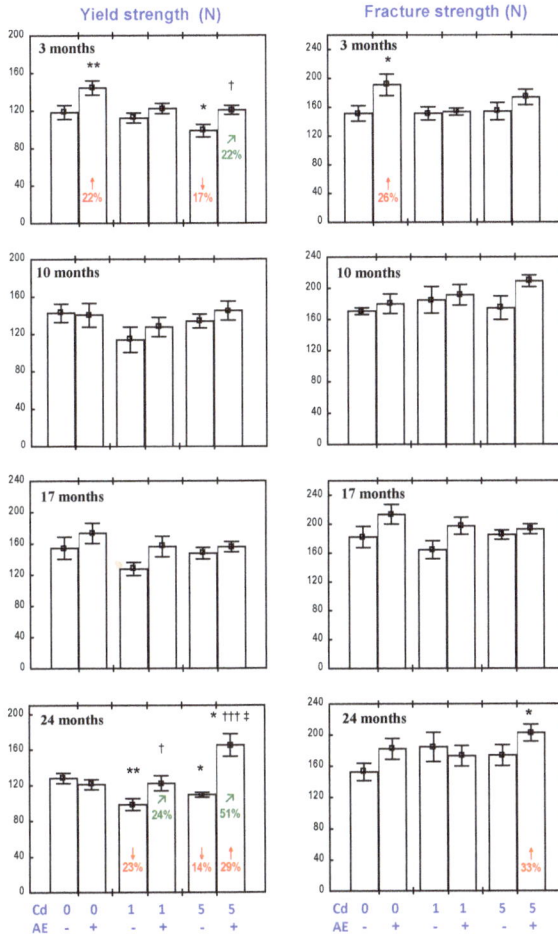

Figure 2. Effect of an extract from the berries of *Aronia melanocarpa* (AE) on the yield and fracture strength of the femoral neck in rats exposed to cadmium (Cd). The rats received 0.1% aqueous AE or not ("+" and "−", respectively) and Cd in diet at the concentration of 0, 1, and 5 mg/kg. Data are represented as mean ± SE for eight rats, except for seven animals in the AE group, and the groups treated with the 1 and 5 mg Cd/kg diet alone after 24 months. Statistically significant differences (Anova, Duncan's multiple range test): * $p < 0.05$, ** $p < 0.01$ vs. control group; † $p < 0.05$, ††† $p < 0.001$ vs. respective group receiving Cd alone; ‡ $p < 0.05$ vs. respective group receiving the 1 mg Cd/kg diet. Numerical values in bars indicate percentage change compared to the control group (↓, decrease; ↑, increase) or the respective group receiving Cd alone (↗, increase).

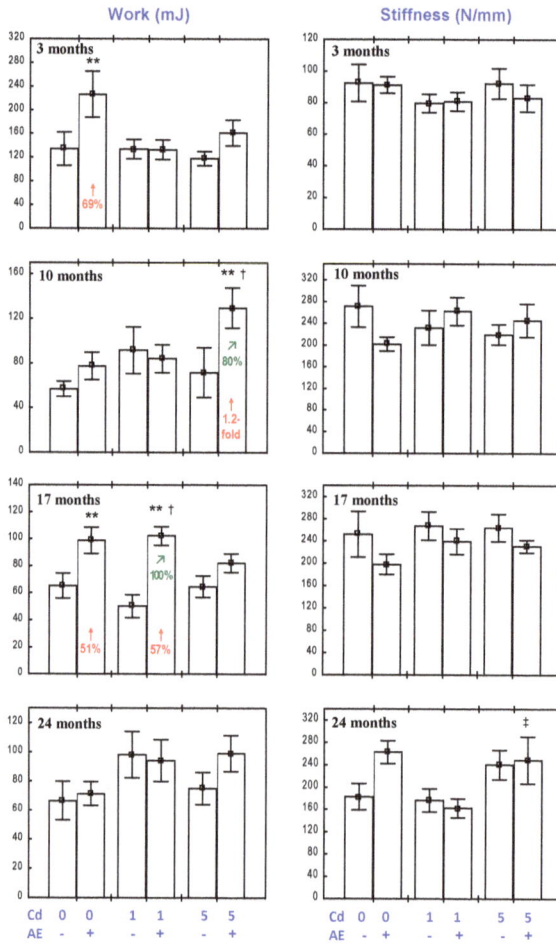

Figure 3. Effect of an extract from the berries of *Aronia melanocarpa* (AE) on the femoral neck stiffness and work to its fracture in rats exposed to cadmium (Cd). The rats received 0.1% aqueous AE or not ("+" and "−", respectively) and Cd in diet at the concentration of 0, 1, and 5 mg/kg. Data are represented as mean ± SE for eight rats, except for seven animals in the AE group, and the groups treated with the 1 and 5 mg Cd/kg diet alone after 24 months. Statistically significant differences (Anova, Duncan's multiple range test): ** $p < 0.01$ vs. control group; † $p < 0.05$ vs. respective group receiving Cd alone; ‡ $p < 0.05$ vs. respective group receiving the 1 mg Cd/kg diet. Numerical values in bars indicate percentage change or a factor of change compared to the control group (↑, increase) or the respective group receiving Cd alone (↗, increase).

The exposure to the 1 mg Cd/kg diet for 3, 10, and 17 months had no impact on the biomechanical properties of the femoral neck; however, after 24 months, the yield strength was decreased (Figures 2 and 3). In the animals treated with the 5 mg Cd/kg diet, the only change in the evaluated biomechanical parameters was a decrease in the yield strength after three and 24 months (Figures 2 and 3).

In the animals receiving the AE under the exposure to the 1 mg Cd/kg diet for 17 months, the work to the neck fracture was higher compared to the control group and the group treated with Cd alone (Figure 3). Moreover, the AE completely prevented the 24-month exposure to Cd-induced decrease in the yield strength (Figure 2). The Anova/Manova analysis revealed that the beneficial impact of the AE consumption under the low treatment with Cd on the yield strength of the femoral neck was an effect of the independent action of this extract's ingredients (F = 4.309, $p < 0.05$) and their interaction with this heavy metal (F = 5.166, $p < 0.05$). The AE administration to the animals treated with 5 mg Cd/kg diet completely prevented the three- and 24-month exposure-induced decrease in the yield strength of the femoral neck (Figure 2), and this effect resulted from the independent action of the extract (F = 10.574, $p < 0.001$) after three months and from its interaction with Cd (F = 17.184, $p < 0.001$) after 24 months. Moreover, the yield strength and fracture strength of the femoral neck in the Cd_5 + AE group after 24 months were higher than in the control group (Figure 2). The extract administration under the 10-month exposure to the 5 mg Cd/kg diet increased the work to the neck fracture compared to the control group and the Cd_5 group (Figure 3), as a result of its independent action (F = 4.362, $p < 0.05$).

3.4. Effect of AE on the Biomechanical Properties of the Femoral Diaphysis in Rats Exposed to Cd

The administration of the AE alone had no impact on the "structural" biomechanical properties (yield strength, fracture strength, stiffness, and work to fracture) of the femoral diaphysis, apart from an increase in the fracture strength after 24 months and a decrease in the stiffness after 10 months, as well as a decrease in the work to fracture after 10 months and its increase after 17 and 24 months (Figures 4 and 5). The only "material" biomechanical property influenced by the consumption of the AE alone was a decrease in the Young modulus of elasticity after 10 months (Figure 6).

The exposure to Cd affected both the "structural" and "material" biomechanical properties of the femoral diaphysis (Figures 4–6). In the rats treated with 1 mg Cd/kg diet, the yield strength, yield stress, and stiffness were decreased after 17 and 24 months (Figures 4–6). Moreover, after 17 months, the fracture strength and fracture stress were decreased, while after 24 months, the work to the diaphysis fracture was increased (Figures 4–6). At the higher exposure to Cd, the yield strength was decreased after 17 and 24 months and the fracture strength and stiffness decreased after 17 months, whereas the work to fracture was increased after 10 and 24 months (Figures 4 and 5). Moreover, the treatment with the 5 mg Cd/kg diet increased the fracture stress after 17 months and decreased the yield stress after 24 months (Figure 6).

The administration of the AE during the exposure to the 1 mg Cd/kg diet completely prevented this heavy metal-induced decrease in the femoral diaphysis yield strength (Figure 4), stiffness (Figure 5), yield stress, and fracture stress (Figure 6). Moreover, the stiffness and fracture strength in the Cd_1 + AE group after 24 months were increased compared to the control group and Cd_1 group (Figures 4 and 5). The Anova/Manova analysis revealed that the impact of the AE consumption under the low-level exposure to Cd on the fracture strength of the femoral diaphysis was an effect of the independent action of this extract's ingredients (F = 8.206, $p < 0.01$) and their interaction with this toxic metal (F = 8.361, $p < 0.01$). Apart from that, the administration of the AE under the 10-month treatment with the 1 mg Cd/kg diet resulted in a decrease in the stiffness of the femoral diaphysis and work to its fracture, and this impact was caused by the interactive action of the extract's ingredients and Cd (F = 6.194, $p < 0.05$ and F = 7.507, $p < 0.05$, respectively). The administration of the AE under the 17-month exposure to the 1 mg Cd/kg diet increased the work to the femoral diaphysis fracture compared to the control group and the Cd_1 group, whereas the extract consumption for 24 months had no impact on the Cd-increased value of this parameter. The consumption of the AE under the higher Cd treatment entirely prevented this heavy metal-caused decrease in the yield strength and fracture strength (Figure 4). The beneficial impact on the yield strength resulted from the independent action of the AE after 17 months (F = 6.643, $p < 0.05$) and its interaction with Cd after 24 months (F = 11.43, $p < 0.01$). The 24-month administration of the extract increased the femoral diaphysis fracture strength (Figure 4) and its stiffness compared to the control group and Cd_5 group (Figure 5), and the diaphysis fracture stress compared to the control group (Figure 6). According to the results of the Anova/Manova analysis, the favourable impact of the AE administration for 24 months on the fracture strength was an effect of its independent action (F = 9.720, $p < 0.01$), whereas the influence on the femoral diaphysis stiffness and yield stress of the bone tissue at the femoral diaphysis resulted from the AE–Cd interaction (F = 5.977, $p < 0.05$ and F = 6.883, $p < 0.05$, respectively). Moreover, this extract administration under the 10-month exposure to the 5 mg Cd/kg diet resulted in a decrease in the work to the diaphysis fracture compared to the control group and Cd$_5$ group, increased the value of this biomechanical parameter compared to the control group after 17 months, and completely prevented its increase after 24 months (Figure 5). The Anova/Manova analysis revealed that the impact of the AE administration on the work to the diaphysis fracture after 10 months was an effect of both its independent (F = 14.03, $p < 0.01$) and interactive action with Cd (F = 53.20, $p < 0.001$), whereas after 17 months, this was only a result of the AE–Cd interaction (F = 18.75, $p < 0.01$). Apart from that, the 10-month consumption of the AE under the exposure to the 5 mg Cd/kg diet decreased the stiffness of the femoral diaphysis (Figure 5) as a result of the interaction with Cd (F = 8.219, $p < 0.01$).

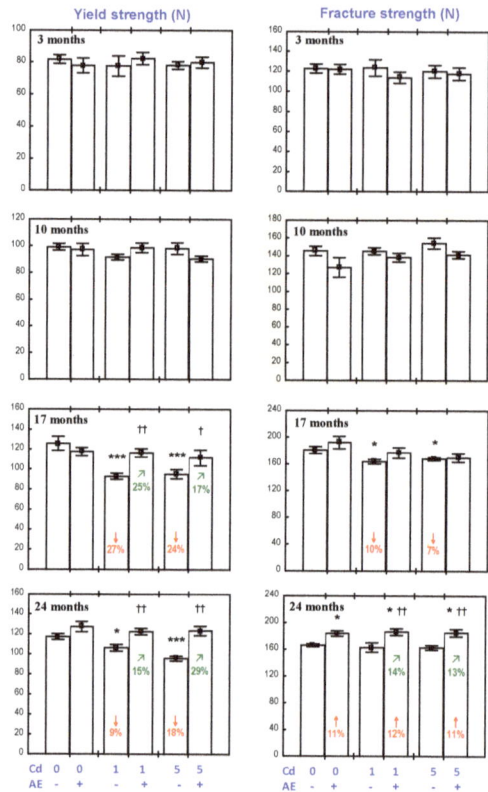

Figure 4. Effect of an extract from the berries of *Aronia melanocarpa* (AE) on the yield and fracture strength of the femoral diaphysis in rats exposed to cadmium (Cd). The rats received 0.1% aqueous AE or not ("+" and "−", respectively) and Cd in diet at the concentration of 0, 1, and 5 mg/kg. Data are represented as mean ± SE for eight rats, except for seven animals in the AE group, and the groups treated with the 1 and 5 mg Cd/kg diet alone after 24 months. Statistically significant differences (Anova, Duncan's multiple range test): * $p < 0.05$, *** $p < 0.001$ vs. control group; † $p < 0.05$, †† $p < 0.01$ vs. respective group receiving Cd alone. Numerical values in bars indicate percentage change compared to the control group (↑, increase; ↓, decrease) or the respective group receiving Cd alone (↗, increase).

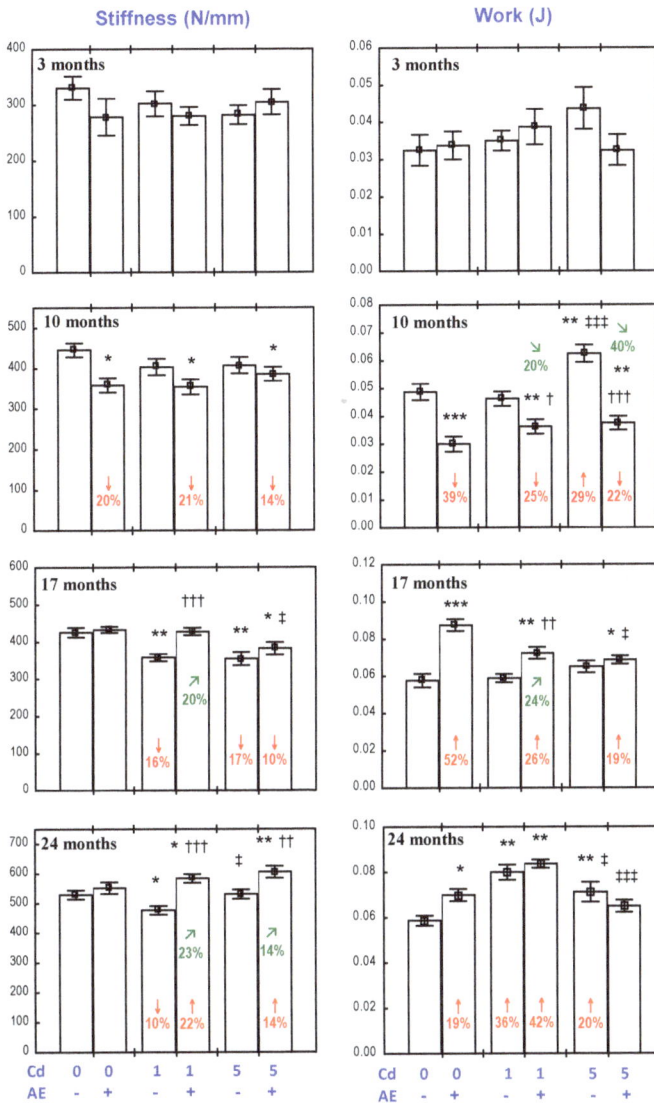

Figure 5. Effect of a polyphenol-rich extract from the berries of *Aronia melanocarpa* (AE) on the femoral diaphysis stiffness and work to its fracture in rats exposed to cadmium (Cd). The rats received 0.1% aqueous AE or not ("+" and "−", respectively) and Cd in diet at the concentration of 0, 1, and 5 mg/kg. Data are represented as mean ± SE for eight rats, except for seven animals in the AE group, and the groups treated with the 1 and 5 mg Cd/kg diet alone after 24 months. Statistically significant differences (Anova, Duncan's multiple range test): * $p < 0.05$, ** $p < 0.01$, *** $p < 0.001$ vs. control group; † $p < 0.05$, †† $p < 0.01$, ††† $p < 0.001$ vs. respective group receiving Cd alone; ‡ $p < 0.05$, ‡‡‡ $p < 0.001$ vs. respective group receiving the 1 mg Cd/kg diet. Numerical values in bars or above the bars indicate percentage change compared to the control group (↑, increase; ↓, decrease) or the respective group receiving Cd alone (↗, increase; ↘, decrease).

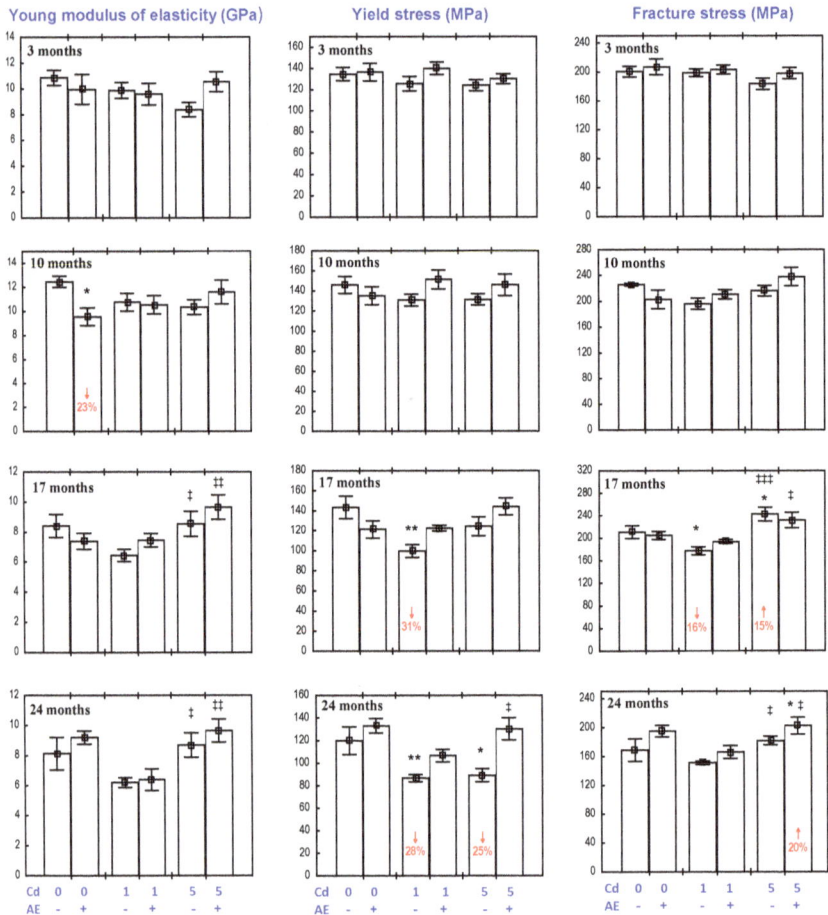

Figure 6. Effect of a polyphenol-rich extract from the berries of *Aronia melanocarpa* (AE) on the "material" biomechanical properties of the femoral diaphysis in rats exposed to cadmium (Cd). The rats received 0.1% aqueous AE or not ("+" and "−", respectively) and Cd in diet at the concentration of 0, 1, and 5 mg/kg. Data are represented as mean ± SE for eight rats, except for seven animals in the AE group, and the groups treated with the 1 and 5 mg Cd/kg diet alone after 24 months. Statistically significant differences (Anova, Duncan's multiple range test): * $p < 0.05$, ** $p < 0.01$ vs. control group; ‡ $p < 0.05$, ‡‡ $p < 0.01$, ‡‡‡ $p < 0.001$ vs. respective group receiving the 1 mg Cd/kg diet. Numerical values in bars indicate percentage change compared to the control group (↑, increase; ↓, decrease).

3.5. Effect of AE on PC I Concentration in the Bone Tissue in Rats Exposed to Cd

The administration of the AE alone for up to 24 months had no impact on the PC I concentration in the bone tissue at the distal epiphysis and diaphysis of the femur (Figure 7).

The exposure to the 1 mg Cd/kg diet for 10, 17, and 24 months resulted in a decrease in the bone tissue concentration of PC I, except for a lack of change in this parameter concentration at the distal femoral diaphysis after 24 months (Figure 7). At the higher exposure to Cd, the concentration of PC I in the bone tissue at the femoral epiphysis was decreased through the whole experiment, while the value of this parameter in the bone tissue at the femoral diaphysis was decreased after the 10th month (Figure 7).

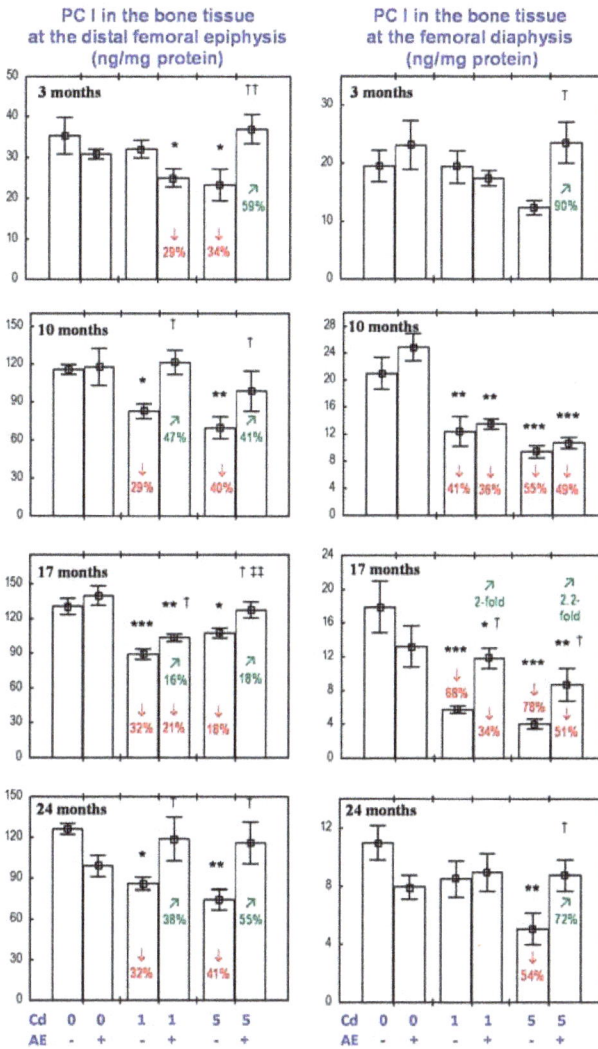

Figure 7. Effect of a polyphenol-rich extract from the berries of *Aronia melanocarpa* (AE) on procollagen I concentration in the bone tissue of rats exposed to cadmium (Cd). The rats received 0.1% aqueous AE or not ("+" and "−", respectively) and Cd in diet at the concentration of 0, 1, and 5 mg/kg. Data are represented as mean ± SE for eight rats, except for seven animals in the AE group, and the groups treated with the 1 and 5 mg Cd/kg diet alone after 24 months. Statistically significant differences (Anova, Duncan's multiple range test): * $p < 0.05$, ** $p < 0.01$, *** $p < 0.001$ vs. control group; † $p < 0.05$, †† $p < 0.01$ vs. respective group receiving Cd alone; ‡‡ $p < 0.01$ vs. respective group receiving the 1 mg Cd/kg diet. Numerical values in bars or above the bars indicate percentage change or a factor of change compared to the control group (↓, decrease) or the respective group receiving Cd alone (↗, increase).

The administration of the AE to the animals fed with the diets containing 1 and 5 mg Cd/kg completely prevented the above-described decrease in the concentration of PC I in the bone tissue at the distal femoral epiphysis, except for a partial protection after 17 months of the exposure to the 1 mg

Cd/kg diet (Figure 7). The effect of the AE on the PC I concentration in the bone tissue at the distal femoral epiphysis in the rats exposed to the 1 mg Cd/kg diet was caused by an independent action of the extract (F = 4.621, $p < 0.05$) after 10 months, whereas the impact after 24 months resulted from the interaction of ingredients of the AE with Cd (F = 10.13, $p < 0.01$). Moreover, the tendency of the AE and Cd to interactively impact the PC I concentration after 10 months (F = 3.832, $p = 0.06$) and the extract alone after 17 months (F = 3.680, $p = 0.06$) was noted. The AE consumption under the three-month treatment with the 1 mg Cd/kg diet decreased the PC I concentration in the bone tissue at the distal femoral epiphysis (Figure 7) as a result of an independent impact of the extract (F = 4.246, $p < 0.05$).

The PC I concentration in the bone tissue at the distal femoral epiphysis of the rats exposed to the 1 mg Cd/kg diet for 10–24 months was, on average, 29–32% lower than in the control group, whereas in the animals receiving the AE during the 10- and 24-month exposure to the 1 mg Cd/kg diet, the concentration of this biomarker of collagen biosynthesis did not differ when compared to the control group (and was higher by 47% and 38%, respectively, than in the Cd_1 group). After 17 months, the value of this parameter was 21% lower than in the control animals (and was 16% higher than in the Cd_1 group; Figure 7). The exposure to the 5 mg Cd/kg diet for 3–24 months decreased the PC I concentration in the bone tissue at the femoral epiphysis by an average of 18–41% compared to the control group, whereas in the animals receiving the AE under the exposure to Cd, the value of this parameter was within the range of the control group and was an average of 18–59% higher compared to the Cd_5 group (Figure 7).

The administration of the AE under the 10-month exposure to the 1 and 5 mg Cd/kg diet had no impact on the PC I concentration at the femoral diaphysis; however, in the case of the 17-month co-administration, partial, but clearly evident, protection, resulting from the AE ingredients–Cd interaction (F = 6.771, $p < 0.05$ and F = 4.513, $p < 0.05$, respectively), was noted (Figure 7). The extract consumption for 24 months completely prevented the exposure to the 5 mg Cd/kg diet-induced decrease in PC I concentration at the femoral diaphysis (Figure 7) as a result of the AE–Cd interaction (F = 9.926, $p < 0.01$). Moreover, the three-month administration of the AE to the rats fed with the 5 mg Cd/kg diet increased the PC I concentration at the femoral diaphysis compared to the Cd_5 group (Figure 7) and the effect resulted from an independent action of the extract's ingredients (F = 5.603, $p < 0.05$).

The exposure to the 1 mg Cd/kg diet for 10 and 17 months decreased the concentration of PC I in the bone tissue at the femoral diaphysis by 41% and 68%, respectively. In the animals receiving the AE during the 17-month exposure to the 1 mg Cd/kg diet, the concentration of PC I in the bone tissue at the femoral diaphysis was two-fold higher compared to the Cd_1 group, but it remained lower (by 34%) than in the control group (Figure 7). In the case of the higher level of Cd exposure (5 mg Cd/kg diet), the PC I concentration in the bone tissue at the femoral diaphysis after 17 and 24 months was 78% and 54% lower, respectively, compared to the control group, whereas in the case of the co-administration of Cd and the AE, the concentration was 2.2-fold and 72% higher, respectively, than in the Cd_5 group. Moreover, after 17 months, the concentration of PC I remained 51% lower than in the control group, while after 24 months, it did not differ compared to the proper values of the control animals.

3.6. Dependence Between the Femur BMD and Its Biomechanical Properties in Rats Exposed to Cd

In the animals receiving the AE under the exposure to Cd, positive correlations were noted between the femur BMD and the yield strength (r = 0.525, $p < 0.001$), fracture strength (r = 0.499, $p < 0.001$), stiffness (r = 0.459, $p < 0.001$), and work to the femoral diaphysis fracture (r = 0.445, $p < 0.001$). Moreover, the femur BMD negatively correlated (r = −0.246, $p < 0.05$) with the Young modulus of elasticity of the bone tissue at the femoral diaphysis. A positive correlation was also noted between the femur BMD and the stiffness of the femoral neck (r = 0.260, $p < 0.05$).

4. Discussion

The present study is the first that investigated and revealed the protective impact of AE consumption under low-level and moderate chronic exposure to Cd on the bone biomechanical properties and collagen biosynthesis in the bone tissue. Although this study was focused mainly on the possibility of the protective influence of the AE on the femur biomechanical properties under chronic exposure to Cd, it has also provided important data on the effect of low-level chronic exposure to Cd on bone vulnerability to fracture.

The study not only confirmed the previously reported results by us [15–18] relating to the unfavourable impact of low exposure to this heavy metal on the bone biomechanical properties, but it also provided evidence that the biomechanical properties of the femur may be weakened at a lower exposure than was previously shown and a very low Cd concentration in the blood and urine (0.185–0.324 µg/L and 0.107–0.285 µg/g creatinine, respectively; such concentrations were reached after 17–24 months of the exposure to the 1 mg Cd/kg diet [25]), comparable to the metal concentrations commonly noted in the general population. Weakening of the bone biomechanical properties at such a low Cd concentration in the blood and urine has been reported in the present paper for the first time. The impact of Cd on the biomechanical properties of the femoral neck and diaphysis evaluated in the current study was relatively subtle, but clearly evident taking into account the fact that the unfavourable effect occurred at low-level exposure, resulting in a blood and urinary Cd concentration comparable to this metal's concentration noted in the general population. The effect of Cd on the femur biomechanical properties in the female rats was less serious than that previously reported by us [15–18], but the investigated levels of exposure were also lower. The decrease in the yield and fracture strength of the femoral diaphysis after 17 months and in the yield strength of the femoral neck after 24 months provide evidence of decreased bone resistance to fracture, resulting in an enhancement in the risk of fracture due to long-term low-level exposure to this heavy metal. However, it should be clearly underlined that the changes in the biomechanical properties of the femur observed in the present study show that long-term, even very low-level, intoxication with this toxic metal has an unfavourable impact on the skeleton. At both levels of exposure, the impact of Cd on the strength of the femur was clearly evident after only 17 months of intoxication. As was reported in detail in our previous papers, the weakening of the biomechanical properties of the femur due to the treatment with Cd results from the unfavourable impact of this heavy metal on the mineral status and organic matrix (formed mainly by collagen) of the bone [15–18,33,34]. The proper amount and structure of collagen fibers play an important role in bone formation and strength [29,30,35]. The results of the present study show that the low exposure to Cd (1 mg Cd/kg diet) inhibited collagen biosynthesis in the bone tissue after 10 months. Because the impact of Cd on the "structural" and "material" biomechanical properties of the femoral diaphysis and the femoral neck susceptibility to fracture was previously reported by us [15–18,33], and the mechanisms leading to an increase in the bone susceptibility to fracture are known and reported, they are not discussed in the present paper. However, the very important finding of the present study regarding the impact of Cd on the femur susceptibility to fracture reveals that this heavy metal may weaken the biomechanical properties of the femoral neck and diaphysis at an exposure lower than has been revealed until now [16,18].

The biomechanical tests performed conclusively revealed that the consumption of the chokeberry extract under long-term low and moderate exposure to Cd improved the femur resistance to fracture. The protective impact of the AE may be explained by the recently reported results by us relating to the beneficial influence of the extract on bone turnover, reflected in an improvement in the femur BMD (Tables S1 and S2) [26] and revealed in the present study's protection from the Cd-induced inhibition of collagen biosynthesis. The possible mechanism of the extract's impact on the bone mineral status has been previously reported by us [26] and it consists of an inhibition of Cd-induced bone resorption and the stimulation of the processes of bone formation. It was also revealed by us that the mechanism of osteoprotective action of the AE extract is mediated by its antioxidative properties, as well as the improvement of the oxidative/antioxidative balance in the bone tissue and protection from oxidative stress and oxidative damage to macromolecules in the bone tissue [27].

The results of the Anova/Manova analysis allow us to recognize that the beneficial impact of the AE administration on the biomechanical properties of the femur resulted from both an independent action of the ingredients of the extract and their interaction with Cd, resulting in a lower body burden of this metal and its lower accumulation in the bone tissue [25–27]. As a result of the AE ingredients–Cd interaction, the direct and indirect damaging impact of this toxic metal on the skeleton has been weakened. The independent impact of the AE ingredients on the skeleton may be explained mainly by the action of polyphenolic compounds, being the most abundant active components of the aronia berries. Polyphenolic compounds are widely known from their osteoprotective impact related with the improvement of BMD, but the data mainly refers to green tea polyphenols [7,24,36]. In the available literature, apart from our recent reports [25–27], there is no data on the impact of the consumption of aronia berries and their products on bone metabolism and bone strength properties. However, our findings in the animals administered the AE alone for 3, 10, 17, and 24 months provide clear evidence for an independent influence of the extract's ingredients on the skeleton, including the impact on the bone turnover, bone mineral status, oxidative/antioxidative status of the bone tissue, and the bone biomechanical properties [22–24]. It seems possible that the main cause of the beneficial impact of the AE under exposure to Cd on the femur biomechanical properties is this extract-caused improvement of the bone mineral status [26]. The positive correlations noted in the current study between the femur BMD and biomechanical properties of the femoral diaphysis (yield and fracture strength, stiffness, work to fracture) in the animals administered with the AE under exposure to Cd confirm the validity of this reasoning. The bone mineral status is one of the main determinants of the bone vulnerability to fracture [28]. Thus, the improvement in the bone mineral status is also related to the improvement in the bone strength properties. Owing to the lack of any literature data on the impact of *A. melanocarpa* on the bone biomechanical properties and the bone susceptibility to fracture, a wider discussion of the results is impossible.

We are aware not only of the achievements, but also of the limitations, of our designed studies on the possible protective impact of AE on the skeleton. At this stage of our investigation, we are unable to explain the exact mechanisms of the beneficial impact of AE on the bone, including the bone susceptibility to fractures, nonetheless our experiment provided unquestionable evidence for this protection. Moreover, because our study was conducted on a female rat model of lifetime environmental exposure, the findings refer to the female skeleton and further study involving an evaluation of AE on the male skeleton is warranted.

5. Conclusions

In summary, the present study provides the first evidence that the consumption of AE under chronic exposure to Cd improves the biomechanical properties of the femur, increasing its resistance to fracture at the neck and diaphysis. Fracture is the most serious consequence of the damaging impact of any factor on bone, thus revealing the fact that chokeberry extract enhances the femur resistance to fracture under exposure to Cd is a very important and practically useful finding of our study. This finding, together with our previous results on the bone impact of AE in the experimental model of the lifetime women exposure to Cd [25–27], provide strong evidence, allowing us to recognize that the consumption of aronia berries and their products under chronic exposure to this heavy metal seems to be a promising natural strategy for preventing skeletal damage. However, the possible use of the *A. melanocarpa* berries as a prophylactic of bone diseases in humans needs further investigation. It seems necessary to analyse the relationship between the consumption of the aronia berries and the bone status in subjects chronically exposed to Cd, including both males and females.

Supplementary Materials: The following are available online at www.mdpi.com/2072-6643/9/6/543/s1, Table S1: Effect of a polyphenol-rich extract from the berries of *Aronia melanocarpa* (AE) on bone turnover in rats exposed to cadmium (Cd), Table S2: Effect of a polyphenol-rich extract from the berries of *Aronia melanocarpa* (AE) on the femur bone mineral density (BMD) in rats exposed to cadmium (Cd), Table S3: Polyphenolic compounds concentration in the extract from the berries of *Aronia melanocarpa*, Table S4: Cadmium (Cd) intake in particular experimental groups, Table S5: The intake of polyphenolic compounds from the extract from *Aronia melanocarpa* berries (AE) in particular experimental groups, Table S6: Effect of the extract from the berries of *Aronia melanocarpa* (AE) on the absolute and relative femur weight of cadmium (Cd)-exposed rats, Table S7: Effect of the extract from the berries of *Aronia melanocarpa* (AE) on the femur length and diameter at the mid-diaphysis in rats exposed to cadmium (Cd).

Acknowledgments: This study was financially supported in part by the Grant (No. N N405 051140) from the National Science Centre (Poland) and Medical University of Bialystok (Poland). The study was conducted with the use of equipment by Medical University of Bialystok as part of the OP DEP 2007–2013, Priority Axis I.3, contract No. POPW.01.00-20-001/12.

Author Contributions: Małgorzata M. Brzóska designed the research, participated in the experiment, interpreted the data, and designed and wrote the paper; Alicja Roszczenko and Joanna Rogalska performed the experiment and statistical analysis, and participated in the manuscript preparation; Małgorzata Gałażyn-Sidorczuk performed the experiment and participated in the manuscript preparation; Magdalena Mężyńska participated in the experiment and manuscript preparation. All authors approved the final version of the manuscript.

Conflicts of Interest: The authors declare no conflict of interest.

Abbreviations

AE, extract from the berries of *Aronia melanocarpa*; A–P, anterior–posterior; BMD, bone mineral density; Cd, cadmium; CSA, cross-sectional area; CSMI, cross-sectional moment of inertia; CV, coefficient of variation; M–L, medial–lateral; PC I, procollagen I; WT, wall thickness.

References

1. Dahl, C.; Søgaard, A.J.; Tell, G.S.; Flaten, T.P.; Hongve, D.; Omsland, T.K.; Holvik, K.; Meyer, H.E.; Aamodt, G. Norwegian Epidemiologic Osteoporosis Study (NOREPOS) Core Research Group. Do cadmium, lead, and aluminum in drinking water increase the risk of hip fractures? A NOREPOS study. *Biol. Trace Elem. Res.* **2014**, *157*, 14–23. [CrossRef] [PubMed]

2. Søgaard, A.J.; Meyer, H.E.; Emaus, N.; Grimnes, G.; Gjesdal, C.G.; Forsmo, S.; Schei, B.; Tell, G.S. Cohort profile: Norwegian Epidemiologic Osteoporosis Studies (NOREPOS). *Scand. J. Public Health* **2014**, *42*, 804–813. [CrossRef] [PubMed]

3. Wong, A.K.O.; Beattie, K.A.; Bhargava, A.; Cheung, M.; Webber, C.E.; Chettle, D.R.; Papaioannou, A.; Adach, J.D. Bone lead (Pb) content at the tibia is associated with thinner distal tibia cortices and lower volumetric bone density in postmenopausal women. *Bone* **2015**, *79*, 58–64. [CrossRef] [PubMed]

4. Shen, C.L.; Yeh, J.K.; Cao, J.J.; Wang, J.S. Green tea and bone metabolism. *Nutr. Res.* **2009**, *29*, 437–456. [CrossRef] [PubMed]

5. Gunn, C.A.; Weber, J.L.; McGill, A.T.; Kruger, M.C. Increased intake of selected vegetables, herbs and fruit may reduce bone turnover in post-menopausal women. *Nutrients* **2015**, *7*, 2499–2517. [CrossRef] [PubMed]

6. Hardcastle, A.C.; Aucott, L.; Reid, D.M.; Macdonald, H.M. Associations between dietary flavonoid intakes and bone health in a Scottish population. *J. Bone Miner. Res.* **2011**, *26*, 941–947. [CrossRef] [PubMed]

7. Shen, C.L.; Chyu, M.C.; Wang, J.S. Tea and bone health: Steps forward in translational nutrition. *Am. J. Clin. Nutr.* **2013**, *98*, 1694S–1699S. [CrossRef] [PubMed]

8. Chen, X.; Wang, K.; Wang, Z.; Gan, C.; He, P.; Liang, Y.; Jin, T.; Zhu, G. Effects of lead and cadmium co-exposure on bone mineral density in a Chinese population. *Bone* **2014**, *63*, 76–80. [CrossRef] [PubMed]

9. Callan, A.C.; Devine, A.; Qi, L.; Ng, J.C.; Hinwood, A.L. Investigation of the relationship between low environmental exposure to metals and bone mineral density, bone resorption and renal function. *Int. J. Hyg. Environ. Health* **2015**, *218*, 444–451. [CrossRef] [PubMed]

10. Wallin, M.; Barregard, L.; Sallsten, G.; Lundh, T.; Karlsson, M.K.; Lorentzon, M.; Ohlsson, C.; Mellström, D. Low-level cadmium exposure is associated with decreased bone mineral density and increased risk of incident fractures in elderly men: The MrOS Sweden study. *J. Bone Miner. Res.* **2015**, *31*, 732–741. [CrossRef] [PubMed]

11. Nawrot, T.S.; Staessen, J.A.; Roels, H.A.; Munters, E.; Cuypers, A.; Richart, T.; Ruttens, A.; Smeets, K.; Clijsters, H.; Vangronsveld, J. Cadmium exposure in the population: From health risks to strategies of prevention. *Biometals* **2010**, *23*, 769–782. [CrossRef] [PubMed]

12. Satarug, S.; Vesey, D.A.; Gobe, G.C. Health risk assessment of dietary cadmium intake: Do current guidelines indicate how much is safe? *Environ. Health Perspect.* **2017**, *125*, 284–288. [CrossRef] [PubMed]

13. Brzóska, M.M.; Moniuszko-Jakoniuk, J. Low-level exposure to cadmium during the lifetime increases the risk of osteoporosis and fractures of the lumbar spine in the elderly: Studies on a rat model of human environmental exposure. *Toxicol. Sci.* **2004**, *82*, 468–477. [CrossRef] [PubMed]

14. Brzóska, M.M.; Moniuszko-Jakoniuk, J. Low-level lifetime exposure to cadmium decreases skeletal mineralization and enhances bone loss in aged rats. *Bone* **2004**, *35*, 1180–1191. [CrossRef] [PubMed]

15. Brzóska, M.M.; Majewska, K.; Moniuszko-Jakoniuk, J. Mechanical properties of femoral diaphysis and femoral neck of female rats chronically exposed to various levels of cadmium. *Calcif. Tissue Int.* **2005**, *76*, 287–298. [CrossRef] [PubMed]

16. Brzóska, M.M.; Majewska, K.; Moniuszko-Jakoniuk, J. Weakness in the mechanical properties of the femur of growing female rats exposed to cadmium. *Arch. Toxicol.* **2005**, *79*, 277–288. [CrossRef] [PubMed]

17. Brzóska, M.M.; Majewska, K.; Kupraszewicz, E. Effects of low, moderate and relatively high chronic exposure to cadmium on long bones susceptibility to fracture in male rats. *Environ. Toxicol. Pharmacol.* **2010**, *29*, 235–245. [CrossRef] [PubMed]

18. Brzóska, M.M. Low-level chronic exposure to cadmium enhances the risk of long bone fractures: A study on a female rat model of human lifetime exposure. *J. Appl. Toxicol.* **2011**, *32*, 34–44. [CrossRef] [PubMed]

19. Olgun, O. The effect of dietary cadmium supplementation on performance, egg quality, tibia biomechanical properties and eggshell and bone mineralisation in laying quails. *Animal* **2015**, *9*, 1298–1303. [CrossRef] [PubMed]

20. Brzóska, M.M.; Borowska, S.; Tomczyk, M. Antioxidants as a potential preventive and therapeutic strategy for cadmium. *Curr. Drug Targets* **2016**, *17*, 1350–1384. [CrossRef] [PubMed]

21. Kopeć, A.; Sikora, A.; Piątkowska, E.; Borczak, B.; Czech, T. Possible protective role of elderberry fruit lyophilizate against selected effects of cadmium and lead intoxication in Wistar rats. *Environ. Sci. Pollut. Res.* **2016**, *23*, 8837–8848. [CrossRef] [PubMed]

22. Borowska, S.; Brzóska, M.M. Chokeberries (*Aronia melanocarpa*) and their products as a possible means for the prevention and treatment of noncommunicable diseases and unfavorable health effects due to exposure to xenobiotics. *Compr. Rev. Food Sci. Food Saf.* **2016**, *15*, 982–1017. [CrossRef]

23. Denev, P.N.; Kratchanov, C.G.; Ciz, M.; Lojek, A.; Kratchanova, M.G. Bioavailability and antioxidant activity of black chokeberry (*Aronia melanocarpa*) polyphenols: In vitro and in vivo evidences and possible mechanisms of action: A review. *Compr. Rev. Food Sci. Food Saf.* **2012**, *11*, 471–489. [CrossRef]

24. Shen, C.L.; Wang, P.; Guerrieri, J.; Yeh, J.K.; Wang, J.S. Protective effect of green tea polyphenols on bone loss in middle-aged female rats. *Osteoporos. Int.* **2008**, *19*, 979–990. [CrossRef] [PubMed]

25. Brzóska, M.M.; Galazyn-Sidorczuk, M.; Jurczuk, M.; Tomczyk, M. Protective effect of *Aronia melanocarpa* polyphenols on cadmium accumulation in the body: A study in a rat model of human exposure to this metal. *Curr. Drug Targets* **2015**, *16*, 1470–1487. [CrossRef]

26. Brzóska, M.M.; Rogalska, J.; Galazyn-Sidorczuk, M.; Jurczuk, M.; Roszczenko, A.; Tomczyk, M. Protective effect of *Aronia melanocarpa* polyphenols against cadmium-induced disorders in bone metabolism: A study in a rat model of lifetime human exposure to this heavy metal. *Chem. Biol. Interact.* **2015**, *229*, 132–146. [CrossRef] [PubMed]

27. Brzóska, M.M.; Rogalska, J.; Roszczenko, A.; Galazyn-Sidorczuk, A.; Tomczyk, M. The mechanism of the osteoprotective action of a polyphenol-rich *Aronia melanocarpa* extract during chronic exposure to cadmium is mediated by the oxidative defense system. *Planta Med.* **2016**, *82*, 621–631. [CrossRef] [PubMed]

28. Follet, H.; Boivin, G.; Rumelhart, C.; Meunier, P.J. The degree of mineralization is a determinant of bone strength: A study on human calcanei. *Bone* **2004**, *34*, 783–789. [CrossRef] [PubMed]

29. Osterhoff, G.; Morgan, E.F.; Shefelbine, S.J.; Karim, L.; McNamarae, L.M.; Augat, P. Bone mechanical properties and changes with osteoporosis. *Inj. Int. J. Care Inj.* **2016**, *47*, S11–S20. [CrossRef]

30. Garnero, P. The role of collagen organization on the properties of bone. *Calcif. Tissue Int.* **2015**, *97*, 229–240. [CrossRef] [PubMed]

31. Kulling, S.E.; Rawel, H.M. Chokeberry (*Aronia melanocarpa*)—A review on the characteristic components and potential health effects. *Planta Med.* **2008**, *74*, 1625–1634. [CrossRef] [PubMed]

32. Kokotkiewicz, A.; Jaremicz, Z.; Łuczkiewicz, M. Aronia plants: A review of traditional use, biological activities, and perspectives for modern medicine. *J. Med. Food* **2010**, *13*, 255–269. [CrossRef] [PubMed]

33. Brzóska, M.M.; Galażyn-Sidorczuk, M.; Rogalska, J.; Roszczenko, A.; Jurczuk, M.; Majewska, K.; Moniuszko-Jakoniuk, J. Beneficial effect of zinc supplementation on biomechanical properties of femoral distal end and femoral diaphysis of male rats chronically exposed to cadmium. *Chem. Biol. Interact.* **2008**, *171*, 312–324. [CrossRef] [PubMed]

34. Galicka, A.; Brzóska, M.M.; Średzińska, K.; Gindzieński, A. Effect of cadmium on collagen content and solubility in rat bone. *Acta Biochim. Polon.* **2004**, *51*, 825–829. [PubMed]

35. Burr, D.B. The contribution of the organic matrix to bone's material properties. *Bone* **2002**, *31*, 8–11. [CrossRef]

36. Hubert, P.A.; Lee, S.G.; Lee, S.K.; Chun, O.K. Dietary polyphenols, berries, and age-related bone loss: A review based on human, animal, and cell studies. *Antioxidants* **2014**, *3*, 144–158. [CrossRef] [PubMed]

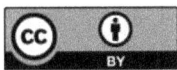

![nutrients logo] *nutrients*

MDPI

Article

Osthole Enhances Osteogenesis in Osteoblasts by Elevating Transcription Factor Osterix via cAMP/CREB Signaling In Vitro and In Vivo

Zhong-Rong Zhang [1], Wing Nang Leung [1], Gang Li [2], Siu Kai Kong [3], Xiong Lu [4], Yin Mei Wong [1] and Chun Wai Chan [1,*]

[1] School of Chinese Medicine, Faculty of Medicine, The Chinese University of Hong Kong, Shatin, Hong Kong, China; zhang_zhongrong@cuhk.edu.hk (Z.-R.Z.); awnleung@gmail.com (W.N.L.); wongyinmei@cuhk.edu.hk (Y.M.W.)

[2] Department of Orthopaedics and Traumatology, Faculty of Medicine, The Chinese University of Hong Kong, Shatin, Hong Kong, China; gangli@cuhk.edu.hk

[3] School of Life Sciences, The Chinese University of Hong Kong, Shatin, Hong Kong, China; skkong@cuhk.edu.hk

[4] Key Lab of Advanced Technologies of Materials, Ministry of Education, School of Materials Science and Engineering, Southwest Jiaotong University, Chengdu 610031, China; luxiong@home.swjtu.edu.cn

* Correspondence: fcwchan@cuhk.edu; Tel.: +852-3943-3768

Received: 28 March 2017; Accepted: 5 June 2017; Published: 8 June 2017

Abstract: Anabolic anti-osteoporotic agents are desirable for treatment and prevention of osteoporosis and fragility fractures. Osthole is a coumarin derivative extracted from the medicinal herbs *Cnidium monnieri* (L.) Cusson and *Angelica pubescens* Maxim.f. Osthole has been reported with osteogenic and anti-osteoporotic properties, whereas the underlying mechanism of its benefit still remains unclear. The objective of the present study was to investigate the osteopromotive action of osthole on mouse osteoblastic MC3T3-E1 cells and on mouse femoral fracture repair, and to explore the interaction between osthole-induced osteopromotive effect and cyclic adenosine monophosphate (cAMP) elevating effect. Osthole treatment promoted osteogenesis in osteoblasts by enhancing alkaline phosphatase (ALP) activity and mineralization. Oral gavage of osthole enhanced fracture repair and increased bone strength. Mechanistic study showed osthole triggered the cAMP/CREB pathway through the elevation of the intracellular cAMP level and activation of the phosphorylation of the cAMP response element-binding protein (CREB). Blockage of cAMP/CREB downstream signals with protein kinase A (PKA) inhibitor KT5720 partially suppressed osthole-mediated osteogenesis by inhibiting the elevation of transcription factor, osterix. In conclusion, osthole shows osteopromotive effect on osteoblasts in vitro and in vivo. Osthole-mediated osteogenesis is related to activation of the cAMP/CREB signaling pathway and downstream osterix expression.

Keywords: osthole; osteoblast; osteogenesis; bone regeneration; fracture repair; cAMP/ CREB signaling

---

1. Introduction

Osteoporosis is a systemic skeletal disease characterized by impairment of bone mineral density, strength, and microstructure, leading to an increased risk of fragility fracture that can cause substantial morbidity and mortality [1]. It has become a major public health problem worldwide along with the aging of the population [2]. Osteoporotic fracture treatment has particular difficulties with high rates of implant fixation failure and increased non-union risk caused by delayed bone formation [3–5]. Apart from novel technology for enhancement of bone healing [6–8], healthy dietary strategies are important modifiable factors for both prevention of osteoporosis and improvement of bone healing [9–11]. It is widely accepted that adequate intake of minerals, proteins, and antioxidants enriched foods benefit bone health [12]. Moreover, numerous bioactive phytochemicals found in functional and medicinal food are suggested to have anti-osteoporotic properties [13–16].

Osthole, a naturally-derived coumarin, is the major bioactive component found in the medicinal herbs *Cnidium monnieri* (L.) Cusson and *Angelica pubescens* Maxim. f., which are commonly used as ingredients in functional foods and herbal medicine formulae [17,18]. Osthole was reported to exert anti-osteoporotic effects in ovariectomy-induced bone loss [19,20]. Moreover, osthole showed in vivo osteoanabolic action by promoting new bone formation in calvaria and endochondral ossification in mice fracture healing [20,21]. Current therapeutic agents of osteoporosis are mainly antiresorptive drugs that inhibit bone resorptive function of osteoclasts, including bisphosphonates, calcitonin, and estrogen analogues. Their efficacy on growth and recovery of bone mass is regarded to be limited [22,23]. On the other hand, bioactive agents that induce osteoblastic bone formation and facilitate fracture repair are suggested more effective and desirable for osteoporosis therapy [24]. Therefore, osthole is a promising potential anabolic agent for osteoporosis and fragility fracture treatment.

The mechanism of the anti-osteoporotic effect of osthole was mainly studied with cell culture models. Previous studies suggested osthole induced osteoblastic differentiation through the bone morphogenetic proteins (BMP)-dependent pathways, which were likely triggered by β-catenin signaling [20,25,26]. More detailed molecular studies are required to enrich the knowledge and to clarify the mechanism of the osteogenic and anti-osteoporotic properties before potential clinical application. On the other hand, multiple studies have demonstrated that cAMP/CREB signaling is the dominant mechanism for the anabolic action of parathyroid hormone (PTH) on bone formation [27–29]. In osteoblastic cells and bone tissues, PTH binds to PTH receptors and produces cyclic adenosine monophosphate (cAMP) from adenosine triphosphate (ATP). It leads to the activation of protein kinase A (PKA) and phosphorylation of the cAMP response element-binding protein (CREB) [27,30]. Activated CREB binds to the cAMP response element (CRE) and triggers the cascade expression of osteogenic-related genes [31,32]. Osthole was reported to elevate cAMP levels in adrenocortical cancer cells, trachea, and corpus cavernosum tissues [33–35]. Although none reported the cAMP-elevating action of osthole in bone cells or osseous tissues, it was highly probable that osthole treatment would increase cellular cAMP levels in osteoblast cultures and regenerating bone. This might be an alternative possible mechanism of the osteopromotive effect of osthole.

Considering the prospects of osthole as an anabolic anti-osteoporotic agent, the objectives of the present study were to investigate the osteopromotive action of osthole in osteoblasts and bone regeneration during fracture repair. We hypothesized that osthole treatment enhanced osteogenesis in osteoblasts and thereby improved fracture repair by increasing bone strength via cAMP-mediated signaling.

2. Materials and Methods

2.1. Chemicals and Cell Culture

Osthole ($\geq$95% high performance liquid chromatography, HPLC grade), PKA inhibitor KT5720, and dimethyl sulfoxide (DMSO) were purchased from Sigma-Aldrich Corporation (St. Louis, MO, USA). Recombinant mouse noggin was purchased from R and D Systems, Inc. (Minneapolis, MN, USA). Vehicle control cells were supplied with solvent DMSO (<0.1%). Cell cultures were pre-treated alone with noggin (100 ng/mL) or KT5720 (4 µM) for 1 h and then co-treated with osthole for pathway blockage. All other reagents were obtained from Sigma-Aldrich unless otherwise indicated.

Mouse preosteoblast cell MC3T3-E1 subclone 14 (ATCC CRL-2594) was purchased from the American Type Culture Collection (Manassas, VA, USA). Cells were routinely maintained in complete growth medium containing alpha minimum essential medium (α-MEM) (Thermo Fisher Scientific, Waltham, MA, USA) supplemented with 10% fetal bovine serum (FBS) (Thermo Fisher Scientific) and

1% penicillin-streptomycin-neomycin antibiotic mixture (Thermo Fisher Scientific), incubated at 37 °C in a humidified 5% CO_2 atmosphere. Cells were differentiated in osteogenic medium supplied with 0.25 mM L-ascorbic acid (L-AA) and 10 mM β-glycerolphosphate (β-GP) in growth medium once reaching 90% confluency. Both growth and differentiation media were renewed every 2 days.

2.2. Mouse Femoral Osteotomy

C57BL/6 mice were obtained from the Laboratory Animal Services Center of the Chinese University of Hong Kong. The animal study was approved by the Animal Experimentation Ethics Committee (Ref. No. 13/010/GRF). All mice were first acclimatized and housed at the research animal laboratory during the experimental period. Open osteotomy at the femur shaft was performed on 12-week-old male C57BL/6 mice. Briefly, mice (weight around 25 to 30 g) were anaesthetized generally with intraperitoneal injection of ketamine (67 mg/kg) and xylazine (13 mg/kg). After shaving and sterilization of the right leg, a lateral incision was made and a 25-gauge needle was inserted retrograde into the intramedullary canal from knee articular surface for internal fixation. Diaphysis of the femur was exposed and an air-driven oscillating saw (Synthes Holding AG, Zuchwil, Switzerland) was used to create a transverse midshaft fracture under irrigation with sterile 0.9% saline solution. Absorbable sutures were used to close the intramuscular septum and skin incision. Osthole reagent was freshly prepared by dissolution with 0.5% (*v/v*) Tween 80 in distilled water. Mice were administrated with 20 mg/kg osthole (dosage derived from previous report [19]) in the osthole treatment group (Ost) and vehicle solvent in the control group (Ctl) through daily oral gavage from post-operative day 7 until euthanasia.

2.3. Cell Viability/Proliferation Assay

Cells were seeded at a density of 1×10^4 per well into a 96-well plate. After 24 h pre-incubation, they were exposed to osthole at concentrations of 0, 10, 20, 50, 100, 200, and 500 μM for 24, 48, and 72 h. At the end of the treatment, cells were washed with phosphate-buffered saline (PBS) and incubated with 0.5 mg/mL 3-(4,5-cimethylthiazol-2-yl)-2,5-diphenyl tetrazolium bromide (MTT) in medium for an additional 3 h. After incubation, 100 μL DMSO was added each well to dissolve the formazan crystals and the optical density at 570 nm (OD_{570}) was measured with a microplate reader (BioTek, Winooski, VT, USA). Cell viability was expressed as the percentage of the control by comparing the viability in the treatment groups to that of the vehicle control group.

2.4. Alkaline Phosphatase (ALP) Enzyme-Cytochemistry and ALP Activity Assay

Cells (4×10^4 per well) were seeded into a 24-well plate and allowed to incubate for 48 h in growth medium, and then exposed to 0–100 μM of osthole in osteogenic medium or growth medium for 12 days. After treatment, cells were washed with PBS and fixed with 70% ethanol. Cells were then equilibrated with ALP buffer (50 mM Tris-HCl, pH 9.5, 100 mM NaCl, 50 mM $MgCl_2$, 0.1% Tween 20) for 10 min, and incubated with ALP staining solution (5 μL 5-bromo-4-chloro-3-indolyl phosphate (BCIP) and 10 μL nitro blue tetrazolium (NBT) (Promega, Fitchburg, WI, USA) in 1 mL of ALP buffer) in dark at 37 °C. Intensity of ALP staining was assessed by both macroscopic and microscopic observations.

Differentiated and control cells in a 24-well plate were washed with PBS and lysed with 150 μL ice cold lysis buffer (50 mM Tris-HCl, pH 7.4, 100 mM NaCl, 2 mM $MgCl_2$, and 0.5% Triton X-100). ALP activities of cell lysate were measured with an ALP-AMP kit (BioSystems Reagents and Instruments, Quezon City, Philippines). Briefly, 50 μL cell lysate was transferred to a 96-well plate, and 150 μL of freshly-prepared substrate working reagent was aliquoted to each well. OD_{405} of the mixture was measured every minute with a microplate reader for 20 min at room temperature. The curve was plotted using absorbance against time, and ΔOD_{405}/min obtained was used to calculate enzyme activity. ALP activity was normalized by protein concentration which was measured with a BCA Protein Assay Kit (Thermo Fisher Scientific) at OD_{562}.

2.5. Calcium Nodule Staining and Quantification

Differentiated and control cells in the 24-well plate were washed with PBS and fixed with ethanol. Cells were stained with 1% alizarin red S (ARS) (pH 4.1) at 37 °C for 30 min. Calcium nodules were visualized by staining with ARS to form an ARS-calcium complex in a chelation process. After washing and removal of free dyes, mineral deposition in the cell culture was assessed and compared by macroscopic and microscopic observation. Quantification of calcium deposits was conducted using an in vitro osteogenesis assay kit (Merck Millipore, Darmstadt, Germany). Briefly, 400 μL of 10% acetic acid was added to each well to extract dyes. Cells and acetic acid were transferred to microcentrifuge tubes and heated to 85 °C for 10 min. Centrifuged supernatant was collected and neutralized with 10% ammonium hydroxide. Samples were then aliquoted to a 96-well plate and measured at OD_{405} along with standards. The linear curve was plotted with ARS concentration against the absorbance of standards, and the ARS concentrations of samples were calculated.

2.6. RNA Extraction and Real-Time RT-PCR

Cells (2×10^5 per well) were seeded into six-well plates and allowed to incubate for 48 h. Cells were exposed to 0–50 μM osthole with or without inhibitors for 12 h or 6 days. Total RNA was extracted from cells with TRIzol reagent (Ambion, Foster City, CA, USA). One microgram of RNA was reverse-transcribed into cDNA using oligo (dT) primers and reverse transcriptase (Promega). Quantitative real-time PCR was performed using a QuantiFast SYBR Green PCR Kit (Qiagen, Hilden, Germany), in a total volume of 20 μL containing 1 μL of reverse-transcription product in the presence of a ribonuclease inhibitor (Takara, Kyoto, Japan) and 0.5 μM of sense and antisense primers of target genes, as below (Tech Dragon Limited, Hong Kong, China). BMP-2 forward: 5′-GCTCCACAAACGAGAAAAGC-3′, reverse: 5′-AGCAAGGGGAAAAGGACACT-3′; FGF-2 forward: 5′-ACACGTCAAACTACAACTCCA-3′, reverse: 5′-TCAGCTCTTAGCAGACA TTGG-3′; IGF-1 forward: 5′-GGACCAGAGACCCTTTGCGGGG-3′, reverse: 5′-GGCTGCTTTTGTA GGCTTCAGTGG-3′; runt-related transcription factor 2 (Runx2) forward: 5′-AAGTGCGGTGCAAAC TTTCT-3′, reverse 5′-TCTCGGTGGCTGGTAGTGA-3′; Osterix (Osx) forward: 5′-ACTGGCTAGGTG GTGGT CAG-3′, reverse: 5′-GGTAGGGAGCTGGGTTAAGG-3′; ALP forward: 5′-AACCCAGACA CAAGCATTCC-3′, reverse: 5′-GAGAGCGAAGGGTCAGTCAG-3; osteocalcin (OCN) forward: 5′-CC GGGAGCAGTGTGAGCTTA-3′, reverse: 5′-TAGATGCGTTTGTAGGCGGTC-3; collagen type I (Col-1) forward: 5′-AGAGCATGACCGATGGATTC-3′, reverse: 5′-CCTTCTTGAGGTTGCCAGTC-3′; glyceraldehyde-3-phosphate dehydrogenase (GAPDH) forward: 5′-ACCCAGAAGACTGTGGAT GG-3′, reverse: 5′-CACATTGGGGGTAGGAACAC-3′. PCR conditions consisted of a 10 min hot start at 95 °C followed by 45 cycles of 15 s at 95 °C and 30 s at 60 °C. The expression levels of the mRNAs were normalized by GADPH levels and compared to the vehicle control.

2.7. Western Blot

Cells were seeded in six-well plates and exposed to 0–50 μM of osthole with or without KT5720 for 6 h. After treatment, cells were lysed in Pierce RIPA lysis buffer (Thermo Fisher Scientific) supplemented with Pierce protease and phosphatase inhibitor mini-tablets (Thermo Fisher Scientific). Equal 30 μg amounts of proteins from the lysate were separated by 10% sodium dodecyl sulfate-polyacrylamide gel electrophoresis (SDS-PAGE) and electrotransferred onto Immun-Blot PVDF membrane (Bio-Rad Laboratories, Hercules, CA, USA). The membrane was blocked with 3% BSA in PBS supplemented with 0.05% Tween-20, followed by overnight incubation at 4 °C with a diluted solution of primary antibody purchased from Cell Signaling (Danvers, MA, USA) against phospho-CREB (p-CREB), CREB, or α-tubulin (loading control). This was followed by incubation with horseradish peroxidase (HRP)-conjugated secondary antibody (Santa Cruz Biotechnology, Dallas, TX, USA) for 1 h at room temperature. The blots were assessed by their enhanced chemiluminescence (ECL) signal using the Pierce ECL Western blotting substrate (Thermo Fisher Scientific). Developed images were captured with Gel Doc molecular imager and ChemiDoc system and analyzed with Image Lab 3.0 software (Bio-Rad).

2.8. cAMP Assay

Intracellular cAMP concentration was quantified with cyclic AMP EIA kit (Cayman Chemical, Ann Arbor, MI, USA) based on the competition between labeled cAMP and non-labeled free cAMP in samples. Briefly, cells were incubated in complete growth medium containing 0–100 µM osthole for 2 h. After drug exposure, cells were lysed in 0.1 M HCl for 20 min with agitation, and the supernatants were collected by centrifuge. 50 µL of samples and standards were added into a 96-well plate followed by incubation with cAMP acetylcholine esterase tracer and cAMP EIA antiserum for 18 h at 4 °C. Each sample was developed with addition of Ellman's reagent and the plate was read at OD_{410} by microplate reader. cAMP concentration was calculated according to the cAMP standard plots and compared to the vehicle control after being normalized with total protein levels.

2.9. Histomorphometry and Immunohistochemistry

Femur specimens were harvested at day 14, and fixed and decalcified with calcium chelating solution (0.5 M EDTA/NaOH, pH 7.5) for two weeks. Decalcified bones were then dehydrated and embedded in paraffin wax using a Leica EG Embedding Center (Leica Microsystem, Wetzlar, Germany). Paraffin blocks were sectioned into 5 µm slices and mounted on glass slides. The sections were deparaffinized and stained with safranin O, fast green, and hematoxylin. The histomorphometry analysis was adapted from our previous study [7]. The bone and cartilage area was measured by a blinded observer using Zen 2012 (Zeiss, Oberkochen, Germany). For immunohistochemistry, deparaffinized sections were rehydrated in PBS and treated with 3% hydrogen perioxide in methanol to quench endogenous peroxidases. Antigen retrieval was performed by incubation in 95 °C 10 mM citrate buffer at pH 6.0 for 10 min. After nonspecific binding blocked with UltraVision protein block (Thermo Fisher Scientific), sections was incubated overnight at 4 °C with diluted solution of primary antibodies against Osx and p-CREB (Abcam, Cambridge, UK) and the solution without antibody as a negative control. The sections were then incubated with secondary antibody for 30 min at room temperature. A colorimetric signal was developed with a Liquid DAB+ Substrate Chromogen System (Dako, CA, USA), counter-stained with hemotoxylin, and subjected to blind evaluation.

2.10. Bone Biomechanical Test

The strength of the fractured and contralateral femur midshaft was measured by a three-point bending test using a mechanical testing machine (Biomomentum Inc., Laval, QC, Canada) [36]. Briefly, the surrounding soft tissue of femur was removed and then kept moisture with PBS-soaked gauze before testing. The span distance between the two end supports was fixed at 7.35 mm, load was applied on the bone femur midshaft with a displacement rate of 5 mm/min, and the ultimate load for each sample was measured.

2.11. Statistical Analysis

Statistical analysis was conducted using GraphPad Prism 5.0 (GraphPad Software, San Diego, CA, USA) and Excel (Microsoft, San Francisco, CA, USA). Mean and standard deviation values (mean ± SD) were calculated for all statistically analyzed parameters. The differences between groups were analyzed using analysis of variance (ANOVA) followed by Turkey's post-hoc test or unpaired Student's *t*-tests. The *p*-value less than 0.05 were considered statistically significant.

3. Results

3.1. Osthole Promoted Osteogenesis in Osteoblasts

MTT results demonstrated that osthole inhibited the proliferation of MC3T3-E1 cells in a time-and concentration-dependent manner from 0 to 500 μM (Figure 1). Osthole did not lead to significant inhibition on cell proliferation at concentrations less than 100 μM. Thus, 100 μM or below of osthole would be applied on the osteoblastic differentiation in the following experiments. Osteoblastic differentiation was assessed with two measurements: ALP activity and calcium nodule formation. The ALP enzyme cyotochemistry showed that the ALP-positive cell colony number increased with osthole concentration (Figure 2A). ALP activity was also significantly increased by osthole in the range of 0–100 μM in a dose-dependent manner (Figure 2B). In ARS staining of calcium nodule formation, the number and area of stained nodules increased dramatically in osthole-treated cells at concentrations of 50 and 100 μM (Figure 2C) compared with the control and low concentration of osthole. Quantitative analysis of ARS concentration was consistent with the qualitative results (Figure 2D).

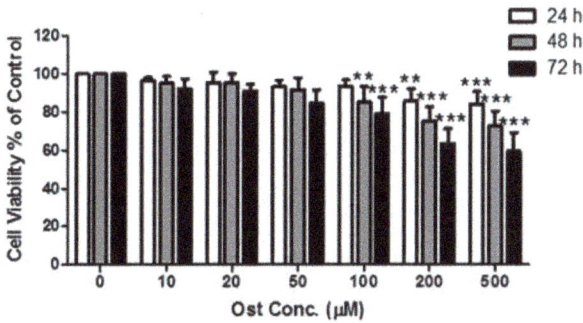

Figure 1. Effect of osthole on proliferation of MC3T3-E1 cells. Cells were treated with 0–500 μM of osthole for 24, 48, and 72 h. The viability was monitored with MTT assay. $n = 6$, One-way ANOVA followed by Tukey's test and compared to the vehicle control, ** $p < 0.01$, *** $p < 0.001$.

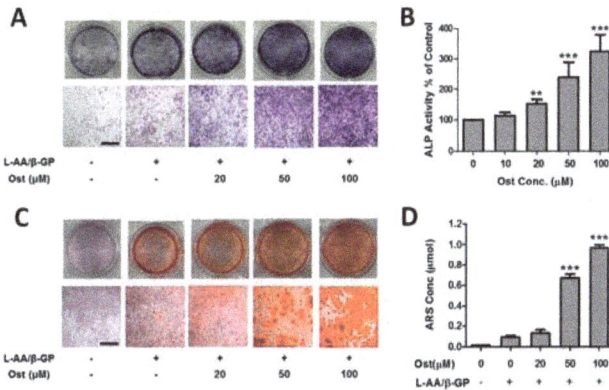

Figure 2. Osthole promoted osteogenic differentiation in osteoblasts. MC3T3-E1 cells were treated with 0–100 μM osthole in growth or osteogenic medium for 12 (**A**,**B**) or 24 days (**C**,**D**). (**A**) Representative macroscopic and microscopic photos of ALP staining cells ($n = 4$); (**B**) ALP activities were measured by ALP-AMP kit ($n = 6$); (**C**) Representative photos of ARS staining cells ($n = 4$); (**D**) cell mineralization was quantified by extraction of ARS dye ($n = 4$). One-way ANOVA was followed by Tukey's test and compared to the vehicle control, ** $p < 0.01$, *** $p < 0.001$. Bar = 500 μm.

3.2. Osthole Promoted Bone Regeneration and Bone Strength

To determine the effect of osthole administration on bone regeneration process in vivo, mice were treated with osthole and vehicle solvent during the fracture repair period. The bone volume of healing fractured callus at day 14 was measured by histomorphometric analysis, and strength of the fractured and contralateral bones was measured at day 28 by a three-point bending test. As shown in Figure 3A, the longitudinal section of calluses in the Ost group contained more bony tissue area and less cartilaginous tissue area than those in Ctl group. Histomorphometric analysis also confirmed the bony callus area in the Ctl group was significantly smaller than Ost group (19.95 ± 3.30 vs. 32.98 ± 4.60); while the cartilaginous callus area was much larger (20.02 ± 2.30 vs. 8.50 ± 2.77), indicating faster growth of bone in the treatment group. Additionally, the maximum load of healing fractured femurs in Ost group (13.96 N) were significantly higher than that in the Ctl group (10.23 N). The maximum load of the contralateral femur in the Ost group was also slightly higher than the Ctl group by 10.76%, but without significant difference (Figure 3B).

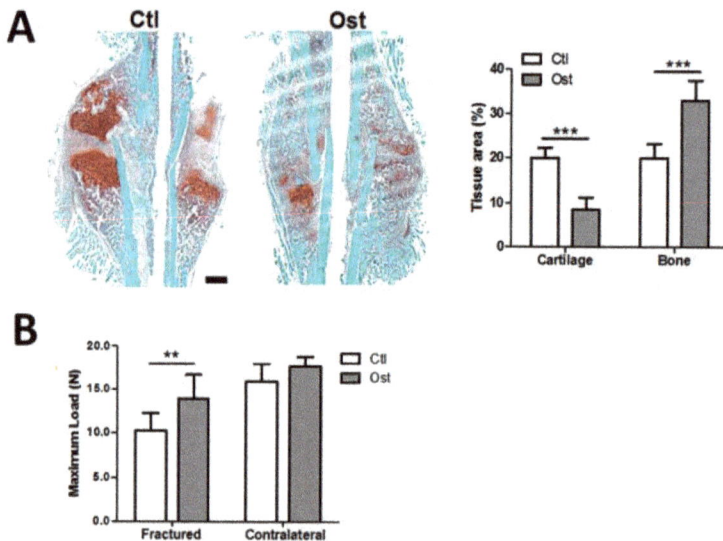

Figure 3. Osthole enhanced bone growth and bone strength during fracture repair. Post-operated fractured and contralateral bones were harvested at day 14 and day 28. (**A**) Callus sections at day 14 were stained with safranin O (cartilage)/fast green and hematoxylin ($n = 4$). Osthole treatment reduced cartilaginous tissue area, but increased bone tissue area; (**B**) the maximum load of femur samples at day 28 was determined by three-point bending ($n = 8$). An unpaired Student *t*-test was compared between control and osthole group, ** $p < 0.01$, *** $p < 0.001$. Bar = 500 µm.

3.3. Osthole Induced Osteogenesis via the BMP-Dependent Signaling Pathway

Expression of osteogenic-related genes was measured in osthole-treated MC3T3-cells to explore the mechanism of the osteopromotive action. The mRNA levels of growth factors (BMP-2, FGF-2 and IGF-1) were measured at 12 h while transcription factors (Runx2 and Osx) and osteogenic maker genes (ALP, OCN and Col-1) were measured at 6 days. Results showed that BMP-2 expression was upregulated in a dose-dependent manner under 0–50 µM of osthole exposure. In contrast, mRNA levels of FGF-2 and IGF-1 did not change significantly (Figure 4A). Both transcription factor genes were upregulated dose-dependently by osthole (Figure 4B). Osthole also significantly activated downstream ALP, OCN, and Col-1, whereas the effect on Col-1 was relatively weak (Figure 4C). To examine the role of BMP signaling in osthole-induced osteogenesis, BMP antagonist noggin was applied to block the BMP-dependent pathway. Osteogenic marker ALP activity, calcium deposits, and osteogenic-related genes were quantified with or without noggin. Application of noggin completely inhibited osthole-induced ALP activation, without a notable change of ALP in vehicle control (Figure 4D). The expression level of osteogenic-related genes Runx2, ALP, and OCN evoked by osthole were also significantly downregulated by co-treatment with noggin (Figure 4E).

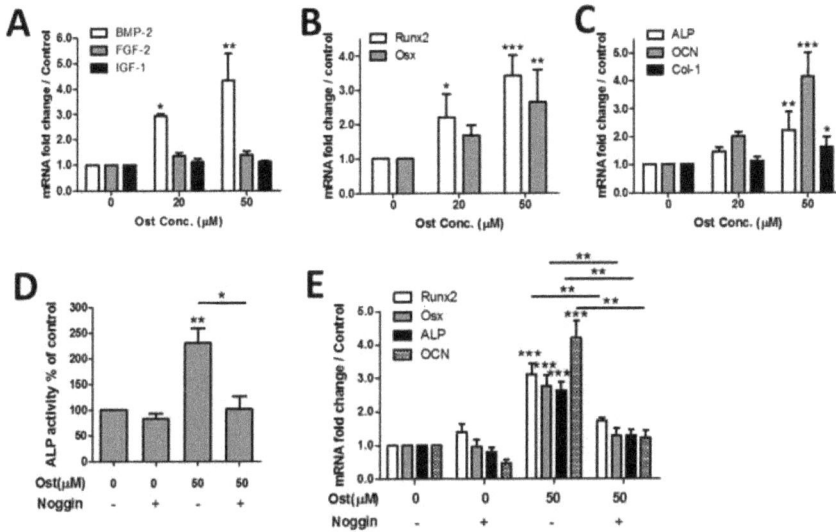

Figure 4. Osthole activated the BMP-2-dependent signaling pathway and BMP antagonist noggin completely inhibited osthole-mediated osteogenesis. MC3T3-E1 cells were treated with 0–50 μM osthole in osteogenic medium in the presence or absence of 100 ng/mL noggin for 12 h (A), 6 days (B,C,E), or 12 days (D). ALP activity was measured by an ALP-AMP kit; gene expression levels were detected by real-time RT-PCR. (A) $n = 5$, (B–E) $n = 4$; one-way ANOVA, followed by Tukey's test, was compared to the vehicle control; unpaired Student t-test was compared between noggin ±, * $p < 0.05$, ** $p < 0.01$, *** $p < 0.001$.

3.4. Osthole Activated cAMP/CREB Signaling Pathway

To testify whether osthole triggered the cAMP/CREB pathway or not, the effect of osthole on cellular cAMP concentration and CREB phosphorylation were evaluated in MC3T3-E1 cells. Quantification of cAMP demonstrated that osthole significantly elevated the intracellular cAMP level dose-dependently from 0 to 100 μM (Figure 5A). In addition, osthole exposure activated phosphorylation of CREB significantly, but not in the total amount of CREB (Figure 5B). Both results suggested that osthole treatment activated cAMP/CREB signaling in osteoblasts. Immunohistochemistry of phosphorylated CREB (p-CREB) was compared between osthole-treated fractured femurs and control. The p-CREB was only found in nuclei. The percentage of p-CREB positive cells was calculated by the average value of six random views in the bony callus. After treatment with osthole, the percentage of p-CREB-positive nuclei in newly-formed bone significantly increased and the signal intensity in the nuclei was also notably enhanced (Figure 5C).

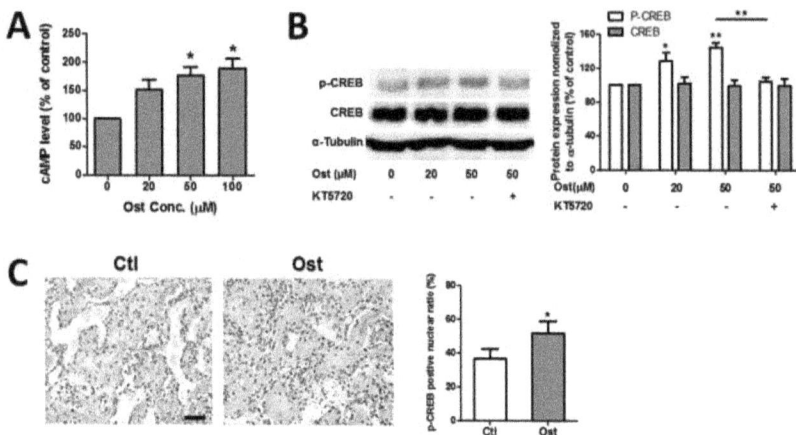

Figure 5. Osthole activated cAMP/CREB pathway. (**A**) MC3T3-E1 cells were incubated with 0–100 μM osthole in growth medium for 2 h, and cellular cAMP levels were quantified with cAMP EIA kit ($n = 3$); (**B**) Cells were treated with 0, 20, or 50 μM osthole in osteogenic medium in the presence or absence of 4 μM KT5720 for 6 h. Proteins were separated by 10% SDS-PAGE and assessed with Western blotting, and the intensity of the bands was quantified ($n = 5$); (**C**) Callus sections at day 14 were blotted with p-CREB antibody and counterstained with hematoxylin. The p-CREB-positive nuclei percentage was counted ($n = 4$). One-way ANOVA, followed by Tukey's test, was compared to the vehicle control; an unpaired Student t-test was compared between KT5720 ± groups, * $p < 0.05$, ** $p < 0.01$. Bar = 50 μm.

3.5. Osthole Enhanced Osteogenesis through Osterix Activiated by cAMP/CREB Signaling

The effects of osthole-activated cAMP/CREB signaling activity was determined by the application of PKA inhibitor KT5720 during osteoblast differentiation. Co-treatment of KT5720 with osthole completely blocked the activation of p-CREB in osthole-mediated cAMP/PKA signaling (Figure 5B). PKA inhibitor markedly suppressed both ALP activation and mineralization mediated by osthole; whereas these two osteogenic markers were still significantly higher than the vehicle control after complete blockage of osthole-induced PKA signaling (Figure 6A,B). Additionally, KT5720 exposure alone did not change the viability or differentiation status of cells. All results suggested that PKA blockage only partially suppressed the osteogenic differentiation activated by osthole. Osteogenic-related gene expressions were measured in the presence or absence of KT5720. Consistent to the results of ALP activity and calcium deposit, ALP and OCN gene expression were evidently downregulated by PKA inhibitor, but they were still higher than control levels by 0.47 and 1.59 folds, respectively (Figure 6C). Expression level of Osx was markedly reduced by PKA inhibition, but BMP-2 and Runx2 levels remained almost unchanged (Figure 6C). Likewise, KT5720 had no significant influence on expression levels of osteogenic-related genes when applied alone. On the other hand, expression of Osx in healing fractured bone was assessed by IHC. The expression of Osx in the Ost group was observably higher than that of the Ctl group in osteogenic cells surrounding newly-formed bone tissue (Figure 6D).

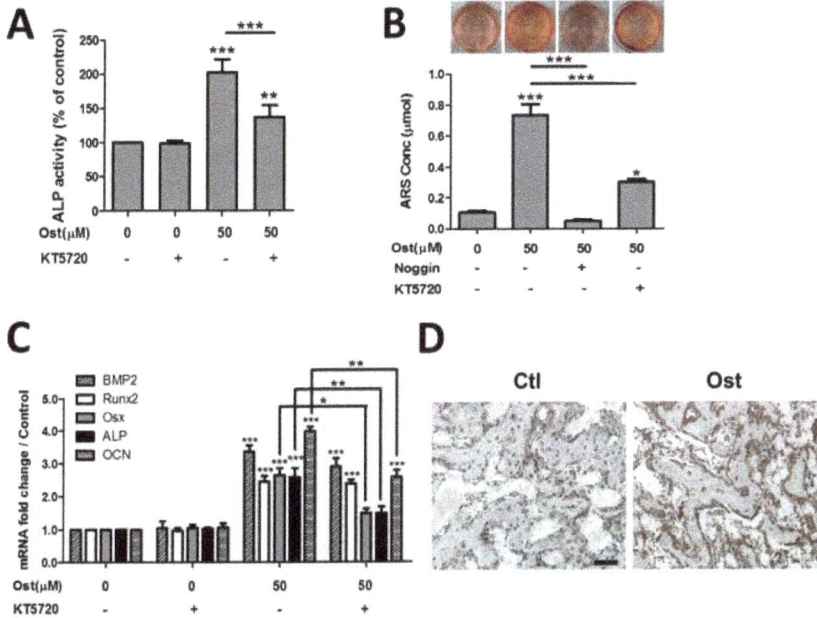

Figure 6. PKA inhibitor partially suppressed osthole-evoked osteogenesis and Osx expression. MC3T3-E1 cells were treated with 0 or 50 μM osthole in osteogenic medium in the presence or absence of 4 μM KT5720 or 100 ng/mL noggin for 12 days (**A**), 24 days (**B**) 12 h or 6 days (**C**). (**A**) ALP activity was measured by ALP-AMP kit (*n* = 5), (**B**) calcium nodules were stained with ARS, and cell mineralization was quantified by extraction of ARS dye (*n* = 3); (**C**) gene expression levels were detected by real-time RT-PCR (*n* = 4); (**D**) callus sections at day 14 were blotted with osterix antibody and counterstained with hematoxylin (*n* = 4). One-way ANOVA was followed by Tukey's test compared to the vehicle control; unpaired Student *t*-test compared between KT5720 ± or noggin ± group, * $p < 0.05$, ** $p < 0.01$, *** $p < 0.001$. Bar = 50 μm.

4. Discussion

Mouse calvarial preosteoblast MC3T3-E1 with a similar cellular response to primary calvarial osteoblasts was used in this study. Previous studies reported that osthole stimulated growth of osteoblast-like UMR106 cells and primary rat osteoblasts [37,38]. However, others found that osthole only stimulated osteoblastic differentiation at the same doses but not cell proliferation [20,25]. Our results showed that 0–50 μM osthole exhibited little effect on cell proliferation at all time points, whereas 100 μM showed slightly inhibited cell growth at 48 h without notable cell death morphology. This was reasonable since temporal arrest in the G1 phase of the cell cycle was regarded as a prerequisite for cell differentiation, and osthole exposure mediated osteogenic differentiation in osteoblasts [39,40]. Additionally, results showed that the mitogenic growth factor FGF-2 level only slightly increased without significant difference and the IGF-1 level remained almost unchanged after osthole treatment. FGF-2 and IGF-1 were both regarded as mitogens of osteoblastic cell proliferation [41,42], which might explain why there was not any promotive effect of osthole on the proliferation of this cell line.

Increasing in ALP activity and calcium nodule formation in osthole-treated cells suggested that it promoted osteogenic differentiation, which was consistent with previous findings in other osteoblastic-like cells. We also found that osthole treatment not only mediated osteogenesis in osteoblasts in vitro, but also enhanced the ossification process in vivo, which resulted in faster bone regeneration during bone repair. Time point day 14 was located in the reparative phase of fracture repair when the bone grew inside the callus and replaced cartilage until bony fusion. At post-operation day 28, the remodeling phase took place when fractured bone was restored to its original shape and strength after the completed fusion of bony callus [21]. Osthole administration resulted in faster bone formation during repair, which led to stronger bone at the end point after bony fusion. This finding echoed with the osteoanabolic effect found in mouse calvaria [20]. Moreover, worth mentioning was that the average bone strength in contralateral intact femur was also increased. This result was consistent with findings of previous studies [19] suggesting osthole exhibited an anti-osteoporotic property by raising the bone mineral density and bone strength. Stronger healing bone in the Ost group should be an achievement resulting from both a faster bone regeneration rate and a higher bone mineral density [21]. Since the bone formation rate in heathy bone was much slower than in repairing bone, the strength difference between Ost and Ctl groups in contralateral bone was much smaller.

Previous studies suggested that osthole stimulated osteogenesis in osteoblasts through BMP-dependent pathway [20,25]. Our results confirmed the effect of osthole on BMP-2 expression. Expression of BMPs triggers osteogenic signaling cascades driving the whole process of differentiation. Both key transcription factors of osteogenesis, Osx, and Runx2, were evoked by osthole and so did three downstream osteogenic marker genes ALP, OCN, and Col-1. Moreover, the influence of BMP pathway in osthole-mediated osteogenesis was examined by the measurement of ALP activity, mineralization, and marker genes in the presence of BMP antagonist noggin. The osteopromotive effect of osthole was abolished by blockage of the BMP pathway, which indicated osthole-mediated osteogenesis was completely BMP-dependent.

On the other hand, osthole was suggested to elevate the cAMP level by inhibition of cAMP phosphodiesterases (PDEs), which hydrolyzes cAMP into AMP in various types of tissues. This was the first time cAMP elevation action of osthole was confirmed in osteoblastic cell culture, suggesting the action should be non-tissue-specific. Osthole also induced phosphorylation/activation of CREB, downstream target of cAMP/PKA signaling It indicated that osthole triggered the cAMP/PKA/CREB pathway, similar to PTH and some other cAMP activators that promote osteogenesis [29,43]. The effect of osthole on phosphorylation of CREB was also found in neural cells [44], which further revealed cAMP/CREB activation by osthole was not tissue-specific and might contribute to its multiple bioactivities. PKA inhibitor KT5720 could completely block the cAMP-mediated phosphorylation of CREB induced by osthole; meanwhile, the inhibitor only partially suppressed osthole-mediated osteogenesis. In addition, ALP activity, mineralization, and the osteogenic gene level treated with KT5720 were still significantly higher than that of vehicle controls, which suggested that osthole-induced osteogenesis was only partially mediated by the cAMP/CREB pathway. This finding supported previous suggestions that osthole-induced cell differentiation operated by both Smad-dependent and -independent pathways [25]. cAMP/CREB activators, such as PTH and db-cAMP, were found to directly stimulate growth factors (especially BMP-2) and their downstream target genes in mesenchymal stem cells [43]. However, our results showed only a slight reduction of BMP-2 expression without significant difference after PKA blockage, which indicated that osthole-activated cAMP/CREB signaling might promote BMP-dependent osteogenesis signaling through other downstream elements rather than only evoking BMP expression in this cell line.

Furthermore, we also found that osthole-activated cAMP/CREB signaling targeted transcription factor Osx rather than Runx2. Although the interaction between Runx2 and Osx remains controversial, both transcription factors have been found indispensable in both in vitro and in vivo osteogenesis/ossification process [45–47]. Previous studies found deficiencies of either Osx or Runx2 genes leading to a complete absence of bone formation at the embryonic stage, but the phenotype of Osx null mice were different from Runx2 null mice at birth [47]. Others reported that Osx and Runx2 regulated distinct gene groups [48]. Both suggested that Osx and Runx2 were critical, but with distinct functions in bone formation progress. Osteogenesis in osteoblasts was mediated through the BMP-dependent pathway while the key transcription factor Osx was further upregulated via cAMP/CREB signaling. Meanwhile, single activation of Osx by cAMP signaling was not sufficient

Nutrients **2017**, *9*, 588

for osteogenic cascade in osteoblasts, probably because it lacked some key elements induced by other transcription factors, such as Runx2. This might be the reason why the blockage of the BMP pathway completely stopped osteogenic differentiation, while inhibition of cAMP/CREB could only partially suppress ALP activity, cell mineralization and osteogenic gene expression. In the mouse bone repair model, we also found that osthole treatment promoted the expression of p-CREB and Osx in osteoblastic cells showing newly-formed woven bone. This indicated that osthole also activated the cAMP/CREB pathway in osteoblasts in vivo. Faster bone formation during repair process might also relate to activation of CREB and Osx in bone forming cells. Thus, apart from the BMP-dependent pathway, osthole also enhanced osteogenesis through cAMP/CREB signaling by upregulating transcriptional factor Osx in osteoblasts.

Several limitations in this study need to be addressed. PKA-specific inhibitor KT5720 was applied for investigation of the influence of osthole-evoked cAMP elevation on osteogenesis. In spite of the wide usage of KT5720 for the inhibition of the cAMP/PKA/CREB pathway, it would be preferable to use RNA interference to specifically knock down the target pathway. Osthole-induced upregulation of p-CREB and Osx in healing bone were insufficient to prove the related mechanism applied in vivo as well. However, these results supported future study of this promising pathway in animal models. Selectively blocking this pathway should be applied to explore the osteoanabolic effect of osthole in vivo.

5. Conclusions

In summary, this study had demonstrated that osthole promoted osteogenic differentiation in osteoblasts by the BMP-dependent pathway, which was enhanced by cAMP/CREB signaling targeting the transcription factor osterix. Osthole treatment upregulated osterix expression and promoted bone regeneration during mice femoral fracture repairing. The findings of the study contribute to the knowledge of the mechanism involved in osteopromotive and anti-osteoporotic effects of osthole. It provides biological evidence for diet supplementary of osthole and osthole-contained functional food or medicine for prevention and therapy of osteoporosis and osteoporotic fracture.

Acknowledgments: This project was supported by General Research Fund, Hong Kong Research Grant Council (Ref. No.: 461113) and direct grant (Ref. No. 2030445 and 4053024). The study was also technically supported by the Institute of Chinese Medicine, the Chinese University of Hong Kong.

Author Contributions: Z.-R.Z., W.N.L., G.L., S.K.K., X.L. and C.W.C. conceived and designed the experiments; Z.-R.Z. and Y.M.W. performed the experiments and analyzed the data; G.L. and S.K.K. contributed cell lines and reagents; and Z.-R.Z. and C.W.C. wrote the manuscript.

Conflicts of Interest: The authors declare no conflict of interest.

References

1. Raisz, L.G. Pathogenesis of osteoporosis: Concepts, conflicts, and prospects. *J. Clin. Investig.* **2005**, *115*, 3318–3325. [CrossRef] [PubMed]
2. Sambrook, P.; Cooper, C. Osteoporosis. *Lancet* **2006**, *367*, 2010–2018. [CrossRef]
3. Nikolaou, V.S.; Efstathopoulos, N.; Kontakis, G.; Kanakaris, N.K.; Giannoudis, P.V. The influence of osteoporosis in femoral fracture healing time. *Injury* **2009**, *40*, 663–668. [CrossRef] [PubMed]
4. Kyllonen, L.; D'Este, M.; Alini, M.; Eglin, D. Local drug delivery for enhancing fracture healing in osteoporotic bone. *Acta Biomater.* **2015**, *11*, 412–434. [CrossRef] [PubMed]
5. Rothberg, D.L.; Lee, M.A. Internal fixation of osteoporotic fractures. *Curr. Osteoporos. Rep.* **2015**, *13*, 16–21. [CrossRef] [PubMed]
6. Chan, C.W.; Qin, L.; Lee, K.M.; Zhang, M.; Cheng, J.C.; Leung, K.S. Low intensity pulsed ultrasound accelerated bone remodeling during consolidation stage of distraction osteogenesis. *J. Orthop. Res.* **2006**, *24*, 263–270. [CrossRef] [PubMed]

7.   Chan, C.W.; Qin, L.; Lee, K.M.; Cheung, W.H.; Cheng, J.C.; Leung, K.S. Dose-dependent effect of low-intensity pulsed ultrasound on callus formation during rapid distraction osteogenesis. *J. Orthop. Res.* **2006**, *24*, 2072–2079. [CrossRef] [PubMed]

8.   Xie, C.; Lu, X.; Wang, K.; Yuan, H.; Fang, L.; Zheng, X.; Chan, C.; Ren, F.; Zhao, C. Pulse electrochemical driven rapid layer-by-layer assembly of polydopamine and hydroxyapatite nanofilms via alternative redox in situ synthesis for bone regeneration. *ACS Biomater. Sci. Eng.* **2016**, *2*, 920–928. [CrossRef]

9.   Hardcastle, A.C.; Aucott, L.; Fraser, W.D.; Reid, D.M.; Macdonald, H.M. Dietary patterns, bone resorption and bone mineral density in early post-menopausal scottish women. *Eur. J. Clin. Nutr.* **2011**, *65*, 378–385. [CrossRef] [PubMed]

10. Hughes, M.S.; Kazmier, P.; Burd, T.A.; Anglen, J.; Stoker, A.M.; Kuroki, K.; Carson, W.L.; Cook, J.L. Enhanced fracture and soft-tissue healing by means of anabolic dietary supplementation. *J. Bone Joint Surg. Am.* **2006**, *88*, 2386–2394. [CrossRef] [PubMed]

11. Yaman, F.; Acikan, I.; Dundar, S.; Simsek, S.; Gul, M.; Ozercan, I.H.; Komorowski, J.; Sahin, K. Dietary arginine silicate inositol complex increased bone healing: Histologic and histomorphometric study. *Drug Des. Dev. Ther.* **2016**, *10*, 2081–2086. [CrossRef] [PubMed]

12. Welch, A.A.; Hardcastle, A.C. The effects of flavonoids on bone. *Curr. Osteoporos. Rep.* **2014**, *12*, 205–210. [CrossRef] [PubMed]

13. Zhang, G.; Qin, L.; Sheng, H.; Yeung, K.W.; Yeung, H.Y.; Cheung, W.H.; Griffith, J.; Chan, C.W.; Lee, K.M.; Leung, K.S. Epimedium-derived phytoestrogen exert beneficial effect on preventing steroid-associated osteonecrosis in rabbits with inhibition of both thrombosis and lipid-deposition. *Bone* **2007**, *40*, 685–692. [CrossRef] [PubMed]

14. Luo, Z.; Liu, M.; Sun, L.; Rui, F. Icariin recovers the osteogenic differentiation and bone formation of bone marrow stromal cells from a rat model of estrogen deficiency-induced osteoporosis. *Mol. Med. Rep.* **2015**, *12*, 382–388. [CrossRef] [PubMed]

15. Park, K.H.; Gu, D.R.; So, H.S.; Kim, K.J.; Lee, S.H. Dual role of cyanidin-3-glucoside on the differentiation of bone cells. *J. Dent. Res.* **2015**, *94*, 1676–1683. [CrossRef] [PubMed]

16. Dou, C.; Cao, Z.; Ding, N.; Hou, T.; Luo, F.; Kang, F.; Yang, X.; Jiang, H.; Xie, Z.; Hu, M.; et al. Cordycepin prevents bone loss through inhibiting osteoclastogenesis by scavenging ros generation. *Nutrients* **2016**, *8*, 231. [CrossRef] [PubMed]

17. Zhang, Z.R.; Leung, W.N.; Cheung, H.Y.; Chan, C.W. Osthole: A review on its bioactivities, pharmacological properties, and potential as alternative medicine. *Evid. Based Complement. Alternat. Med.* **2015**, *2015*, 919616. [CrossRef] [PubMed]

18. An, J.; Yang, H.; Zhang, Q.; Liu, C.; Zhao, J.; Zhang, L.; Chen, B. Natural products for treatment of osteoporosis: The effects and mechanisms on promoting osteoblast-mediated bone formation. *Life Sci.* **2016**, *147*, 46–58. [CrossRef] [PubMed]

19. Li, X.X.; Hara, I.; Matsumiya, T. Effects of osthole on postmenopausal osteoporosis using ovariectomized rats; comparison to the effects of estradiol. *Biol. Pharm. Bull.* **2002**, *25*, 738–742. [CrossRef] [PubMed]

20. Tang, D.Z.; Hou, W.; Zhou, Q.; Zhang, M.; Holz, J.; Sheu, T.J.; Li, T.F.; Cheng, S.D.; Shi, Q.; Harris, S.E.; et al. Osthole stimulates osteoblast differentiation and bone formation by activation of beta-catenin-BMP signaling. *J. Bone Miner. Res.* **2010**, *25*, 1234–1245. [CrossRef] [PubMed]

21. Zhang, Z.; Leung, W.N.; Li, G.; Lai, Y.M.; Chan, C.W. Osthole promotes endochondral ossification and accelerates fracture healing in mice. *Calcif. Tissue Int.* **2016**, *99*, 649–660. [CrossRef] [PubMed]

22. Rodan, G.A.; Martin, T.J. Therapeutic approaches to bone diseases. *Science* **2000**, *289*, 1508–1514. [CrossRef] [PubMed]

23. Sandhu, S.K.; Hampson, G. The pathogenesis, diagnosis, investigation and management of osteoporosis. *J. Clin. Pathol.* **2011**, *64*, 1042–1050. [CrossRef] [PubMed]

24. Lane, N.E.; Kelman, A. A review of anabolic therapies for osteoporosis. *Arthritis Res. Ther.* **2003**, *5*, 214–222. [CrossRef] [PubMed]

25. Kuo, P.L.; Hsu, Y.L.; Chang, C.H.; Chang, J.K. Osthole-mediated cell differentiation through bone morphogenetic protein-2/p38 and extracellular signal-regulated kinase 1/2 pathway in human osteoblast cells. *J. Pharmacol. Exp. Ther.* **2005**, *314*, 1290–1299. [CrossRef] [PubMed]

26. Ming, L.G.; Zhou, J.; Cheng, G.Z.; Ma, H.P.; Chen, K.M. Osthol, a coumarin isolated from common cnidium fruit, enhances the differentiation and maturation of osteoblasts in vitro. *Pharmacology* **2011**, *88*, 33–43. [CrossRef] [PubMed]

27. Qin, L.; Partridge, N.C. Stimulation of amphiregulin expression in osteoblastic cells by parathyroid hormone requires the protein kinase a and camp response element-binding protein signaling pathway. *J. Cell. Biochem.* **2005**, *96*, 632–640. [CrossRef] [PubMed]

28. Yang, D.; Singh, R.; Divieti, P.; Guo, J.; Bouxsein, M.L.; Bringhurst, F.R. Contributions of parathyroid hormone (PTH)/PTH-related peptide receptor signaling pathways to the anabolic effect of pth on bone. *Bone* **2007**, *40*, 1453–1461. [CrossRef] [PubMed]

29. Zhang, R.; Edwards, J.R.; Ko, S.Y.; Dong, S.; Liu, H.; Oyajobi, B.O.; Papasian, C.; Deng, H.W.; Zhao, M. Transcriptional regulation of BMP2 expression by the PTH-CREB signaling pathway in osteoblasts. *PLoS ONE* **2011**, *6*, e20780. [CrossRef] [PubMed]

30. Tyson, D.R.; Swarthout, J.T.; Partridge, N.C. Increased osteoblastic c-fos expression by parathyroid hormone requires protein kinase a phosphorylation of the cyclic adenosine 3′,5′-monophosphate response element-binding protein at serine 133. *Endocrinology* **1999**, *140*, 1255–1261. [CrossRef] [PubMed]

31. Huang, W.C.; Xie, Z.; Konaka, H.; Sodek, J.; Zhau, H.E.; Chung, L.W. Human osteocalcin and bone sialoprotein mediating osteomimicry of prostate cancer cells: Role of cAMP-dependent protein kinase a signaling pathway. *Cancer Res.* **2005**, *65*, 2303–2313. [CrossRef] [PubMed]

32. Takai, H.; Nakayama, Y.; Kim, D.S.; Arai, M.; Araki, S.; Mezawa, M.; Nakajima, Y.; Kato, N.; Masunaga, H.; Ogata, Y. Androgen receptor stimulates bone sialoprotein (BSP) gene transcription via camp response element and activator protein 1/glucocorticoid response elements. *J. Cell. Biochem.* **2007**, *102*, 240–251. [CrossRef] [PubMed]

33. Chiou, W.F.; Huang, Y.L.; Chen, C.F.; Chen, C.C. Vasorelaxing effect of coumarins from cnidium monnieri on rabbit corpus cavernosum. *Planta Med.* **2001**, *67*, 282–284. [CrossRef] [PubMed]

34. Teng, C.M.; Lin, C.H.; Ko, F.N.; Wu, T.S.; Huang, T.F. The relaxant action of osthole isolated from angelica pubescens in guinea-pig trachea. *Naunyn Schmiedebergs Arch. Pharmacol.* **1994**, *349*, 202–208. [CrossRef] [PubMed]

35. Pan, Z.; Fang, Z.; Lu, W.; Liu, X.; Zhang, Y. Osthole, a coumadin analog from *Cnidium monnieri* (L.) cusson, stimulates corticosterone secretion by increasing steroidogenic enzyme expression in mouse y1 adrenocortical tumor cells. *J. Ethnopharmacol.* **2015**, *175*, 456–462. [CrossRef] [PubMed]

36. He, Y.X.; Zhang, G.; Pan, X.H.; Liu, Z.; Zheng, L.Z.; Chan, C.W.; Lee, K.M.; Cao, Y.P.; Li, G.; Wei, L.; et al. Impaired bone healing pattern in mice with ovariectomy-induced osteoporosis: A drill-hole defect model. *Bone* **2011**, *48*, 1388–1400. [CrossRef] [PubMed]

37. Meng, F.; Xiong, Z.; Sun, Y.; Li, F. Coumarins from *Cnidium monnieri* (L.) and their proliferation stimulating activity on osteoblast-like umr106 cells. *Pharmazie* **2004**, *59*, 643–645. [PubMed]

38. Zhang, Q.; Qin, L.; He, W.; Van Puyvelde, L.; Maes, D.; Adams, A.; Zheng, H.; De Kimpe, N. Coumarins from cnidium monnieri and their antiosteoporotic activity. *Planta Med.* **2007**, *73*, 13–19. [CrossRef] [PubMed]

39. Damien, C.J.; Parsons, J.R. Bone graft and bone graft substitutes: A review of current technology and applications. *J. Appl. Biomater.* **1991**, *2*, 187–208. [CrossRef] [PubMed]

40. Li, V.C.; Kirschner, M.W. Molecular ties between the cell cycle and differentiation in embryonic stem cells. *Proc. Natl. Acad. Sci. USA* **2014**, *111*, 9503–9508. [CrossRef] [PubMed]

41. Dupree, M.A.; Pollack, S.R.; Levine, E.M.; Laurencin, C.T. Fibroblast growth factor 2 induced proliferation in osteoblasts and bone marrow stromal cells: A whole cell model. *Biophys. J.* **2006**, *91*, 3097–3112. [CrossRef] [PubMed]

42. Radcliff, K.; Tang, T.B.; Lim, J.; Zhang, Z.; Abedin, M.; Demer, L.L.; Tintut, Y. Insulin-like growth factor-i regulates proliferation and osteoblastic differentiation of calcifying vascular cells via extracellular signal-regulated protein kinase and phosphatidylinositol 3-kinase pathways. *Circ. Res.* **2005**, *96*, 398–400. [CrossRef] [PubMed]

43. Siddappa, R.; Martens, A.; Doorn, J.; Leusink, A.; Olivo, C.; Licht, R.; van Rijn, L.; Gaspar, C.; Fodde, R.; Janssen, F.; et al. cAMP/PKA pathway activation in human mesenchymal stem cells in vitro results in robust bone formation in vivo. *Proc. Natl. Acad. Sci. USA* **2008**, *105*, 7281–7286. [CrossRef] [PubMed]

44. Hu, Y.; Wen, Q.; Liang, W.; Kang, T.; Ren, L.; Zhang, N.; Zhao, D.; Sun, D.; Yang, J. Osthole reverses beta-amyloid peptide cytotoxicity on neural cells by enhancing cyclic amp response element-binding protein phosphorylation. *Biol. Pharm. Bull.* **2013**, *36*, 1950–1958. [CrossRef] [PubMed]

45. Javed, A.; Afzal, F.; Bae, J.S.; Gutierrez, S.; Zaidi, K.; Pratap, J.; van Wijnen, A.J.; Stein, J.L.; Stein, G.S.; Lian, J.B. Specific residues of Runx2 are obligatory for formation of BMP2-induced Runx2-smad complex to promote osteoblast differentiation. *Cells Tissues Organs* **2009**, *189*, 133–137. [CrossRef] [PubMed]

46. Lee, M.H.; Kwon, T.G.; Park, H.S.; Wozney, J.M.; Ryoo, H.M. BMP-2-induced osterix expression is mediated by Dlx5 but is independent of Runx2. *Biochem. Biophys. Res. Commun.* **2003**, *309*, 689–694. [CrossRef] [PubMed]

47. Nakashima, K.; Zhou, X.; Kunkel, G.; Zhang, Z.; Deng, J.M.; Behringer, R.R.; de Crombrugghe, B. The novel zinc finger-containing transcription factor osterix is required for osteoblast differentiation and bone formation. *Cell* **2002**, *108*, 17–29. [CrossRef]

48. Matsubara, T.; Kida, K.; Yamaguchi, A.; Hata, K.; Ichida, F.; Meguro, H.; Aburatani, H.; Nishimura, R.; Yoneda, T. BMP2 regulates osterix through Msx2 and Runx2 during osteoblast differentiation. *J. Biol. Chem.* **2008**, *283*, 29119–29125. [CrossRef] [PubMed]

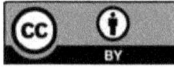

nutrients

MDPI

Review

The Role of AOPP in Age-Related Bone Loss and the Potential Benefits of Berry Anthocyanins

Melissa M. Melough , Xin Sun and Ock K. Chun *

Department of Nutritional Sciences, University of Connecticut, Storrs, CT 06269, USA;
melissa.melough@uconn.edu (M.M.M.); xin.sun@uconn.edu (X.S.)
* Correspondence: ock.chun@uconn.edu; Tel.: +1-860-486-6275

Received: 31 May 2017; Accepted: 19 July 2017; Published: 22 July 2017

Abstract: Age-related bone loss is a major factor in osteoporosis and osteoporotic fractures among the elderly. Because bone homeostasis involves a balance between bone formation and resorption, multiple mechanisms may induce age-dependent changes in bone. Oxidative stress is one such factor that contributes to the pathology of aging-associated osteoporosis (AAO). Advanced oxidation protein products (AOPP) are a biomarker of oxidant-mediated protein damage, and can also act to increase the production of reactive oxygen species (ROS), thereby perpetuating oxidative damage. AOPP is a relatively novel marker of oxidative stress, and its role in bone aging has not been fully elucidated. Furthermore, it has been theorized that dietary antioxidants may decrease AOPP levels, thereby reducing AAO risk, but a limited number of studies have been specifically targeted at addressing this hypothesis. Therefore, the objective of this review is to examine the findings of existing research on the role of AOPP in age-related bone loss, and the potential use of dietary antioxidants to mitigate the effects of AAOP on age-related bone loss. Cross-sectional studies have delivered mixed results, showing that AOPP levels are inconsistently associated with bone loss and aging. However, in vitro studies have documented multiple mechanisms by which AOPP may lead to bone loss, including upregulation of the JNK/p38 MAPK signaling pathways as well as increasing expression of sclerostin and of receptor activator of NFκB ligand (RANKL). Studies also indicate that antioxidants—especially berry anthocyanins—may be an effective dietary agent to prevent aging-associated bone deterioration by inhibiting the formation of AOPP and ROS. However, the understanding of these pathways in AAO has largely been based on in vitro studies, and should be examined in further animal and human studies in order to inform recommendations regarding dietary anthocyanin use for the prevention of AAO.

Keywords: AOPP; bone; aging; osteoporosis; antioxidants; berry anthocyanins

1. Introduction

Age-related bone loss is a primary contributor to osteoporosis and osteoporotic fractures in the elderly. Osteoporosis is considered a major public health threat for an estimated 44 million Americans, or 55% of the population aged 50 years and older [2]. Numerous studies employing various methods have dealt with the pathophysiology of postmenopausal osteoporosis [3], but aging-associated osteoporosis (AAO) has not been as well studied [4]. AAO is thought to be a type of low-turnover osteoporosis resulting from aging-associated calcium deficiency and an imbalance between bone resorption and formation [5].

Oxidative stress plays a central role in human aging and accelerates the aging process [6,7]. Bone density is maintained by two phases of bone remodeling: bone resorption by osteoclasts and bone formation by osteoblasts [8]. Emerging evidence indicates that the increased production of reactive oxygen species (ROS) in bone cells may activate bone resorption, resulting in a gradual decline in bone mass and density with aging [7]. Studies have shown that oxidative stress results in reduced bone formation, increased osteoblast and osteocyte apoptosis, and decreased bone mineral density (BMD) in aged mice [9]. Reduced BMD is one of the defining characteristics of osteoporosis, and correlates with bone strength and fracture risk [2]. Induced oxidative stress in young mice and rats has also been shown to reduce osteoblastogenesis and to increase osteoclast number and activity [10,11]. Loss of sex steroids potentiates the effects of aging by weakening defense mechanisms against oxidative stress [10]. Previous studies have clearly demonstrated that the bone turnover pattern remains relatively steady in advanced aging [12]. Based on this pattern, there is a reduction in bone formation as a result of a decreased recruitment of osteoblasts and an elevation of bone resorption that might result from enhanced activity of osteoclasts, which is the primary underlying mechanism of AAO [12].

Advanced oxidation protein products (AOPP) arise from the reaction between plasma proteins and chlorinated oxidants (e.g., hypochlorous acid, HOCl) by the H_2O_2-myeloperoxidase (MPO) system, and are di-tyrosine-containing cross-linking protein products considered to be novel markers of oxidant-mediated protein damage [13–15]. AOPP are mainly carried by albumin in the circulation, and oxidized albumin is rapidly cleared mainly through the uptake by the liver and spleen [16]. Like advanced glycation end products (AGEs), AOPP signal via the receptor for AGE (RAGE) in endothelial cells and induce endothelial dysfunction [17]. Increased plasma levels of AOPP have been found in many diseases, such as diabetes, uremia, obesity, coronary artery disease, and inflammatory bowel diseases. Evidence indicates that AOPP increase with age, and that AOPP can trigger cytosolic superoxide generation via the activation of nicotinamide adenine dinucleotide phosphate (NADPH) oxidase (NOX), which is a major source of ROS [18] (Figure 1). Therefore, AOPP may serve not only as markers of oxidant-mediated protein damage, but also as potential inducers of oxidative stress [15].

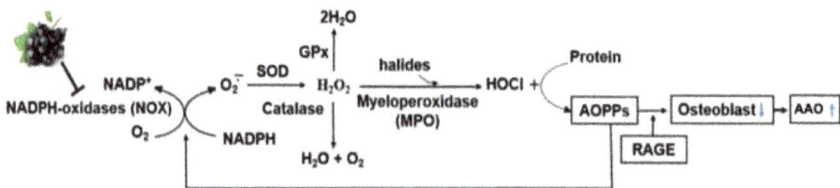

Figure 1. Potential mechanism of anthocyanins in lowering aging-associated osteoporosis (AAO) risk through inhibiting nicotinamide adenine dinucleotide phosphate (NADPH) oxidase (NOX)-mediated advanced oxidation protein products (AOPP) formation. GPx: glutathione peroxidase; RAGE: receptor for advanced glycation end products; SOD: superoxide dismutase.

Due to the public health relevance of AAO and the emerging evidence demonstrating the role of oxidative stress in bone aging, it is of great importance to characterize the ways in which AOPP may affect bone health and homeostasis. It has also been hypothesized that due to their antioxidant capacity, anthocyanins found in plants such as berries may prevent or reduce bone resorption and deterioration. Therefore, the purpose of this review is to examine the current state of knowledge regarding the role of AOPP in age-related bone loss and to assess the potential for the use of berry anthocyanins to reduce the formation of AOPP and improve bone-related outcomes in aging.

Articles included in this review were identified using PubMed and Web of Science. To examine the role of AOPP in bone loss, databases were searched for "AOPP bone loss". Other keywords added to this search were osteoporosis, osteoblasts, and osteoclasts. To find studies investigating the effects of anthocyanins on bone loss, databases were searched for "berry anthocyanin bone loss", and the following terms were added to expand the search: AOPP, antioxidant, osteoporosis. All articles for this review were published by May 2017. Publications identified by these methods were then limited to those describing cross-sectional analyses of AOPP and bone health in humans and animals, in vitro studies of cells treated with AOPP, and clinical trials or observational studies seeking to examine the effects of dietary antioxidants on AOPP and bone outcomes.

2. Aging-Associated Osteoporosis

Osteoporosis is a skeletal disease characterized by the deterioration of bone mass and microarchitecture, leading to increased fragility and predisposition to bone fractures [2]. While postmenopausal osteoporosis is related to estrogen deficiency and affects trabecular bone, aging-associated osteoporosis (AAO) primarily affects cortical bone and has many contributing factors including genetics, nutrition, physical activity, and physiological changes to bone [5]. Because bone loss appears to begin near age 40 and accelerates after age 60, age-related bone loss affects a growing number of men and women as the global population of older individuals increases [19].

One well-established physiological effect of bone aging is decreased bone mineral content, which is associated with increased brittleness and decreased fracture resistance [20]. Aging is also associated with morphological changes to bone such as thinning of the cortical walls and the overall slimming of the bones, as well as changes to proteins in bone, including collagen [20]. Increased bone resorption in aging may also contribute to reduced bone mineral density (BMD), and can be exacerbated by reductions in bone formation related to reduced osteoblastogenesis and increased adipogenesis in the bone marrow, which affects matrix formation and mineralization [21]. The etiology of osteoporosis is multifactorial and influenced by both genetic and environmental factors. Of particular interest to this review is the effect of oxidative stress.

3. AOPP as a Marker of Oxidative Stress in Bone

Studies indicate that oxidative stress may enhance bone resorption and disturb the coupling of bone resorption to bone formation, contributing to AAO [19,22]. Oxidative stress increases with age, as ROS production rises and the activities of antioxidant enzymes such as superoxide dismutase (SOD) and glutathione peroxidase simultaneously decrease [19,23]. The oxidative stress resulting from this imbalance can stimulate apoptosis of osteoblasts and osteocytes [24,25], and may reduce osteoblastogenesis [26] while also increasing the formation and activation of osteoclasts [10].

AOPP is a novel marker of oxidative stress that may be particularly important in the context of bones, both as a biological driver and a biomarker of bone degradation. Several cross-sectional studies have examined the relationship between bone status and AOPP in both humans and animals (Table 1). Zhang et al. demonstrated that among male Wistar rats, AOPP levels in both plasma and femurs increased with age, while SOD activity decreased [19]. AOPP was also associated with decreases in BMD, bone volume, trabecular thickness, and the rate of bone formation. Similarly, a 2015 study showed that plasma AOPP was associated with reduced BMD and increased markers of bone turnover among postmenopausal women [27]. Importantly, this study did not adjust for potential cofounding factors such as age, body mass index, diet, or smoking. Recent studies by a group in Italy linked lipid hydroperoxides—one marker of oxidative stress—to reduced BMD in postmenopausal women, but did not find significant relationships between AOPP and BMD [28]. Differences between these studies could reflect differences in study populations as well as the progression of bone disease or oxidative damage. The currently available cross-sectional study data provide weak evidence to support the link between AOPP and bone health. Given these mixed findings and important limitations to each study, alternative study designs that illuminate potential mechanisms of AOPP in bone are essential for understanding the relationship between AOPP and osteoporosis.

Table 1. Cross-sectional studies of AOPP and bone status in humans and animals.

Study	Population	Observations	Limitations
Zhang (2011) [19]	Young, adult, and old (*n* = 26 each) male Wistar rats	AOPP in plasma and femur increased with aging and were negatively associated with femur BMD	Sample size; potentially limited translatability to humans
Wu (2015) [27]	60 postmenopausal women with osteoporosis, 60 without osteoporosis	AOPP was associated with reduced BMD and increased bone turnover markers	Sample size; no adjustment for factors such as BMI, diet, or smoking; BMD assessed only at lumbar spine
Cervellati (2013) [28]	98 pre- and 93 post-menopausal women	No significant association between AOPP and bone status	Potential for residual confounding; AOPP assessed only in serum
Cervellati (2014) [22]	167 postmenopausal women	No significant association between AOPP and bone status	Potential for residual confounding; AOPP assessed only in serum

AOPP: advanced oxidation protein products; BMD: bone mineral density; BMI: body mass index.

Few interventional trials in animals have investigated the actions of AOPP on bone. One study showed that AOPP administration accelerated bone deterioration in aged male rats and that the AOPP-induced changes in bone turnover markers, trabecular BMD, and microstructural parameters could be completely prevented by the oral administration of the NOX inhibitor apocynin, suggesting that AOPP induced bone deterioration via the activation of NAPDH oxidase [4]. Another study showed that administration of the radical scavenger antioxidant melatonin reduced AOPP levels and other markers of oxidative stress in streptozotocin-induced diabetic male rats, leading to beneficial effects on bone healing in a short-term study [29]. Although not specific to osteoporosis, this suggests that AOPP may inhibit bone formation.

4. Mechanisms of Action of AOPP in Bone

Several in vitro studies that have challenged cells with AOPP have helped to clarify the mechanisms by which AOPP may impact bone (Table 2). A recent study using an osteocyte-like cell line (MLO-Y4) demonstrated that when cultured with AOPP-modified mouse serum albumin (AOPP-MSA), AOPP increased ROS generation and activated the c-Jun N-terminal kinase (JNK) and p38 mitogen-activated protein kinase (p38 MAPK) signaling pathways in a ROS-dependent manner, leading to apoptosis of these cells [30]. Upregulation of the JNK/p38 MAPK signaling pathways by AOPP also increased the expression of the protein sclerostin [30], which inhibits osteoblast function and bone formation by antagonizing the Wnt signaling pathway [31]. Through the JNK/p38 MAPK pathway, AOPP also upregulated the expression of receptor activator of NFκB ligand (RANKL) [30], which can upregulate osteoclastogenesis upon binding to its receptor [32].

A study using rat mesenchymal stem cells (MSC, which give rise to osteoblasts and osteocytes) demonstrated that exposure to AOPP-modified bovine serum albumin (AOPP-BSA) inhibited MSC proliferation, reduced alkaline phosphatase (ALP) activity, decreased collagen I mRNA levels, and inhibited bone nodule formation [33]. AOPP also increased ROS generation and upregulated the expression of RAGE [33]. In rat osteoblast-like cells, AOPP-modified rat serum albumin (AOPP-RSA) induced many of the same effects and provided evidence that AOPP may inhibit the proliferation of osteoblast-like cells through the ROS-dependent NFκB pathway [34].

Table 2. In vitro studies of the effect of AOPP on bone cells.

Study	Cell Type	Treatments	Outcome
Yu (2016) [30]	Osteocytic MLO-Y4 cells	Cultured with AOPP-MSA (25, 50, 100, or 200 μg/mL for 24 h or 200 μg/mL for 3, 6, 12, or 24 h)	AOPP triggered apoptosis and upregulated expression of sclerostin and RANKL in a JNK/p38 MAPK-dependent manner
Sun (2013) [33]	Rat MSC	Cultured with AOPP-BSA (50, 100, 200, or 400 μg/mL for 3 days or 200 μg/mL for 24, 48, or 72 h)	AOPP inhibited proliferation, reduced ALP activity and ALP and collagen I mRNA, increased ROS generation, upregulated RAGE expression
Zhong (2009) [34]	Rat osteoblast-like cells	Cultured with AOPP-RSA (50, 100, or 200 μg/mL for 24 h or 100 μg/mL for 24, 48, or 72 h)	AOPP inhibited proliferation, reduced ALP activity, downregulated expression of osteocalcin, induced ROS generation and NFκB phosphorylation

AOPP: advanced oxidation protein products; MLO-Y4: murine osteocyte-like cell line Y4; AOPP-MSA: AOPP-modified mouse serum albumin; RANKL: receptor activator of NFκB (nuclear factor κB) ligand; JNK: c-Jun N-terminal kinase; p38 MAPK: p38 mitogen-activated protein kinase; MSC: mesenchymal stem cells; AOPP-BSA: AOPP-modified bovine serum albumin; ALP: alkaline phosphatase; ROS: reactive oxygen species; RAGE: receptor for advanced glycation end products; AOPP-RSA: AOPP-modified rat serum albumin.

Taken together, these in vitro studies indicate that AOPP may act through the NFκB, JNK, and p38 MAPK signaling pathways to inhibit bone formation while promoting resorption. Previous reports have shown that the binding of RANKL to RANK causes recruitment of TNF receptor-associated factor 6 (TRAF6), which in turn activates NFκB, JNK, and MAPK, which induce nuclear factor of activated T cells (NFAT)c1, a key transcription factor for osteoclastogenesis [35,36]. Therefore, AOPP may disturb the balance between bone formation and resorption by upregulating osteoclastogenesis through these pathways.

Furthermore, it has also been documented that AGE-RAGE interaction induces the generation of ROS through the NOX pathway, resulting in the apoptosis of osteoblasts/MSC [37] and in the inhibition of the proliferation and differentiation of osteoblasts/MSC [38]. RAGE overexpression by lentiviral transfection has been shown to inhibit osteoblast proliferation through the suppression of the Wnt, phosphoinositide 3-kinase (PI3K), and extracellular signal-related kinase (ERK) pathways [38]. It has also been reported that RAGE plays a critical role in osteoclast maturation and activation [39], and RAGE expression in osteoclasts is age-dependent [40]. Studies using RAGE knockout mice have also shown that bone mass and bone biomechanical strength are increased with a decreased number of osteoclasts compared with wild-type mice [41]. Therefore, based on observations from the current literature, AOPP may inhibit osteoblastic activity and differentiation through the AOPP-RAGE-ROS pathway via the activation of NOX, which may be an important mechanism involved in the development of AAO.

5. Antioxidant Intake and Bone Health: Potential Benefits of Berry Anthocyanins

Because of the potential role of AOPP in aging-associated bone turnover, it is plausible that increased consumption of dietary antioxidants could reduce the formation of AOPP by inhibiting the NOX pathway, thereby lowering AAO risk. Two studies that support this hypothesis showed that murine osteoblastic MC3T3-E1 cells cultured with 2-deoxy-D-ribose (dRib) to induce oxidative damage could be rescued from dRib toxicity by the addition of the flavonoid antioxidants hesperetin [41] and myricetin [42], and that these antioxidant treatments markedly reduced AOPP along with other markers of oxidation. Melatonin is a well-studied antioxidant [43], and has also been shown to protect against H_2O_2-induced apoptosis of MSC [44]. The positive effects of dietary antioxidants on BMD and bone status have also been demonstrated in multiple cross-sectional investigations [45–47]. However, due to the inherent limitations of cross-sectional studies, this hypothesis should be further investigated using cohort studies or interventional trials.

Recently, considerable attention has been directed to the potential favorable effects of berries in enhancing bone health due to the antioxidant properties of anthocyanins in berries. Several studies indicate that blackcurrant anthocyanins exhibit a range of health benefits, including antioxidant [48,49] and anti-inflammatory effects [50,51], which could potentially improve bone remodeling. Several studies have utilized ovariectomized (OVX) animals to mimic the estrogen deficiency of menopause, and have found that supplementation with blueberry or blackcurrant attenuated the OVX-induced bone loss (Table 3) [52–54].

Table 3. Animal studies of the impact of berry antioxidants on ovariectomy-induced bone loss.

Study	Population	Treatments	Duration	Outcome
Li (2014) [52]	Female Sprague Dawley rats (total $n = 30$)	Randomized to sham operation, OVX control, and OVX blueberry treatment (10% w/w freeze-dried blueberry powder)	12 weeks	Blueberry inhibited bone resorption, bone loss, and the reduction of bone strength of OVX rats
Zheng (2016) [53]	Female C57BL/6J mice (total $n = 54$)	Randomized to sham operation or OVX, then further divided into control diet or diet containing 1% blackcurrant extract	4, 8, or 12 weeks	Blackcurrant attenuated OVX-induced bone loss as measured by BMD and trabecular volume; blackcurrant reduced bone resorption activity
Devareddy (2008) [54]	Female Sprague Dawley rats ($n = 30$)	Randomized to sham operation, OVX control, and OVX blueberry treatment (5% w/w dried blueberry powder)	100 days	Blueberry prevented OVX-induced loss of whole-body BMD; blueberry treatment group had lower serum osteocalcin

OVX: ovariectomized; BMD: bone mineral density.

However, evidence of bone-protective effects of berries outside of an estrogen-deficient model is still limited. In recent in vitro experiments using murine bone marrow macrophages, anthocyanins from blackcurrant, blackberry, and blueberry suppressed NOX (NOX1 and NOX2) mRNA expression by over 60% [51]. This reduction consequently downregulated nuclear factor (erythroid-derived 2)-like 2 (Nrf2) mRNA expression, suggesting that the NOX pathway was the major source of ROS production and that berry anthocyanins effectively inhibited the NOX pathway, thus reducing ROS production (Figure 1). In cultured RAW 264.7 macrophages, anthocyanins from blackcurrant, blueberry, and blackberry significantly inhibited lipopolysaccharide-induced inflammation as indicated by lower mRNA levels of TNFα and interleukin-1β, and lowered nuclear p65 levels, indicating decreased NFκB activity [51]. TNFα plays a central role in inflammation-mediated bone loss by augmenting osteoblastic RANKL-induced osteoclastogenesis and directly stimulates osteoclast formation [55,56]. These results indicate that berry anthocyanins may be an effective dietary agent in preventing aging-associated bone deterioration directly by inhibiting NOX-mediated AOPP formation and indirectly by reducing bone resorption through lowering ROS formation.

6. Conclusions

Oxidative stress contributes to the universal phenomenon of bone aging, and is a key factor in the development of AAO. AOPP is a biomarker of oxidative damage to protein and has been associated with lower BMD in both humans and animals in some observational studies. While not all observational studies confirmed the role of AOPP in AAO, the association between AOPP and bone loss is supported by several mechanistic studies elucidating the signaling pathways by which AOPP may reduce bone formation and/or increase bone resorption. Relatively little work has specifically examined how dietary antioxidants may impede bone aging through the reduction of AOPP. Studies that have addressed this hypothesis indicate that antioxidant consumption may be an effective method of inhibiting AOPP formation and lowering ROS formation in bone. Importantly, these findings are largely based on in vitro studies and should be expanded in future research examining how long-term consumption of dietary antioxidants reduces AOPP formation and mitigates aging-associated bone loss in older adulthood. This type of research may serve as a basis for future human clinical studies, which may ultimately lead to the development of dietary recommendations and strategies for the prevention of AAO.

Acknowledgments: This study was supported by the USDA National Institute of Food and Agriculture (NIFA) Seed Grant (Award Number 2016-67018-24492) to Ock K. Chun.

Conflicts of Interest: The authors declare no conflict of interest.

References

1. Yamagishi, S. Role of Advanced Glycation End Products (AGEs) in Osteoporosis in Diabetes. *Curr. Drug Targets* **2011**, *12*, 2096–2102. [CrossRef] [PubMed]
2. Alejandro, P.; Constantinescu, F. A Review of Osteoporosis in the Older Adult. *Clin. Geriatr. Med.* **2017**, *33*, 27–40. [CrossRef] [PubMed]
3. Raisz, L.G. Science in medicine Pathogenesis of osteoporosis: Concepts, conflicts, and prospects. *J. Clin. Investig.* **2005**, *115*, 3318–3325. [CrossRef] [PubMed]
4. Zeng, J.H.; Zhong, Z.M.; Li, X.D.; Wu, Q.; Zheng, S.; Zhou, J.; Ye, W.B.; Xie, F.; Wu, X.H.; Huang, Z.P.; et al. Advanced oxidation protein products accelerate bone deterioration in aged rats. *Exp. Gerontol.* **2014**, *50*, 64–71. [CrossRef] [PubMed]
5. Duque, G.; Troen, B.R. Understanding the mechanisms of senile osteoporosis: New facts for a major geriatric syndrome. *J. Am. Geriatr. Soc.* **2008**, *56*, 935–941. [CrossRef] [PubMed]
6. Wei, Y.H.; Lee, H.C. Oxidative Stress, Mitochondrial DNA Mutation, and Impairment of Antioxidant Enzymes in Aging. *Exp. Biol. Med.* **2002**, *227*, 671–682. [CrossRef]
7. Wauquier, F.; Leotoing, L.; Coxam, V.; Guicheux, J.; Wittrant, Y. Oxidative stress in bone remodelling and disease. *Trends Mol. Med.* **2009**, *15*, 468–477. [CrossRef] [PubMed]
8. Parfitt, A.M.; Chir, B. Bone remodeling and bone loss: Understanding the pathophysiology of osteoporosis. *Clin. Obstet. Gynecol.* **1987**, *30*, 789–811. [CrossRef] [PubMed]
9. Atashi, F.; Modarressi, A.; Pepper, M.S. The role of reactive oxygen species in mesenchymal stem cell adipogenic and osteogenic differentiation: A review. *Stem Cells Dev.* **2015**, *24*, 1150–1163. [CrossRef] [PubMed]
10. Garrett, I.R.; Boyce, B.F.; Oreffo, R.O.C.; Bonewald, L.; Poser, J.; Mundy, G.R. Oxygen-derived free radicals stimulate osteoclastic bone resorption in rodent bone in vitro and in vivo. *J. Clin. Investig.* **1990**, *85*, 632–639. [CrossRef] [PubMed]
11. Suzuki, T.; Katsumata, S.; Matsuxaki, H.; Suzuki, K. Dietary zinc deficiency induces oxidative stress and promotes tumor necrosis factor-α- and interleukin-1β-induced RANKL expressio in rat bone. *J. Clin. Biochem. Nutr.* **2016**, *58*, 122–129. [CrossRef] [PubMed]
12. Almeida, M.; Han, L.; Martin-Millan, M.; Plotkin, L.I.; Stewart, S.A.; Roberson, P.K.; Kousteni, S.; O'Brien, C.A.; Bellido, T.; Parfitt, A.M.; et al. Skeletal Involution by Age-associated Oxidative Stress and Its Acceleration by Loss of Sex Steroids. *J. Biol. Chem.* **2007**, *282*, 27285–27297. [CrossRef] [PubMed]
13. Hazen, S.L.; Hsu, F.F.; Heinecke, J.W. p-Hydroxyphenylacetaldehyde Is the Major Product of L-Tyrosine Oxidation by Activated Human Phagocytes. *J. Biol. Chem.* **1996**, *271*, 1861–1867. [CrossRef] [PubMed]
14. Heinecke, J.W.; Li, W.; Daehnke, H.L.; Goldstein, J.A. Dityrosine, a Specific Marker of Oxidation. *J. Biol. Chem.* **1993**, *268*, 4069–4077. [PubMed]
15. Witko-Sarsat, V.; Friedlander, M.; Capeillère-Blandin, C.; Nguyen-Khoa, T.; Nguyen, A.T.; Zingraff, J.; Jungers, P.; Descamps-Latscha, B. Advanced oxidation protein products as a novel marker of oxidative stress in uremia. *Kidney Int.* **1996**, *49*, 1304–1313. [CrossRef] [PubMed]
16. Iwao, Y.; Anraku, M.; Hiraike, M.; Kawai, K.; Nakajou, K.; Kai, T.; Suenaga, A.; Otagiri, M. The structural and pharmacokinetic properties of oxidized human serum albumin, advanced oxidation protein products (AOPP). *Drug Metab. Pharmacokinet.* **2006**, *21*, 140–146. [CrossRef] [PubMed]

17. Guo, Z.J.; Niu, H.X.; Hou, F.F.; Zhang, L.; Fu, N.; Nagai, R.; Lu, X.; Chen, B.H.; Shan, Y.X.; Tian, J.W.; et al. Advanced oxidation protein products activate vascular endothelial cells via a RAGE-mediated signaling pathway. *Antioxid. Redox Signal.* **2008**, *10*, 1699–1712. [CrossRef] [PubMed]
18. Sherman, S.S.; Tobin, J.D.; Hollis, B.W.; Gundberg, C.M.; Roy, T.A.; Plato, C.C. Biochemical parameters associated with low bone density in healthy men and women. *J Bone Min Res.* **1992**, *7*, 1123–1130. [CrossRef] [PubMed]
19. Zhang, Y.B.; Zhong, Z.M.; Hou, G.; Jiang, H.; Chen, J.T. Involvement of oxidative stress in age-related bone loss. *J. Surg. Res.* **2011**, *169*, e37–e42. [CrossRef] [PubMed]
20. Boskey, A.L.; Coleman, R. Aging and Bone. *J. Dent. Res.* **2010**, *89*, 1333–1348. [CrossRef] [PubMed]
21. Demontiero, O.; Vidal, C.; Duque, G. Aging and bone loss: New insights for the clinician. *Ther. Adv. Musculoskelet. Dis.* **2012**, *4*, 61–76. [CrossRef] [PubMed]
22. Cervellati, C.; Bonaccorsi, G.; Cremonini, E.; Romani, A.; Fila, E.; Castaldini, M.C.; Ferrazzini, S.; Fifanti, M.; Massari, L. Oxidative stress and bone resorption interplay as a possible trigger for postmenopausal osteoporosis. *Biomed. Res. Int.* **2014**, *2014*, 1–8. [CrossRef] [PubMed]
23. Sánchez-Rodríguez, M.A.; Ruiz-Ramos, M.; Correa-Muñoz, E.; Mendoza-Núñez, V.M. Oxidative stress as a risk factor for osteoporosis in elderly Mexicans as characterized by antioxidant enzymes. *BMC Musculoskelet. Disord.* **2007**, *8*, 1–7. [CrossRef] [PubMed]
24. Östman, B.; Michaëlsson, K.; Helmersson, J.; Gedeborg, R.; Melhus, H. Oxidative stress and bone mineral density in elderly men: Antioxidant activity of alpha-tocopherol. *Free Radic. Biol. Med.* **2009**, *47*, 668–673. [CrossRef] [PubMed]
25. Huang, C.; Lv, B.; Wang, Y. ProteinpPhosphatase 2A mediates oxidative stress induced apoptosis in osteoblasts. *Mediat. Inflamm.* **2015**, *2015*, 1–8. [CrossRef]
26. Almeida, M.; Han, L.; Martin-Millan, M.; O'Brien, C.A.; Manolagas, S.C. Oxidative stress antagonizes Wnt signaling in osteoblast precursors by diverting β-catenin from T cell factor- to forkhead box O-mediated transcription. *J. Biol. Chem.* **2007**, *282*, 27298–27305. [CrossRef] [PubMed]
27. Wu, Q.; Zhong, Z.M.; Pan, Y.; Zeng, J.H.; Zheng, S.; Zhu, S.Y.; Chen, J.T. Advanced Oxidation Protein Products as a Novel Marker of Oxidative Stress in Postmenopausal Osteoporosis. *Med. Sci. Monit.* **2015**, *21*, 2428–2432. [CrossRef] [PubMed]
28. Cervellati, C.; Bonaccorsi, G.; Cremonini, E.; Bergamini, C.M.; Patella, A.; Castaldini, C.; Ferrazzini, S.; Capatti, A.; Picarelli, V.; Pansini, F.S.; et al. Bone mass density selectively correlates with serum markers of oxidative damage in post-menopausal women. *Clin. Chem. Lab. Med.* **2013**, *51*, 333–338. [CrossRef] [PubMed]
29. Yildirimturk, S.; Batu, S.; Alatli, C.; Olgac, V.; Firat, D.; Sirin, Y. The effects of supplemental melatonin administration on the healing of bone defects in streptozotocin-induced diabetic rats. *J. Appl. Oral Sci.* **2016**, *24*, 239–249. [CrossRef] [PubMed]
30. Yu, C.; Huang, D.; Wang, K.; Lin, B.; Liu, Y.; Liu, S.; Wu, W.; Zhang, H. Advanced oxidation protein products induce apoptosis, and upregulate sclerostin and RANKL expression, in osteocytic MLO-Y4 cells via JNK/p38 MAPK activation. *Mol. Med. Rep.* **2016**, *15*, 543–550. [CrossRef] [PubMed]
31. Baron, R.; Kneissel, M. WNT signaling in bone homeostasis and disease: From human mutations to treatments. *Nat. Med.* **2013**, *19*, 179–192. [CrossRef] [PubMed]
32. Boyce, B.F.; Xing, L. Biology of RANK, RANKL, and osteoprotegerin. *Arthritis Res. Ther.* **2007**, *9*, S1. [CrossRef] [PubMed]
33. Sun, N.; Yang, L.; Li, Y.; Zhang, H.; Chen, H.; Liu, D.; Li, Q.; Cai, D. Effect of advanced oxidation protein products on the proliferation and osteogenic differentiation of rat mesenchymal stem cells. *Int. J. Mol. Med.* **2013**, *32*, 485–491. [CrossRef] [PubMed]
34. Zhong, Z.M.; Bai, L.; Chen, J.T. Advanced oxidation protein products inhibit proliferation and differentiation of rat osteoblast-like cells via NF-κB pathway. *Cell. Physiol. Biochem.* **2009**, *24*, 105–114. [CrossRef] [PubMed]
35. Naito, A.; Azuma, S.; Tanaka, S.; Miyazaki, T.; Takaki, S.; Takatsu, K.; Nakao, K.; Nakamura, K.; Katsuki, M.; Yamamoto, T.; et al. Severe osteopetrosis, defective interleukin-1 signalling and lymph node organogenesis in TRAF6-deficient mice. *Genes Cells* **1999**, *4*, 353–362. [CrossRef] [PubMed]
36. Takayanagi, H. The role of NFAT in osteoclast formation. *Ann. N. Y. Acad. Sci.* **2007**, *1116*, 227–237. [CrossRef] [PubMed]

37. Wautier, M.; Chappey, O.; Corda, S.; Stern, D.M.; Schmidt, A.M.; Wautier, J. Activation of NADPH oxidase by AGE links oxidant stress to altered gene expression via RAGE. *Am. J. Physiol. Endocrinol. Metab.* **2001**, *280*, E685–E694. [PubMed]

38. Li, G.; Xu, J.; Li, Z. Receptor for advanced glycation end products inhibits proliferation in osteoblast through suppression of Wnt, PI3K and ERK signaling. *Biochem. Biophys. Res. Commun.* **2012**, *423*, 684–689. [CrossRef] [PubMed]

39. Zhou, Z.; Immel, D.; Xi, C.X.; Bierhaus, A.; Feng, X.; Mei, L.; Nawroth, P.; Stern, D.M.; Xiong, W.C. Regulation of osteoclast function and bone mass by RAGE. *J. Exp. Med.* **2006**, *203*, 1067–1080. [CrossRef] [PubMed]

40. Cui, S.; Xiong, F.; Hong, Y.; Jung, J.U.; Li, X.S.; Liu, J.Z.; Yan, R.; Mei, L.; Feng, X.; Xiong, W.C. APPswe/AB regulation of osteoclast activation and RAGE expression in an age-dependent manner. *J. Bone Miner. Res.* **2011**, *26*, 1084–1098. [CrossRef] [PubMed]

41. Choi, E.M.; Kim, Y.H. Hesperetin attenuates the highly reducing sugar-triggered inhibition of osteoblast differentiation. *Cell Biol. Toxicol.* **2008**, *24*, 225–231. [CrossRef] [PubMed]

42. Lee, K.H.; Choi, E.M. Myricetin, a naturally occurring flavonoid, prevents 2-deoxy-d-ribose induced dysfunction and oxidative damage in osteoblastic MC3T3-E1 cells. *Eur. J. Pharmacol.* **2008**, *591*, 1–6. [CrossRef] [PubMed]

43. Reiter, R.J.; Tan, D.X.; Mayo, J.C.; Sainz, R.M.; Leon, J.; Czarnocki, Z. Melatonin as an antioxidant: Biochemical mechanisms and pathophysiological implications in humans. *Acta Biochim. Pol.* **2003**, *50*, 1129–1146. [PubMed]

44. Wang, F.W.; Wang, Z.; Zhang, Y.M.; Du, Z.X.; Zhang, X.L.; Liu, Q.; Guo, Y.J.; Li, X.G.; Hao, A.J. Protective effect of melatonin on bone marrow mesenchymal stem cells against hydrogen peroxide-induced apoptosis in vitro. *J. Cell. Biochem.* **2013**, *114*, 2346–2355. [CrossRef] [PubMed]

45. Rivas, A.; Romero, A.; Mariscal-Arcas, M.; Monteagudo, C.; López, G.; Lorenzo, L.; Ocaña-Peinado, F.M.; Olea-Serrano, F. Association between dietary antioxidant quality score (DAQs) and bone mineral density in Spanish women. *Nutr. Hosp.* **2012**, *27*, 1886–1893. [CrossRef] [PubMed]

46. Zhang, J.; Munger, R.G.; West, N.A.; Cutler, D.R.; Wengreen, H.J.; Corcoran, C.D. Antioxidant intake and risk of osteoporotic hip fracture in Utah: An effect modified by smoking status. *Am. J. Epidemiol.* **2006**, *163*, 9–17. [CrossRef] [PubMed]

47. De Franca, N.A.; Camargo, M.B.; Lazaretti-Castro, M.; Martini, L.A. Antioxidant intake and bone status in a cross-sectional study of Brazilian women with osteoporosis. *Nutr. Health* **2013**, *22*, 133–142. [CrossRef] [PubMed]

48. Shen, C.L.; von Bergen, V.; Chyu, M.C.; Jenkins, M.R.; Mo, H.; Chen, C.H.; Kwun, I.S. Fruits and dietary phytochemicals in bone protection. *Nutr. Res.* **2012**, *32*, 897–910. [CrossRef] [PubMed]

49. McGhie, T.K.; Walton, M.C.; Barnett, L.E.; Vather, R.; Martin, H.; Au, J.; Alspach, P.A.; Booth, C.L.; Kruger, M.C. Boysenberry and blackcurrant drinks increased the plasma antioxidant capacity in an elderly population but had little effect on other markers of oxidative stress. *J. Sci. Food Agric.* **2007**, *87*, 2519–2527. [CrossRef]

50. Kumazawa, Y.; Kawaguchi, K.; Takimoto, H. Immunomodulating Effects of Flavonoids on Acute and Chronic Inflammatory Responses Caused by Tumor Necrosis Factor α. *Curr. Pharm. Des.* **2006**, *12*, 4271–4279. [CrossRef] [PubMed]

51. Lee, S.G.; Kim, B.; Yang, Y.; Pham, T.X.; Park, Y.K.; Manatou, J.; Koo, S.I.; Chun, O.K.; Lee, J.Y. Berry anthocyanins suppress the expression and secretion of proinflammatory mediators in macrophages by inhibiting nuclear translocation of NF-κB independent of NRF2-mediated mechanism. *J. Nutr. Biochem.* **2014**, *25*, 404–411. [CrossRef] [PubMed]

52. Li, T.; Wu, S.M.; Xu, Z.Y.; Ou-Yang, S. Rabbiteye blueberry prevents osteoporosis in ovariectomized rats. *J. Orthop. Surg. Res.* **2014**, *9*, 56–62. [CrossRef] [PubMed]

53. Zheng, X.; Mun, S.; Lee, S.G.; Vance, T.M.; Hubert, P.; Koo, S.I.; Lee, S.K.; Chun, O.K. Anthocyanin-Rich Blackcurrant Extract Attenuates Ovariectomy-Induced Bone Loss in Mice. *J. Med. Food* **2016**, *19*, 390–397. [CrossRef] [PubMed]

54. Devareddy, L.; Hooshmand, S.; Collins, J.K.; Lucas, E.A.; Chai, S.C.; Arjmandi, B.H. Blueberry prevents bone loss in ovariectomized rat model of postmenopausal osteoporosis. *J. Nutr. Biochem.* **2008**, *19*, 694–699. [CrossRef] [PubMed]

55. Komine, M.; Kukita, A.; Kukita, T.; Ogata, Y.; Hotokebuchi, T.; Kohashi, O. Tumor necrosis factor-alpha cooperates with receptor activator of nuclear factor kappaB ligand in generation of osteoclasts in stromal cell-depleted rat bone marrow cell culture. *Bone* **2001**, *28*, 474–483. [CrossRef]
56. Fox, S.W.; Evans, K.E.; Lovibond, A.C. Transforming growth factor-β enables NFATc1 expression during osteoclastogenesis. *Biochem. Biophys. Res. Commun.* **2008**, *366*, 123–128. [CrossRef] [PubMed]

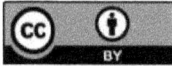

MDPI AG

St. Alban-Anlage 66

4052 Basel, Switzerland

Tel. +41 61 683 77 34

Fax +41 61 302 89 18

http://www.mdpi.com

Nutrients Editorial Office

E-mail: nutrients@mdpi.com

http://www.mdpi.com/journal/nutrients

www.ingramcontent.com/pod-product-compliance
Lightning Source LLC
Chambersburg PA
CBHW051853210326
41597CB00033B/5876